ISO 13485

A Complete Guide to
Quality Management
in the
Medical Device
Industry

ISO 13485

A Complete Guide to Quality Management in the Medical Device Industry

Itay Abuhav

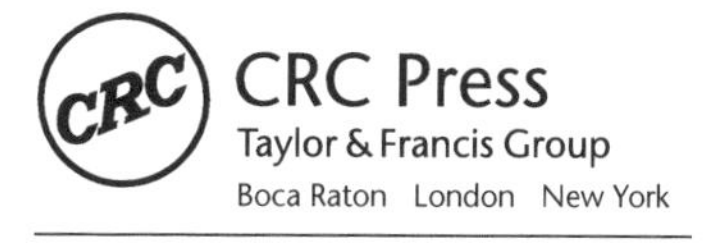

CRC Press is an imprint of the
Taylor & Francis Group, an **informa** business

CRC Press
Taylor & Francis Group
6000 Broken Sound Parkway NW, Suite 300
Boca Raton, FL 33487-2742

Version Date: 20110707

International Standard Book Number: 978-1-4398-6611-5 (Hardback)

Library of Congress Cataloging-in-Publication Data

Abuhav, Itay.
ISO 13485 : a complete guide to quality management in the medical device industry / Itay Abuhav.
p. ; cm.
Includes bibliographical references and index.
ISBN 978-1-4398-6611-5 (hardback : alk. paper)
1. Medical instruments and apparatus--Standards--Handbooks, manuals, etc. 2. Medical instruments and apparatus industry--Quality control--Standards--Handbooks, manuals, etc. I. Title.
[DNLM: 1. Equipment and Supplies--standards. 2. Equipment Design--standards. 3. Manufactured Materials--standards. 4. Quality Control. W 26]

R856.15.A28 2012
610.284--dc23 2011022826

Visit the Taylor & Francis Web site at
http://www.taylorandfrancis.com

and the CRC Press Web site at
http://www.crcpress.com

Contents

Preface

Two years ago, I noticed that there was an unfulfilled need in the quality management world—a documented and structured clarification and interpretation of the ISO 13485 Standard. As a consultant I decided to do something about this. The task was a challenging one: it included thousands of hours of research and consultation with other great people. Today you are holding the result—a unique document that gathers, analyses, and demonstrates the standard requirements. This book was designed by a quality manager for quality managers (as well as for other organizational parties). I am acquainted with the challenges and issues that readers face. Overcoming these challenges requires sophistication, creativity, and dedication, and this book is a valuable tool in assisting the reader to do this. In order to present the reader with a practical and useful guide, I have provided a definition of my quality policy and objectives.

My Quality Policy

Presenting and reviewing the ISO 13485 Standard requirements through analysis, interpretation, and demonstration, with explanations, insightful examples, and events from the industry.

My Quality Objectives

- Commitment to the highest level of consulting regarding the ISO 13485 Standard.
- Reviewing all the topics and issues related to the realization of a medical device, with reference to various types of processes and products in the industry.
- Providing support in the implementation of an effective quality management system.
- Facilitating the documentation of processes.
- Providing reference to the extraordinary characteristics of the ISO 13485 Standard; that is, the specific procedures, specific documentations and records, regulatory requirements, and risk management.

However, a policy and related objectives are ineffective without also having in place designed and structured tactics and methods to achieve them:

- The book is designed and structured to mirror the standard's table of contents in order to simplify navigation and use.
- Each clause and subclause of the standard are discussed and analyzed through quality perspectives, such as: the implications for an organization—its processes, management, human resources, infrastructures, work environment, control and effectiveness, and documentation and records.

- Each chapter refers to the alignment with regulatory requirements and the association to the risk management.
- The ISO 13485 Standard acts like a complicated web of prerequisites with relations between them. A full and comprehensive reference to the inter-relations between the different clauses and subclauses has been included.
- Putting words into actions—the book will assist in translating the requirements and objectives into feasible activities and tasks. It visualizes situations with everyday events from the different sectors, branches, and the products in the sectors.
- The book compares, using a table, every ISO 13485 to the ISO 9001—requirement versus requirement. This feature is an effective method which enables you to position your quality management status concerning the implementation.

List of Exclusions

I decided to exclude Chapter 0 of the standard from this book since it mainly provides explanations regarding the ISO 13485 that are already covered elsewhere in this book. In Chapter 3, the terms and definitions that appear in clauses 3.1–3.8 have also been excluded, both because the standard is very clear, and these are also mentioned elsewhere in the book.

My biggest wish is that you, as a reader, will refer to this book as a consulting session, and that you will read and explore it, draw information and knowledge that suits you and your organization, and that you will introduce this information to your quality management system and processes.

Acknowledgments

I wish to thank all the people—consultants, co-workers, auditors, mentors, bosses, and friends—that introduced me to the quality world, and that have aided, supported, taught, lectured, consulted, and provided valuable knowledge and information during the undertaking of this book and also in my professional career. You have helped give an edge to this book. The list of names is too extensive to include here, but you know who you are.

I wish to thank my dear family for their warm support throughout the years.

I also wish to thank my wife Angela for pushing, believing, and supporting me up in the hard times.

Thank you.

1 Scope

Welcome to the ISO 13485 Standard. That is the meaning of chapter 1 of the ISO 13485 Standard—Scope. This chapter reviews the ISO 13485 Standard's aims and concepts and defines the scope of application of the standard to your quality management system. The following are presented in this chapter:

- The goals and purposes of the standard
- The intended application
- The approach and reference to regulatory requirements
- The approach and reference to customer requirements
- Restrictions, principles, constraints, and limitations regarding the implementation of the various standard requirements
- The resolution of uncertainties concerning the relation to the ISO 9001 Standard

It may be boring and I bet that most of you have not even bothered to look through it, but I can guarantee you that the information in this chapter will assist you and might even ease the certification process once properly understood and applied.

1.1 GENERAL

The ISO 13485 international standard specifies requirements for a quality management system for organizations that realize and deliver medical devices or related services. The principles presented in chapter 1.1 (General) define which organizations the standard is targeted and applicable to (Table 1.1).

Differentiation from Other Quality Management Standards (the ISO 9001 Standard)

The ISO 13485 Standard has definite objectives, which are distinct and unique. These concern all aspects of a quality management system. This fact will be demonstrated over and over again throughout this book. In this chapter however, the principles of the standard are detailed; they reflect an entire quality management architecture, policy, objective processes, documentation, and records.

- The ISO 13485 Standard is basically aimed at a certain type of organization and the requirements for procedure, documentations, and records are designed and planned to support manufacturers that design, develop, realize, and market medical devices and related services. It refers to specific issues and matters relevant to this sector.
- The ISO 9001 Standard is aimed to satisfy customers by fulfilling its requirements along with applicable international and national regulations. The ISO 13485 Standard has another objective. It is not that customer satisfaction does

TABLE 1.1
Standard Requirements of Clause 1.1

ISO 13485	ISO 9001
The ISO 13485 international standard specifies requirements for the implementation and maintenance of a quality management system for organizations that provide medical devices and related services with the goal and objective of meeting customer and regulatory requirements consistently	The ISO 9001 international standard specifies requirements for the implementation and maintenance of quality management systems. The goal and objective of the standard is to initiate a quality management system that will act to consistently meet customer requirements as well as applicable regulatory requirements The requirements of the ISO 9001 Standard apply to the final product or service delivered to the customer and not to intern or intermediate products
The requirements of this standard initiate harmonization between a quality management system of the organization and applicable regulatory requirements	The requirements suggested in the ISO 9001 Standard will facilitate a continual improvement of processes included in the quality management system
The standard includes specific requirements related to medical devices and related service and thus excludes certain requirements of the ISO 9001 Standard that do not apply to the harmonization with the relevant regulations. Organizations that implement and maintain the ISO 13485 Standard requirements and were certified may not claim compatibility to the ISO 9001 unless they were audited and certified	

not interest or concern it; it just measures it in another way with other goals and objectives (feedback) that are appropriate to its concept and purposes.

- Another substantial difference is the fact the ISO 13485 demands the maintenance of effectiveness or processes (while the ISO 9001 Standard supports continual improvement of processes). The difference, the reason and the implementation will be discussed many times in this book; this I can assure you.
- The ISO 13485 sets applicable regulatory requirements front and center and demands that such applicable requirements shall be harmonized with the quality management system.

Harmonization with Regulations and External Requirements

One of the main objectives of the ISO 13485 Standard is to harmonize regulatory requirements with quality management system requirements. Utopia! What is the meaning of harmonizing in this context? To harmonize is to bring several things into correspondence or to make several areas compatible. In the quality management case, it is required to bring the applicable and relevant international, national, local, and regulatory requirements into consonance with quality management system aspects: the planning and implementation of designated processes and activities, design of documentation, training qualification of human resources, and relation to the safety of the user of the medical device. These should be planned and performed in collaboration with the regulatory requirements. Legal requirements refer to any requirements issued by a legal authorization or an authority that have an impact or effect on the design, development, production, storage, delivery, provision, installation, and after-sale activities of the medical device. These may appear as legislation, statutory regulations, regional directives, permits, licenses, authorizations, legal orders or decrees, tribunals, and laws and rules. The first step is to identify the applicable ones and then refer to them in the quality management system.

1.2 APPLICATION

Chapter 1.2 (Application) defines the basic principles for the determination of the scope and extent of the quality management system in an organization (Table 1.2).

The purpose and objective of the application is the identification and inclusion of

- The main products and services that the organization offers its customers
- The activities, main sites, technologies, functions, and processes that constitute the core business of the organization

The second point derives from the first. The determination of the application will frame the scope of your quality management system and will define which of the standard requirements, appearing in Chapter 7 (Product Realization), are applicable to your organization. A quality management system (QMS) is a combination of various activities and processes—marketing, design and development, production, technical activities, storage, and distribution—operated by various functions and roles that demand certain qualifications. Determining what is to be included under the QMS will define which organizational aspects will be designed, managed, and controlled under the quality requirements: products, processes, activities, sites, information and data, tools and equipment, and human resources. The scope of the application directly affects the definitions of authorities and responsibilities relevant to the quality management system.

A description of the scope and a detailed list of the standards requirements related to the QMS will be included in the quality manual where it is required to include a list of the operations, processes, and products that are included. The objective is to describe all the quality operations and processes that are applicable to the organization: planning of product realization, customer related processes, purchasing, etc.

Size and Type of the Organization

The first statement of this clause defines the appointment and adequacy of the ISO 13485 Standard requirements to organizations that provide medical devices. The statement indicates that size and type of an organization do not affect the application of the standard. In other words, when you are defining the application of the standard requirements to your processes, activities, and products, the size and type of the organization are not factors for consideration.

TABLE 1.2
Standard Requirements of Clause 1.2

ISO 13485	ISO 9001
The requirements of this international standard are specific for all kinds, extents, and sizes of organizations providing medical devices and/or related services	The requirements of this international standard are generic requirements that are appropriate and applicable for all kinds and sizes of organizations and appropriate and applicable for any kind of product
Where regulatory requirements allow exclusions of design and development controls (as specified in chapter 7.3), the organization may exclude these requirements. These regulations may serve as the justifications for the exclusions. The exclusion is conditioned such that the regulations define substitute control requirements for design and development. The organization shall ensure that the alternatives suggested by the regulations are applicable to and adequate for the controls and documentations as specified in clauses 4.2.2-a and 7.3 of this standard	
The organization may not include some of this standard's requirements when they cannot be applied to the organization due to the nature of its processes and products. The organization may "not include" requirements only from chapter 7 (product realization) and when it is beyond any doubt and provable that the noninclusion does not affect the product's quality. The organization shall provide the reason for the nonapplicability and a justification for the noninclusion, as specified in chapter 4.2.2-a	The organization may exclude some of this standard's requirements when these cannot be applied to the organization due to the nature of its processes and products. The organization may exclude requirements only from chapter 7 (product realization) and when it is beyond any doubt and provable that the exclusions do not affect the product's quality
Where "if appropriate" or "where appropriate" are indicated throughout the ISO 13485 Standard and the organization chooses to exclude these requirements, it must justify the exclusion. These requirements may not be excluded when: • The requirements support corrective action process and are necessary for meeting the medical device requirements • The requirements support and are necessary for the execution of the corrective action process	

Application of Regulations and Other Requirements

It is necessary to identify and document other requirements that are applicable to the operations, processes, and realization of the products: regulatory requirements, other international standards, or internal standards. The objective is to identify all the requirements that may affect or implicate elements that are related to the product: processes, activities, human resources, documentation, and risk management. These may have special demands regarding the extent, structural activities, and documentation of the QMS. This is the practical harmonization mentioned earlier.

Exclusions and Noninclusions

Exclusions and noninclusions mean that certain standard requirements (one or more) are not applicable to the organization due to the nature of its activities, processes, or products, and the organization decided not to implement these requirements in its QMS. The implication of the exclusion and noninclusion is that certain quality activities specified in the standard will not be applied. What is the difference between exclusion and noninclusion? Exclusion of a requirement will be motioned and stated on the certification of the manufacturer while noninclusion will not. But both will be referred to and justified in the quality manual. The organization is allowed to exclude and not include only requirements that appear in Chapter 7 (Product Realization). All other Chapters (1–6 and 8) are obligatory for meeting the ISO 13485 Standard requirements and will be implemented. The documentation and approval of the exclusions and noninclusions will be documented in the quality manual. Each standard requirement that was left out will be justified or will be referred to another documented justification. The justification shall confirm that the exclusion does not affect the quality of the activities, processes, and products.

The organization must strongly consider which standard requirements do not apply. It is very tempting to not include and exclude, but the experience, the reality, and above all the external audit show that exclusions and noninclusions are often mistakenly applied. For example:

- The company manufactures, markets, and delivers a medical device. The design and the development are done by an external company. The company may not exclude the design and the development requirements (7.3) since it holds the responsibility for the medical device, its functionality, performance, safety, and intended use.
- The company manufactures the medical device, but the purchasing is done by the parent company. The company may not exclude the purchase requirements (7.4) since it handles information regarding the purchase: type, product, supplier, schedules, and quantities.
- The company designs and develops a medical device according to the customer specifications. The company may not exclude the customer's property requirements (7.5.4) since it manages the customers' documents, diagrams, and technical specifications.

It can be very confusing and each case shall be evaluated on its own merits. I advise you to consult the auditor regarding the exclusions and see what they have in mind and expect.

Exclusion of Design and Development

A developing and designing organization may exclude the requirements presented in chapter 7.3 when other regulation allows the exclusion of these requirements. Nevertheless, this regulation must submit alternative design and development controls. There is no doubt that designing and developing the medical device must be controlled. However, it may be that the manufacturer designs and develops its medical devices in a region with certain regulatory systems and controls of the processes that have already been implemented. There is no logic in maintaining two sets of controls. Thus, the ISO 13485 Standard allows the organization to implement other regulatory controls and to exclude the controls specified in clause 7.3. For example, if the organization is developing the medical device while implementing the requirements of the FAD QSR21 CFR820.30: Design Controls, it may exclude the controls of clause 7.3. The exclusion must be documented and justified.

Outsourced Processes

The application of the standard requirements includes processes related to the medical device but that are performed outside the organization. Such processes are applicable to the quality management system and must be identified, documented (if and where appropriate), controlled, and verified. This does not relate to purchased goods, materials, or components, but to the provision of core processes needed for the realization of the product supplied by suppliers or contractors: design and development, production, assembly, sterilization, cleaning, accreditation, storage, and transportation. The standard does rule out the fact that in today's business reality organizations must outsource processes due to specialization. Nevertheless, such processes and the communication with the suppliers will be included under the purchase control requirements (7.4):

- These processes will be identified and included in the quality manual and in the description of the interrelations between other processes of the quality system.
- These processes will be implemented and the necessary realization requirements shall be defined and allocated: production means, human resources, verification, and validations.
- These processes will be appropriately controlled and the manufacturer shall acquire the minimal knowledge and technical abilities to control these processes: necessary documented evidence, the requirement for certifications, and suppliers' audits.

If and Where Appropriate

Some of the requirements in the ISO 13485 Standard are indicated as "if appropriate" or "where appropriate." These requirements can be not included and implemented in the QMS only when it can be proved and justified that these are not appropriate. For example, in clause 7.5.1.2.2 (Installation Activities) it is indicated that the organization shall maintain documented procedures "if appropriate"—if it maintains installation activities. In this case it would be pretty easy to prove that the manufacturer does not install the medical device, installation is not covered by the quality management system, and thus it is not appropriate to maintain documented procedures on this matter.

- "If appropriate": clauses 6.4-d, 7.5.1.2.2, 8.5.2
- "Where appropriate": clause 7.4.2

2 Normative References

Chapter 2 (Normative References) is one of the most unread chapters in the history of the ISO Standards. You must admit that I am right. But I read it and here is my interpretation (Table 2.1).

The meaning and purpose of the normative references is to indicate that terminology and nomenclature specified in this standard is not open for debate or an interpretive discussion. The ISO 13485 refers us to a specific document, "ISO 9000:2000: Quality management systems—Fundamentals and vocabulary," in case questions or misunderstandings arise during the implementation and application of the standard requirements. The ISO 13485:2003 Standard refers us to the 2000 edition, but a documented Technical Corrigendum 1 was released on 01.08.2009 with the purpose of declaring that the ISO 13485 Standard is related to the ISO 9001 Standard (not ISO 9001:2000). This indirectly indicates that the normative reference of the ISO 13485 Standard is ISO 9000:2005 (and not 2000). Aside from that, the standard encourages the organization to investigate and examine the validity and applicability of a document by reviewing its revisions.

TABLE 2.1
Standard Requirements of Chapter 2

ISO 13485	ISO 9001
Documents mentioned in this chapter are essential for the scope and application of the ISO 13485 Standard	Documents mentioned in this chapter are essential for the scope and application of the ISO 9001 Standard
Documents with dates indicating the validity or revision of the document: only the last date cited is to be applied	Documents with dates indicating the validity or revision of the document: only the last date cited is to be applied
Documents without dates: only the last version is to be applied including appendix or supplements	Documents without dates: only the last version is to be applied including appendix or supplements
The requirement applies the subsequent amendments, appendix, or supplements of the document	The requirement applies the subsequent amendments, appendix or supplements of the document
Referred document: ISO 9000:2000: Quality management systems—Fundamentals and vocabulary	Referred document: ISO 9000:2005: Quality management systems—Fundamentals and vocabulary

3 Terms and Definitions

In order to clarify matters and disputes, the standard presents its interpretations and explanations regarding terms and definitions presented throughout the standard. These are inseparable and an integral part of the standard. Although the explanations provided are very descriptive and clear, there are some points that I would like to focus on:

Reference to the ISO 9000

Term and definitions mentioned and discussed in the ISO 9000 Standard are applicable to this standard along with the other definitions mentioned in chapter 3. Misunderstanding and arguments will be solved there.

Definition of the Supply Chain Management

The standard relates to the following flowchart as the acceptable supply chain model: supplier → organization → customer. In this flowchart:

- External bodies that provide you with products, materials, services, or any other element used by you to realize the product have the role of the supplier.
- You, who maintain relations with customer, have the role of the organization (as a manufacturer, distributor, or service supplier).
- The end user and operator of the medical device, who receives goods from you, are considered as the customer.

Product = Service

The term "product" appears in the standard over and over again. In addition to the medical device as a tangible product, this term applies to services and activities that the organization supplies as a product: software, plans, data, processes, services, and processed products such as liquids or oils. Sterilization or cleanliness services are supplied as activities rather than a product, for example.

Medical Device as a Complex of Activities

Throughout the standard, the term "medical devices" appears countless times. However, the standard considers the medical device as a complex of elements and actions that constitute its characteristics and attributes. The term "medical devices" applies to all additional services, activities, accessories, or supplements that are provided with the medical device. If it is an implementable device, the packaging and the delivery activities are included under the requirements, and when it is a medical imaging device, the installation and the maintenance are included.

Regulatory Requirements

Clauses 3.1–3.8 of the standard present definitions of types of medical devices. These are considered as generic terms and definitions. But you as a manufacturer need to detect the international, national, local, or statutory regulations appropriate to your activities and to relate to the specific terms and definitions presented there that are relevant to your product. These definitions have consequences regarding the requirements and conditions that are to be applied to your quality management system. One classic example is the classification of the medical device according to the type of the device and the assignment to regulatory classes dictated by the FDA. Harmonization; rings a bell? For the specific terms and definitions (clauses 3.1–3.8) please refer to the standard.

4 Quality Management System

4.1 GENERAL REQUIREMENTS

Chapter 4.1 is a general chapter. In this chapter the general requirements and main principles of a quality management systems are presented. The specific requirements appear throughout the following chapter 4.2. This chapter can be regarded as a foundation for self-evaluation of whether the organization's quality management system follows the general requirements. First let me review the basics requirements (Table 4.1)...

The Main Goal: Implementing a Quality Management System

Clause 4.1 refers to the concept of quality management in an organization. The standard requires definition of the main principles of the quality management system in the quality manual, definition of the scope of your quality management system by identifying the processes, and its support with activities described in the quality procedures. Next, the standard specifies...

Identification of Processes Included in the Quality Management System

The processes for product realization are the basis of a quality management system (QMS). But what are the processes? The processes need to be identified first, in order to understand where to invest and control resources. Otherwise you may find yourself documenting and controlling processes that have no relation to your medical device. It is advisable to first draw the general flowchart of the process, describing how the product will be realized (Figure 4.1).

From this process the subprocesses will be derived that will be included under the quality management system. Another technique is to divide activity into different areas according to the standard suggestions and identify which processes are related in each area:

- Work environment
- Review of requirements related to the product
- Validation of processes
- Preservation of property
- Control of purchasing

At the end of the process there will be a list of processes that will be included in the QMS as follows:

- Planned according to the ISO 13485 Standard requirements
- Controlled according to the ISO 13485 Standard requirements
- Contributes to the effectiveness of the quality management system

The list will be included in the quality manual.

TABLE 4.1
Standard Requirements of Clause 4.1

ISO 13485	ISO 9001
The organization shall establish and maintain the quality management system documented and implemented within the organization with conformity to the requirements of the ISO 13485 Standard	The organization shall establish and maintain the quality management system documented and implemented within the organization with conformity to the requirements of the ISO 9001 Standard
The organization is required to maintain the effectiveness of the quality management system	The organization is required to act continually to improve the effectiveness of the quality management system
While establishing the quality management system the organization shall refer to the following issues:	While documenting its quality management system, the organization shall refer to the following issues:
The main processes of the quality management system shall be identified and documented according to the application of the standard (chapter 1.2). The identified processes must be implemented	The main processes of the quality management system shall be identified and documented according to the application of the standard (chapter 1.2). The identified processes must be implemented
The relations, applications, and sequences between the processes will be defined and implemented	The relations, applications, and sequences between the processes will be defined and implemented
Methods and criteria for effective monitoring and control of the processes will be defined and applied	Methods and criteria for effective monitoring and control of the processes will be defined and applied
Any resources and information needed for supporting these processes shall be adequate and available	Any resources and information needed to support these processes shall be adequate and available
The processes will be controlled, monitored, measured, and analyzed according to prior specifications	The processes will be controlled, monitored, measured, and analyzed according to prior specifications
The organization will implement specific measures for obtaining improvement: achievement of objectives and maintenance of effectiveness	The organization will implement specific measures for obtaining improvement: achievement of objectives and maintenance of effectiveness
The processes will be planned, implemented, and realized according to the requirements of the ISO 13485 Standard	The processes will be planned, implemented, and realized according to the requirements of the ISO 9001 Standard
Outsourced processes that have a direct affect on the product's quality shall be included in the quality management system and shall be submitted to control and monitoring as well as for continual improvement	Outsourced processes that have a direct affect on the product's quality shall be included in the quality management system and shall be submitted to control and monitoring as well as for continual improvement

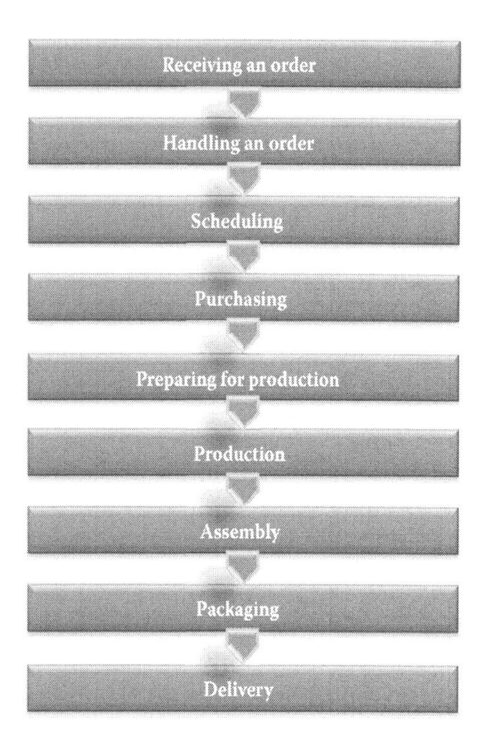

FIGURE 4.1 General process.

Interrelation between Processes

What does "the relation and sequences between the main processes" mean? The best way to demonstrate this is to present an example (Figure 4.2).

In Figure 4.2 one can see that these main processes are required to realize the product:

1. Order transfer
2. Product realization processes
3. Purchasing
4. Goods delivery

The diagram presents the relations and interfaces between these processes and the process of the quality management system:

- Management responsibility
- Resource management
- Measurement, analysis, and improvement

Activities related to sources from outside the organization are mentioned as well:

- Purchase evaluation
- Feedback activities

This kind of diagram helps people to associate themselves and their activities with the structure of the QMS. The ISO 13485 Standard requires reference to the

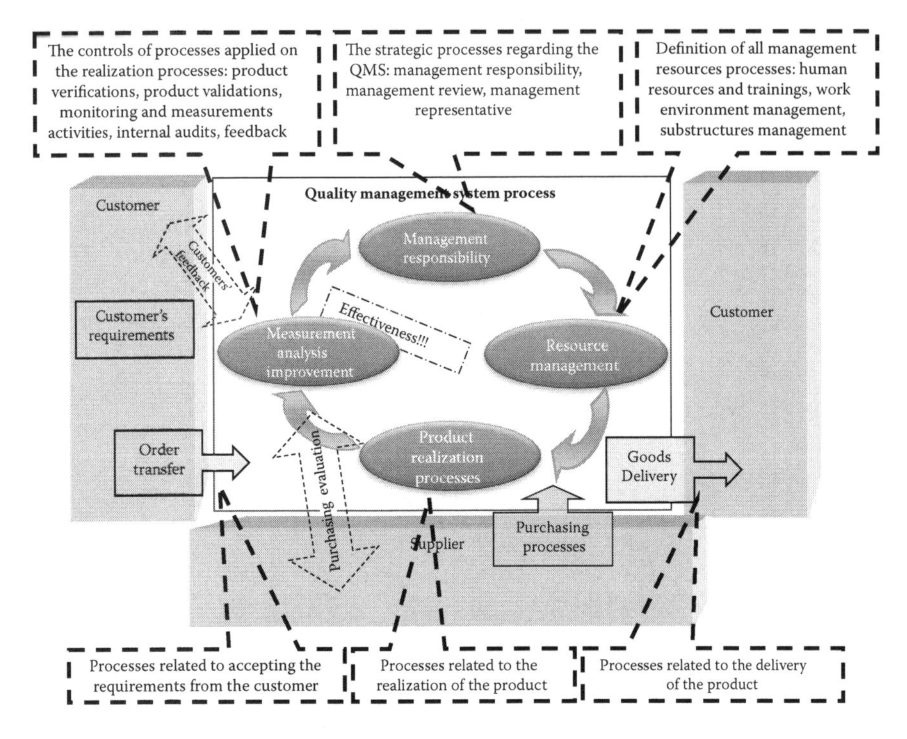

FIGURE 4.2 Interrelation between processes.

defined and documented tools and means used to realize and demonstrate these interrelations; process flowchart diagrams, routing cards or forms, and procedures. These means will be defined. This is the link to the list of processes mentioned above, explaining the relation between the different processes and activities and the quality management processes. This diagram will be placed in the quality manual.

Maintenance of Effectiveness

What does effectiveness mean exactly? Effectiveness is the extent to which planned activities are realized and planned results achieved. Something is planned and the extent of the results are tested against the expected objectives. This is performed in order to achieve systematic improvement.

The ISO 13485 Standard requires constant maintenance of the effectiveness of the quality management system (while the ISO 9001 Standard requires continual improvement of the effectiveness). The requirement is for maintaining processes and documented systems that allow the organization to constantly assess whether its quality management system is effective or not and when it is necessary to replan its further steps. These will be accomplished through the definition of quality objectives. Obtaining these objectives will achieve improvement of the quality management system. Objectives may include schedules, defined time frames for responses, results of processes, reductions of returned goods, etc. The objectives are to be measurable in order to be compared to criteria.

Availability of Resources

Resources and information needed to support the processes are required to be available. The specific requirements regarding resource management are well covered in chapter 6 (Resource Management). Definition for information, however, is divided into two types:

- Defining the required information and data needed to perform activities and operate processes. This shall be available to the relevant parties. Here we may encounter documentation that supports operations of processes, process diagrams, standard operation procedures, and work instructions. First you must define the processes and then document them.
- Defining the communication channels regarding information that flows between different organizational elements. The purpose is to ensure that the information required for the quality management system and the realization processes is transferred correctly and the information that flows reaches its destination. This relates directly to the interrelations mentioned earlier.

Processes regarding information are required to be identified and included under the QMS.

Monitoring, Measurement, and Analysis of Processes

The organization is required to monitor and measure processes defined under the QMS in order to examine whether it achieves its quality objectives and whether the medical device meets its requirements. The ISO 13485 Standard requires maintaining the effectiveness of the QMS while the ISO 9001 Standard requires "only" improving it. By defining the activities and actions for monitoring, measurement, and analysis and implementing them systematically throughout your processes, the effectiveness may be maintained. The activities and actions for monitoring, measurement, and analysis must relate to predefined *acceptance criteria* in order to evaluate the level of achievement. **A tip:** A "Cockpit" system is a good example for maintaining the effectiveness of the quality management system. A "Cockpit" (or a Business Process Management System) is a system that reports data in real time. The name is a metaphor from the aviation world. The management can control in real time the achievement of objectives, just like a pilot controls his parameters. The "Cockpit" allows the management to track, in real time, defined quality management objectives and to determine whether the quality management system is effective or not.

Within the "Cockpit" systems, the quality objectives, the criteria, and processes (in some cases) are defined, and measured per product, per day, per hour—according to the definition. This kind of system allows the management to detect trends and patterns in product provision and to react immediately, in order to improve. As a result, the effectiveness of the quality management system is maintained continually instead of being analyzed once in every period.

A highly recommended system. In fact, I believe that this is the future of management. There will no longer be shouting and anger once every quarter when the reports arrive. From now on, there will be shouting and anger every hour. I have implemented this kind of system in some organizations. The employees there feared me...

Yearning for Improvement: Actions Necessary for the Achievement of Planned Results

Until now processes have been defined, interrelations have been determined, objectives have been set, and activities for monitoring, measurement, and analysis have been implemented. But something is missing. The loop has not yet been closed. The organization must initiate actions for improvements. The organization will systematically identify situations and processes where planned results, quality objectives, or criteria were not met. These situations will be analyzed, the root cause will be recognized, and actions for improvement will be applied.

Outsourced Processes

The organization is responsible for outsourced processes as if the processes were conducted within the organization's facilities. Medical regulations hold the manufacturer responsible for any parameters of the medical device (intended use, performance, safety, and functionality). That means that whether outputs were generated within the organization or within its supplier's facilities, the organization is responsible. In order to submit the outsourced processes to the quality management system, the organization must identify these processes as part of the quality management system. For example, when a manufacturer is realizing a medical device, but the packaging activities are carried out by a supplier, the following are required:

- To include these packaging activities under the quality management system
- To include these processes in the quality manual
- To monitor, measure, and analyze them and to control their effectiveness

4.2 DOCUMENTATION REQUIREMENTS

4.2.1 General

Subclause 4.2.1 is a general paragraph presenting the main documentation requirements of a quality management system according to the ISO 13485 Standard. The specific documentation requirements are mentioned in subclauses 4.2.2–4.2.4 of the standard. This subclause discusses the general requirements for documentation of the ISO 13485. The different types of documentations that will be included in the QMS are as in Table 4.2.

You can use this chapter as a basis for evaluation of your documentation against the standard's requirements:

- Check what is already documented.
- Check which documentations are missing.
- Chart your documentation system and refer it to the standard's requirements.

The purposes of the documentations are as follows:

- The achievement of quality objectives
- The prevention of nonconformities throughout the processes
- The achievement of unity and equality between all the organizational units

The extent, scope, and size of documentation in organizations are affected by the following factors:

- The size of the organization: The more departments included under the QMS, the more documentation is needed.

TABLE 4.2
Standard Requirements of Subclause 4.2.1

ISO 13485	ISO 9001
A quality policy or other statement demonstrating the commitment of the organization to the implementation of the quality management system and to the improvement of its effectiveness	A quality policy or other statement demonstrating the commitment of the organization to the implementation of the quality management system and to the improvement of its effectiveness
Quality objectives	Quality objectives
Quality manual	Quality manual
Documented procedures as required by the ISO 13485	Procedures as required by the ISO 9001
Documents that serve the organization for the purpose of effective planning, operations, performance, and control of processes	Documents that serve the organization for the purpose of effective planning, operations, performance, and control of processes
Records and evidence required by the ISO 13485 Standard	Records and evidence required by the ISO 9001 Standard
Any kind of additional documentation (such as procedures or records) required by any applicable regulatory requirement (national or international)	
Where the standard uses the word "documented" for a particular requirement, process, activity, or an arrangement, it will be established, documented, implemented, and controlled	
Each model, type, or other category of the medical device will have a designated file containing or referring to specific and relevant documentation that describes the medical device specifications and realization processes including servicing and installation activities	

- The level of complicity, functionality, and interrelations between its processes: The more complex and demanding the processes are, the more intense and acute the documentation will be.
- The qualifications of the employees: The less qualified and trained employees are, the more excessive and detailed documentation will need to be.
- Quality objectives: The more quality objectives refer to organizational units and roles, the more the documentation will assist in achieving these objectives.

How can it be determined when a procedure is needed and when a process should be charted? The extent of the documentation of a process will be determined according to the parameters mentioned above. Sample a process and evaluate the following:

- What is the level of its complexity? Do I need only to document the principles and main stages of the process or do I need to document each subprocess?

- What is the level of the personnel's qualifications? Do I need to provide them with a general guideline or do I need to describe a detailed work instruction?
- Does the documentation assist me in achieving quality objectives?
- How many departments and organizational units are included under the quality management system?

Quality Manual

The documentation will include the documented quality manual of the organization, and form and structure of the QMS. The content of the quality manual will be discussed in chapter 4.2.2 (Quality Manual).

Quality Policy

The documentation of the quality management system will include the quality policy of the organization. Usually the policy is documented in the quality manual, although this is not required. It is very useful because there is a direct relation between the two. But the requirement is for a documented statement: a message to communicate the intentions and guidelines set by the top management regarding the quality management system (with reference to the requirements of subclause 5.3 (Quality Policy).

Quality Objectives

The documentation will include the documented quality objectives of the organization. There are various ways and technologies to implement, document, and set the objectives in an organization. A lot of organizations make the mistake of referring to the quality objectives in the quality manual and not elaborating on them. This is not satisfactory. The principle is to define where they will be determined and documented: management review, designated systems, or Excel charts.

Documented Procedures Required by the ISO 13485 Standard

Throughout the standard there are several requirements for documented procedures. They start with the words: "the organization shall establish documented procedure..." When you see this, you know a documented procedure is requested on the subject. Please review Table 4.3. It specifies the ISO 13485 documentation requirements for procedures.

This table will save a lot of trouble. The procedures are divided into three kinds of documents:

- Quality manual. A document specifying the form and structure of the QMS.
- Quality procedure. The quality activities which the standard demands be described and controlled on a documented procedure: control of documents, control of records, internal audit, control of nonconforming product, corrective action, and preventive actions.
- Procedures. Documents that are required from the manufacturer in order for them to ensure effective planning, operations, and control of its processes: procedures, organizational charts, specifications, work instructions, production plans, test protocols, quality plans, purchasing plans.

TABLE 4.3
Documented Procedures Required by the ISO 13485 Standard

Clause	Description	Document Type
4.2.2	Quality manual	Manual
4.2.3	Control of documents	Quality procedure
4.2.4	Control of records	Quality procedure
7.3.1	Design and development planning	Procedure
7.4.1	Purchasing process	Procedure
7.5.1.2.1	Cleanliness of product and contamination control	Procedure
7.5.1.2.2	Installation activities	Procedure
7.5.1.2.3	Servicing activities	Procedure
7.5.2.1	Validation of computer software	Procedure
7.5.2.2	Validation of sterile processes	Procedure
7.5.3.1	Product identification	Procedure
7.5.3.1	Returned product identification	Procedure
7.5.3.2.1	Product traceability	Procedure
7.5.5	Preservation of product (processing)	Procedure
7.5.5	Preservation of product (shelf life)	Procedure
7.6	Control of monitoring and measuring devices	Procedure
8.2.1	Feedback system	Procedure
8.2.2	Internal audits	Quality procedure
8.3	Control of nonconforming product	Quality procedure
8.4	Analysis of data	Procedure
8.5.1	Issue and implementation of advisory notices Notification of adverse events to the regulatory authorities	Procedure
8.5.2	Corrective action	Quality procedure
8.5.3	Preventive action	Quality procedure

The Word "Documented"

Where the standard uses the word "documented" for a particular requirement, process, activity, or an arrangement, it will be established, documented, implemented, and controlled. I did a little research and found which standard clauses and subclauses mention the word "documented":

- 5.5.1: Documentation of responsibilities of the QMS
- 6.2.2: Documentation required by national or regional regulations regarding competence, awareness, and training of human resources
- 6.3: Documented requirements for the operations and maintenance of infrastructures
- 6.4: Documented requirements for health, cleanliness, and clothing
- 7.1: Documented requirements for risk management
- 7.2.2: Documented product requirements
- 7.5.1.1: Documented procedures defining the manner of production

- 8.1: Documented procedures required by national or regional regulations for implementation and control of the application of statistical techniques
- 8.3: Documented procedure for rework

On these topics organizations are required to present documentation that will assist in obtaining these requirements. It is not a recommendation but requirement. Where "documented requirements" is specified, it can be forms, checklists, routing cards, protocols, and maintenance plans. Where "documented procedure" is written, a documented procedure is expected.

Regulatory Requirements for Documentations

When regulation requires maintenance of any kind of certain documentation, it should be planned, established, implemented, and maintained under the requirements of chapter 4.2. For example, if the office of health (in your country or region) requires maintenance of a special form for the registrations of toxicants held in the factory, it is necessary to implement this form in the quality management system.

The ISO organization is aware that there are many regulations for producing medical devices throughout the world and the ISO 13485 Standard gives their requirements the same scale as any standard requirement for documentation. Identify these documentation requirements and include them in the QMS.

Device Master Records (DMR)

For each model, type, or other category of the medical device, the organization must maintain a specific file describing the documents for the medical device specifications. Such a file is often referred to as a Technical File or Device Master Record (DMR). This file will serve as a table of contents of specific documentations required for obtaining materials, components, and specifications for manufacturing, and realization evaluation and control of a specific medical device.

This file has a direct relation to the requirements set out in clause 7.1 (Planning of Product Realization) and will support them in a documentary manner:

- The quality objective of the medical device
- The requirements for procedures, specifications, and instructions
- The need for controls, verifications, and validations
- The requirements for records and evidence

The objective of such a file is to refer each of the organizational participants to one definite location or file that contains master records and specifications relevant to the medical device ("records" here does not mean exclusively quality records of processes). Try to imagine that there is an argument between the quality control inspector and the production manager (not so far from the truth). This file will be the arbitrator; they will go to the file, open the documents, and settle the dispute.

Another objective is to define the scope of the quality management system regarding the control of the medical device: what is required to control, when, how much, by whom, and how long. What kind of documents can we expect to see there?

- Product specifications: Characteristics of the product, product descriptions, specifications of functions, specifications for raw materials, lists of parts, engineering drawings, product drawings, specifications of components, specifications of functions

- Process specifications: Equipment, machinery, and tools specifications and operations, production methods, work instructions, assembly plans, cleanliness and sterilization processes, quality plans
- Quality requirements: Outputs of risk management activities, acceptance criteria, test instructions, inspection procedures, validation plans, packaging validations
- Packaging requirements: Packaging instructions, labeling instructions, delivery instructions
- Installation activities and processes
- Service and maintenance activities and processes

The definition of such a file will assist the control and verification that all the required documentation exists and is available. One way to implement it is to maintain a checklist describing the necessary records and documents. Conservatives will establish a documented procedure although it is not required. I would too. Framing specifications on a procedure never hurt anybody and can only be of help. Each document determined in this file will be submitted to the documents control process as required by subclause 4.2.3 (Control of Documents).

4.2.2 Quality Manual

Let us review the ISO 13485 Standard documentation requirements for quality manuals (Table 4.4). The quality manual is a document with a clear goal: to introduce and communicate the intentions, scope, and structure of a quality management system in an organization. Imagine that a new employee arrives at the organization. He would take the quality manual, read it through, and could immediately answer questions such as: What are the main products and services? How do the

TABLE 4.4
Standard Requirements of Subclause 4.2.1

ISO 13485	ISO 9001
The organization is required to maintain and control the document as a quality manual	The organization is required to maintain a controlled document as a quality manual
The quality manual will specify the scope of the quality management system	The quality manual will specify the scope of the quality management system
The quality manual will specify a list of the exclusions and nonapplications as required in clause 1.2. The list will include justifications for the exclusions or nonapplications	The quality manual will specify a list of the exclusions as required in clause 1.2. The list will include justifications for the exclusions
The quality manual will specify the procedures included under the quality management system or refer to a list that specifies them	The quality manual will specify the procedures included under the quality management system or refer to a list that specifies them
The quality manual will describe the interactions between the processes and the QMS	The quality manual will describe the interactions between the processes and the QMS
The quality manual shall describe the structure of the documentation system used by the quality management system	

main processes flow? What does the organizational structure look like? What are the quality policy and objectives of the firm? The organization may use the manual as a training tool and communication channel regarding quality policy and quality objectives to its employees. I used to get each employee to sign a form indicating that they had read it through, understood the policy and the objectives, and were familiar with the quality procedures. This is the minimum that is required from employees.

I have seen a lot of quality manuals in my life. Most have been collections of superficial statements not related to the real status of the quality management system. I can say that I appraise a quality management system and its effectiveness according to the form and content of its quality manual and so your auditor; the quality manual, its structure and content may tell great deal about the QMS and its effectiveness.

The extent and the size of the quality manual are determined according to organizational parameters: geographic locations, organization structure, areas of activity, and scope of certification. It may be that an organization will request a certification for only one of its products. It may be requested that only one division will be certified. This is where the quality manual clarifies what is included in the QMS. It describes the organization, its activities and profile, in which technologies it is active, and what the processes and products are.

Guidance on development of quality manuals can be found in the ISO 10013 Standard: Guidelines for Quality Management System Documentation.

Organization's Profile

It is common to include the company's profile in the quality manual although it is not requested. The requirement is to present and describe the main technologies and products that the manufacturer works with. The company's profile may serve this purpose. It may be that the quality manual will be distributed to customers for review and then the top management would like to present some nice photos and text along with it. The profile may include details such as:

- The ranges and industries where the firm is active
- The different products and services that the company provides (this is not yet the scope)
- Historical details such as year of establishment
- Geographical areas where the firm is active
- The address of the organization that the quality manual refers to

Scope of the Quality Management System

The scope of the quality management system will be defined in the quality manual. The scope of the quality management system defines and describes which services, operations, and products the quality system applies to. Here are some examples of wordings from certificates I have seen:

- Design, manufacture, and sales of patient monitors
- The design, development, and manufacture of IVD for specimen preparation
- The design and manufacture of medical, surgical, and laparoscopic devices and accessories

- Manufacture of nonsterile respiratory products including aerosol masks and handheld nebulizers
- Design, development, production servicing and marketing, and installation of patient monitoring equipment

Defining the scope correctly is crucial because the scope determines which of your products and services are included under the quality management system and that determines the processes and activities that need to be controlled. The scope will relate to the following issues:

- The product that will be included under the quality management system
- All the applicable realization activities that will be under the quality management system: research and development, production, marketing, installation, service
- Locations of the organizational units that will be under the quality management system (if applicable)

Determining the scope is discussed thoroughly in clause 1.2 (Application). But let us take an example and assume that the scope is already defined and documented. The organization is, however, developing a brand new product with new processes and activities. As long as the product is not included in the scope of the quality manual (and thus the scope of the ISO 13485 certificate), it is not officially included in the quality management system, although the development and realization were done under the appropriate controls and all the records are maintained, etc.

Organizational Structure

Although it is not mentioned, I recommend including the organizational structure in the quality manual. The organizational structure is the definition of hierarchy in the organization. The structure defines who is superior to whom and who reports to whom. The structure will relate to the working processes and scope of the QMS. This will help in charting the QMS. The organizational structure will include all the departments and organizational units or entities that the QMS controls. The emphasis will be on the organizational dependence. The organizational structure is the most basic definition of your QMS. This definition is very important to the charting of the processes and their interactions and helps to position all the participants of the QMS in the organization. I have prepared a very basic diagram as an example (Figure 4.3).

Quality Policy and Quality Objectives

The quality policy and quality objective or a reference to them will be included in the quality manual. Developing the quality policy will be discussed in chapter 5.3 (Quality Policy).

A list of the quality objectives or reference to them will be included as well. It is highly important to mention and indicate in the quality manual the commitment of top management to the definition of effective quality objectives and their communication throughout the different organizational levels.

List of Processes and Reference to the standard Requirements

The quality manual will include the procedures or list of procedures that are included in the QMS. These are the procedures that describe the processes that the manufacturer uses to maintain the quality management system and realize the medical device: standard operating procedures as well as quality procedures.

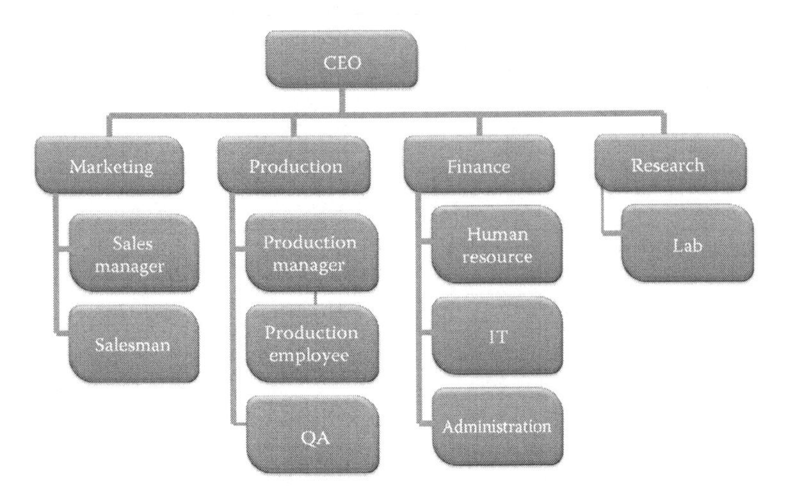

FIGURE 4.3 Example for organizational structure.

One option is to include the procedures in the quality manual itself. I am not fond of this method as I believe that each procedure is entitled to a document on its own. Procedures may be dynamic and frequently changed. Every time a procedure is changed, the whole quality manual will have to be changed, revised, printed, and signed; not very effective.

I prefer separating the quality manual and the procedures and managing a list of procedures. This list will be in the quality manual or the quality manual will refer to it. The list will refer each procedure to its relevant standard requirements. This way it will be possible to ensure that all the standard requirements for documented procedures are covered. I suggest a simple table (Table 4.5). Purchasing processes will be included as well. The purchasing processes include purchasing from internal suppliers such as other department or company divisions.

List of Exclusions and Nonapplications

The quality manual will include the list of the standard requirement exclusions and nonapplications: the standard requirements that the organization for some reason have chosen to exclude and not implement. The reason for the exclusions and nonapplications

TABLE 4.5
List of Processes and Reference to the Standard Requirements

ISO 13485 Standard Requirement	Nr.	Procedure
4.2.3—Control of documents	QP-001-0112	Control of documents
7.6—Control of monitoring and measuring devices	SOP-005-0342	Control of monitoring and measuring devices
8.2.1—Feedback	SOP-004-0121	Handling of customer complaints
	SOP-004-0122	Operating recalls
	SOP-004-0123	Publishing advisory notices

TABLE 4.6
List of Exclusions and Noninclusions

ISO 13485 Standard Requirement	Reason for Exclusion	Reference for Documented Justification (If Appropriate)
7.5.1.3—Particular requirements for sterile medical devices 7.5.2.2—Particular requirements for sterile medical devices	The manufacturer does not apply the medical device to sterilization processes	Product specifications

is that these do not apply to its operations, products, or services. For example, organizations that manufacture nonactive, nonsterile components for use in medical applications, do not perform any installation or services activities, and need not apply the devices to sterilization processes may exclude the following requirements:

- 7.5.1.2.2: Installation activities
- 7.5.1.2.3: Servicing activities
- 7.5.1.3: Particular requirements for sterile medical devices
- 7.5.2.2: Particular requirements for sterile medical devices
- 7.5.3.2.2: Particular requirements for active implantable medical devices and implementable medical devices

Exclusions and nonapplications will be according to the requirements presented in clause 1.2 (Application). But in the quality manual it is necessary to specify what is being excluded and include the justifications. I suggest another table (Table 4.6).

Reference to Regulatory Requirements

A definition of all relevant applicable regulatory requirements is to be documented, mentioned, or referred to in the quality manual. The introduction will be a list or a reference to a list. This is the time to identify all the regulations that apply to the quality management system. Introducing them in the quality manual declares that the organization is committed to implementing them fully throughout its processes and quality management system. The following issues will be referred to:

- Identification of relevant and applicable regulations
- Implementation of requirements throughout the realization processes
- Establishment and maintenance of the required documentation
- Maintenance of the required records
- Promotion of awareness throughout the organization, especially among human resources

A Structure of the Documentation

The quality manual must include a structure of the documentation system used in the quality management system. The idea is to provide a documented description that explains and demonstrates the relations and interrelations between the various documents throughout the QMS; some documents relate to other documents, outputs of one document are the inputs for another document, and so on. But try to define it effectively, present the relations between documents, and make it possible to trace back processes through the documents.

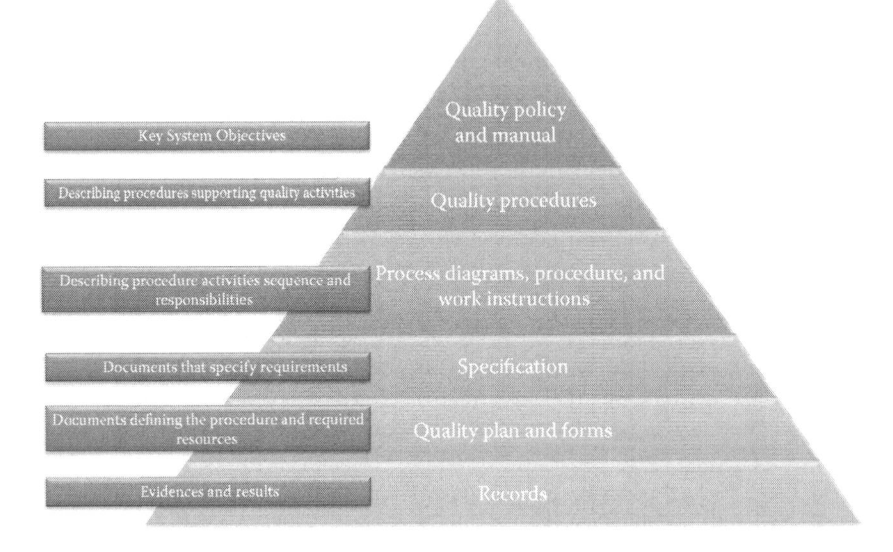

FIGURE 4.4 Documentation pyramid.

How to implement?

- Prepare a chart or a diagram presenting the relations between the various documentations: procedures relating to work instructions, checklists, routing cards.
- Plan a table or a matrix specifying the documents according to subject, issue or range of activities; realization processes, packaging activities, handling customer's complaints. Each subject will include the documents that are relevant to it.
- Use the classic method to present the documentation system as a pyramid (Figure 4.4).

Interaction between the Processes and the Quality Management System

The objectives are as follows:

- To present the relations and interactions between the core business processes of the organization and its QMS processes
- To help people associate themselves with the structure of the QMS

This is the link to the list of processes mentioned above, explaining the relation between the different processes and activities, and the quality management processes. A good example is given in chapter 4.1 (General Requirements).

A Reviewed, Approved, and Controlled Document

The quality manual will be submitted to the process of document control as required in subclause 4.2.3 (Control of Documents). But here are some critical aspects of the control:

- The manual's version and status will be indicated in the manual.
- Changes and revisions will be documented in a way that allow the following changes that were initiated.

TABLE 4.7
Approval of the Quality Manual

Authorized by (Name and Role)	Date	Signature

- The manual will be approved and signed by a defined person (usually the head of top management: president or CEO). The identity of the approver and date of review and approval will be documented. Use this simple table (Table 4.7).
- The accessibility and distribution of the manual to all relevant parties in the organization will be defined in the manual. In other words, where the manual will be stored and how the employees of the organization may review it.

4.2.3 Control of Documents

Documents must be controlled. This is a key element of a quality management system. In order to achieve document control, a method must be maintained. The main idea is to provide control over the documents under the quality management system and to eliminate any confusions and mix ups of different documents from different sources. This method must be one of the organization's quality procedures (Table 4.8).

A Documented Method

The standard demands a method for controlling the documentation that serves the organization for the purpose of effective planning, operations, performance, and control of processes. In subclause 4.2.1 we were given the requirements for the different types of documentation that will support our quality management system. Now it is required to define a method for controlling them. The method will refer to any kind of media: paper printed, magnetic, electronic, or models.

The method will be documented as a procedure. I am used to naming this procedure: document control. I wonder why??? This procedure will be submitted to its own control as required in subclause 4.2.3 (Control or Documents).

Since the topic of controlling your documents refers to a lot of different types and kinds of documents with various characters, I recommend managing the controls using tables. In addition to description of activities, the definitions regarding the documents will be charted on tables according to the issues that the method will cover: table of updates, table of distribution, table of editions, table of revisions, table of changes, table of control, etc. Throughout the chapter I provide you with some examples.

Definition of Document

The organization needs to distinguish between documents that will be controlled and documents that will not be included under the QMS. I suggest you define which documents will be included in your quality management system and will be controlled by this method and procedure. In order not to have too many documents "swirling" around, let's clarify. Allow me to define what a document is:

- Plans, requirements, or specifications for realization or activities
- Input for a process

TABLE 4.8
Standard Requirements of Subclause 4.2.3

ISO 13485	ISO 9001
The organization shall control the documentation of the quality management system	The organization shall control the documentation of the quality management system
A method for controlling the documents shall be defined and documented in a procedure. The methods shall include the following issues:	A method for controlling the documents shall be defined and documented in a procedure. The methods shall include to the following issues:
Each document shall be reviewed and approved for suitability before release for use	Each document shall be approved for suitability before release for use
According to a defined necessity, all documents will bear a validation period, and be reviewed, updated, and approved before the release for use	According to a defined necessity all documents will bear a validation period, and be reviewed, updated, and approved before the release for use
Each document will bear identification regarding the status revision and changes that have occurred on the document	Each document will bear identification regarding the status revision and changes that have occurred on the document
Documents will be distributed and available to relevant parties at the appropriate locations	Documents will be distributed and available to relevant parties at the appropriate locations
The documents will be protected and preserved from damage and will remain usable and readable	The documents will be protected and preserved from damage and will remain usable and readable
External documents will be identified, controlled, and appropriately distributed	External documents will be identified, controlled, and appropriately distributed
Plans and activities for the prevention of use of obsolete or unupdated documents will be established	Plans and activities for the prevention of use of obsolete or unupdated documents will be established
Such documents will be identified and appropriate measures will be planned to handle and control them	Such documents will be identified and appropriate measures will be planned to handle and control them
Changes of documents will be reviewed and approved by a defined function or authority	
The function or authority will be the author of the document or will have precise relevancy to the activity with which the document is associated	
At least one copy of each edition or revision of obsolete documents will be retained according to the following:	
The retention time will be defined	
The copy will be retained for at least the lifetime of its relevant medical device according to the manufacturer's specifications	
In case regulatory requirements demand other retention periods, they will be applied	
The retention time of the obsolete document will cohere to the requirements of record retention (relevant to this document) as specified in subclause 4.2.4 or other regulatory requirements	

- Communication of information
- Sharing of knowledge, information, or data

Unlike a record that is considered as evidence for performance of a process and records the output of a process, the document presents a specification or input for a process. Types of documents in an organization include: diagrams, drawings, process charts, technical specifications, product plans, DMR, quality plans, forms, checklists, routing cards, customer's specifications, manufacturing specifications, process flow diagrams, production plans, standard procedures, quality work procedures, bills of materials, computer files, instructions, test instructions, test protocols, agreements with suppliers, approved lists of suppliers, material specifications, regulations or directives, assembly plans, internal audit plans, corrective action forms, reports of nonconformity, and international standards.

The method will relate to external documents as well. External documents will be distinguished, registered, and controlled. The method shall first identify these external documents that are part of the realization processes of the product and thus require control, for example, a drawing or product received from a customer. This is a classic external document that must be controlled for edition or revision. Examples of external documents may be drawings, packaging instructions, diagrams of production tools, quality requirements, design files, and customer's approvals or agreements. External documents include regulatory requirements. It is necessary to verify that the updated edition of the regulations is available.

I suggest a table that will specify all the documents under the QMS. The fields of the table are:

- Identification number
- Description or name
- Relevant process/relevant department
- Responsible for review
- Responsible for approval
- Media
- Location
- Internal/external
- Other characteristics such as public or classified

Approval and Release of Documents

Each document used by the organization must be supervised, reviewed, and approved before submission for use. The objective is to ensure that the document was appropriately designed, is suitable for working, and will assist the organization in meeting the medical device objectives as well as regulatory requirements. For each document the role, function, or authority that reviews, approves, and releases it will be defined. The definition will be in the procedure.

The function or authority that reviews and approves the document must have some degree of relevancy to the document and the related activity. The standard specifically demands the following:

- The function or person that designed or planned the document
- Other function or person relevant to the activity of the document

How is relevancy determined? You need to review qualifications, experience, and background of the subject and their relevancy to the activities. This requirement will ensure that documents will be checked by appropriate functions or roles and all important aspects will be accounted for. For example, when you are designing a routing card for a production process, the production manager is responsible for reviewing that all the required fields are on the form and then approving it. But if you are planning a process validation form, there are other parties that would like to share their opinion about it: the development guys and the QA guys. The authority for the review and approval is related to the activities that the document specifies. There are situations when more than one function would need to review and approve the document. This may occur when more than one process will be documented in one document, for example packaging instructions. Then the storage and the production manager will need to discuss the matter and together create the optimal document.

The activity of approval and release of a document will be defined, where approval is given. I used to print a master copy, signed the responsible party, and store in a master documents folder. But today you can achieve this with the help of document control computer systems that provide digital approvals. Usually these systems are designed according to the standard requirements. When purchasing such a system, make sure that it is designed according to the ISO 13485 Standard requirements. If you do not have this option, a simple table describing the document and the authority for review and approval will be enough.

Identification of Documents

Any document (internal or external) must be identified. Documents must have a name, catalogue number, or other means of identification: an element that can identify it and submit it to the control. Anyone in the organization that picks the document will know where to assign it. The ISO 13485 Standard requires maintaining a method for identification of documents. The following example is quite primitive but will hold in an audit:

Take a look at the following number: SOP-004-002: Clean room procedure

- SOP: Stands for "standard operating procedure."
- 004: The first three digits represent the process.
- 002: The second three digits represent the subprocess.
- Clean room procedure: The name of the procedure.

And to it I add document FO-004-002-003: Clean room checklist

- FO: Stands for form.
- 004: The first three digits represent the process related to this form.
- 002: The second three digits represent the subprocess related to this form.
- 003: Represents the third form related to this subprocess.
- Clean room checklist: The name of the form.

Together they combine an identification number, maintain the interrelation between each other, but most importantly they provide identification of the documents.

Securing Documents and Their Use

The method shall ensure that documents will remain safe and available for use. The method will define what the appropriate maintenance conditions of the document are. What are the appropriate conditions? The document will remain legible and it would be possible to identify it.

In practice it is necessary to identify what environmental conditions may affect the document. Pay a visit to the different rooms, take a look, and try to review the parameters that might affect the safety of the documents. On the procedure, mention them and what actions are required in order to avoid them. For example, water and heat may damage a paper document and therefore in such environment work instructions and procedures should be laminated, placed in a heatproof pouch, and kept away from hazards. This is a kind of small-scale risk analysis regarding the safety of a document. Backup systems for the company's server are another example of protection.

Another aspect is human resource behavior with documents. Define for the employees how they shall handle documents and where shall they be stored. I found myself printing diagrams again and again, just because they were lost all the time.

Updated and Revised Documents (and Their Status)

The method must ensure that the latest version is always the version in use—and not an older one. Therefore you must define a method for maintaining updated versions and elimination of use of older versions. How does one know what the latest version is? Usually organizations manage a table list of editions and updates for documents. But more important is to indicate it on the document itself. This way it will be clear to any employee that he holds the latest edition. Managing editions must include:

- Date of last update
- The reason/description for the update/comment
- The function that demanded the update
- The function that authorized the update
- Expiry date of the document

It is important to document the history of a document and specify what has been changed and why. I would implement an independent table to manage the editions or revisions:

On the new form the new revision will be indicated: FO-004-002-003(003) or FO-004-002-003 (01/01/2010). Cross-checking between the table and the document will indicate what update revision it is (Table 4.9).

TABLE 4.9
List of Updated and Revised Documents

Doc Nr.	Edition	Change Requested By	Reason	Approved By	Date	New Edition
FO-004-002-003	002	Mr. White	As a request of production employee a field was added: Time of break	Mr. Frank	01/01/2010	003

Changes as a Necessity

The standard demands that documents will be periodically reviewed and reapproved according to need. Which need? The needs are different events or requests regarding changes in documents (internal as well as external). For example:

- Employee's request for a change on a form
- A change in a procedure or a process due to a customer complaint
- A request from a customer for a change in the product specifications
- A change in a regulatory requirement

You need to identify these events and request initiation of a change, review the change and its consequences, and reapprove the document. The method will determine:

- Identification of events or requests for change
- Identification of the relevant documents
- Identification of parties, roles, and authorities needed for the review and approval
- Method of review: what are the inputs, where and when will the review take place
- Approval and records
- Submission to the process of removing obsolete editions, and distributing and implanting the new one

Apropos records, what details are expected to be recorded?

- Date of the review
- Identification of the relevant document, its editions or revision
- The reason and cause for the change
- What was changed
- Who reviewed
- Remarks
- Consequences for regulatory requirements
- Parties present at the occasion
- Approval

This may appear on a designated form that follows all the changes referring to one document or in the table mentioned above.
A tip: MS word change review is not considered a change control.

Document Removal

The method will ensure the use of updated documents throughout the organization, in work stations, departments, or any other locations where the documents are stored. It will be achieved with the removal of invalid documents and their replacement with the updated ones. The input for the removal activity will be a change on a document. The method will include the following steps:

- The document to be replaced will be identified. Whenever a change on a document is initiated, it will result in a removal of the old edition.
- The second stage is the evaluation of the removal: where or which organizational units use the document.
- The physical removal itself: from the work station or from a server.
- The introduction of the new edition to the relevant parties.

The method will refer to computerized or electronic documents as well as printed. To complete the cycle effectively you are required to develop a periodical control that ensures the use of relevant versions only. My recommendation is to design and implement the test on the internal audit.

Availability and Distribution of Documents

Each document will be available to the relevant role or function at the point of use. Defining the availability and distribution of documents must include the following:

- User authorization: Who is authorized to use a document
- Location of the document: Where must a document be kept before and after use
- Form of availability. Paper, magnetic, system form, a product model

A tip: Most of today's process management systems (such as ERP or Business Process Management) provide a document control system relevant to the process it handles. The system presents the user with a screen (a screen on a computer system is a document like any other document) with defined information for input. Most of these systems also have an authorization module installed. In other words, the availability of a document is managed through the system. If you are using such a system to manage your realization processes or some of them, you may describe this in the method.

But when a system like the one mentioned above does not exist in the organization, it must provide the employees with relevant updated documents. That means the latest editions or revision. The issue will be defined in the procedure. In order to remove any doubt, I recommend describing it in Table 4.10.

Archiving

Activities for archiving old documents and obsolete editions will be determined. It is necessary to define what is to be done with old versions that are not updated, how one handles them, and whether they are to be disposed of or archived. Invalid documents that are not disposed of are to be indicated or marked. The mark will ensure beyond any doubt that no one will use them. If you print out several documents and they are now invalid, you have two options: destroy them or mark each one with a stamp. If the documents are saved on the company's server, an authority will be appointed for deleting or archiving the obsolete ones and replacing them with updated ones. You are responsible for implementing the awareness of this issue throughout the organization.

The storage of unupdated documents will be defined. The activities will define the location of the archiving, the retention time, and in which media. Once again I suggest

TABLE 4.10
Specification of Availability and Distribution of Documents

Type of Document	Folder	Responsibility	Location
Quality manual Quality procedures SOP Process diagrams	Folder on the server	Quality manager	I:\Public Quality\ Quality procedures ISO 13485 (a computer file path)
Work instructions	DMR	Production manager Quality manager	Quality department —shelf number 5
Quality instructions	DMR	Quality manager	Quality department —shelf number 5

TABLE 4.11
Retention Time of Documents

Type	Location	Media	Retention Time
Quality procedures	I:\Public Quality\Quality Archive\Quality procedures (a computer file path)	Electronic	7 years
Drawings	I:\Public Quality\Quality Archive\Drawings (a computer file path)	Electronic (must be scanned to the computer)	7 years
Purchasing forms	I:\Public Quality\Quality Archive\Forms (a computer file path)	Electronic	7 years
Employee absence form	Disposal	N/A	N/A

managing a table that describes the archiving parameters for each type of document (Table 4.11).

Retention Time

For obsolete editions of a document, it is necessary to define the retention time according to the following conditions:

- The retention time will be as short as the lifetime of the relevant medical device (the medical device that the document relates to) as defined by the manufacturer.
- When regulatory requirements set retention time for obsolete documents, according to the type of the relevant medical device, the retention time will be set accordingly.
- In any case, retention time of an obsolete edition of a document will not be less than the lifetime of records that relate to this obsolete edition of a document.

I have prepared a visual example in order to make this clearer. Let us assume:

- The defined lifetime of the medical device is one year since it has been delivered.
- Regulatory requirement Nr. 1: The organization is required to retain documents referring to the medical device for at least two years after delivery.
- Regulatory requirement Nr. 2: The organization is required to retain records referring to the medical device for at least four years after delivery.

So, on one beautiful morning the manufacturer delivers the medical device and on the same day one of the documents was changed from edition 1000 to 1001. Edition 1000 became obsolete. The count begins. Refer to the timeline (Figure 4.5).

a. The organization is not allowed to dispose of edition 1000—the medical device is still valid and functioning.
b. The organization is not allowed to dispose of edition 1000—it has not been two years since the release date (regulatory requirement Nr. 1).
c. The organization is not allowed to dispose of edition 1000—it has already been two years, but regulatory requirement Nr. 2 demands keeping records for at least

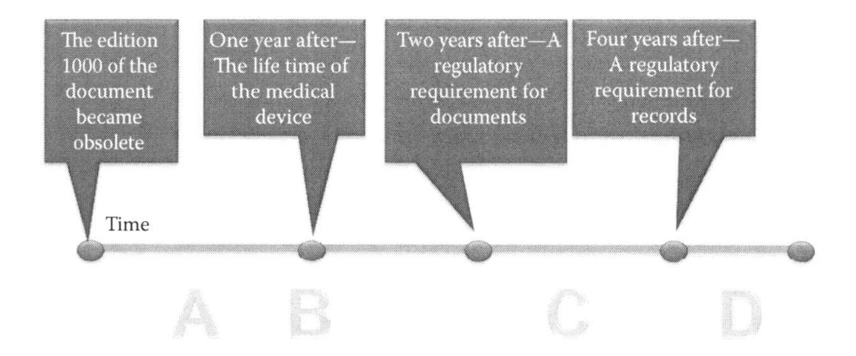

FIGURE 4.5 Retention time of documents.

four years. These records refer to edition 1000. The manufacturer must hold edition 1000 until the records are disposed of.

d. The organization is allowed to dispose of edition 1000.

4.2.4 Control of Records

Directly related to document control, I will now discuss record control requirements. The ISO 13485 Standard requires definition of what records are included in the quality management system and how they are controlled (Table 4.12).

Relationship between Records and the Quality Management System

Why is it so important to define which records to control? Let's presume that tomorrow morning a customer complains about a medical device—let us hope that it will never happen. In order to examine the case thoroughly, the records must be approached and investigated. Then, and only then, can the true story about the medical device be found. In other words, the documentation is the statement of defense (and let us hope that we will never have to use it). But, if tomorrow morning we find ourselves in a certain situation or if any question arises, the records will be our savior.

Documented Procedure

A documented procedure defining the control of the records is required. The procedure will describe the methods, activities, and technologies used to implement the control of the records and the required evidence. The procedure will be submitted to the document control process in the organization as required in subclause 4.2.3 (Control of Documents).

Type of Records

A record is evidence of performing a process or activity or an output of a process. According to the standard, records will serve two main purposes:

- Verification of execution. Records are used to prove conformity to requirements or specifications. A procedure, specification, or other documented requirement demands the execution of a process or activity. With records it is possible to

TABLE 4.12
Standard Requirements of Subclause 4.2.4

ISO 13485	ISO 9001
The organization shall maintain records to demonstrate and prove its conformity to the standard's requirements, processes requirements, and the effectiveness of the quality management system	The organization shall maintain records to demonstrate and prove its conformity to the standard's requirements, processes requirements, and the effectiveness of the quality management system
The organization shall maintain a documented procedure describing the method and activities of controlling records	The organization shall maintain a documented procedure describing the method and activities of controlling records
The methods shall ensure that records are appropriately stored, protected, and retentive	The methods shall ensure that records are appropriately stored, protected, and retentive
The method shall describe activities for the disposal of records	The method shall describe activities for the disposal of records
The method shall ensure that records will remain legible, readably identifiable, and retrievable	The methods shall ensure that records will remain legible, readably identifiable, and retrievable
The method shall define retention of records according to the following:	
The retention time will be defined for each type of record.	
Records shall be retained for at least the lifetime of their relevant medical device according to the manufacturer's specifications but not less than two years since the medical device was released.	
In case regulatory requirements demand other retention periods, they will be applied	

verify that it was done according to the specification: time, sequence, responsibility, and activities.

- Evaluation of effectiveness. With the records one can review the effectiveness of an activity and appraise the results against criteria.

Examples for records and evidence related to the effectiveness of the quality management system may include:

- Changes and justifications for the changes
- Project estimations regarding the objectives of the project
- Meeting summaries

Such records provide evidence that objectives were (or were not) met. Records are logically the last level of your documentations in your quality management system and relate to processes, procedures, work instructions, specifications, and plans. Each of the above is assigned to a function or a role that is responsible for it. This is a standard requirement. So why not records as well? Although the standard does not require a responsible party to be assigned to a record, this is recommended.

Issues that may be covered with records include records of processes, purchasing, regulatory requirements, and customer's records.

TABLE 4.13
List of Different Types of Records

Type of Record	Name	Nr.	Media	Location	Responsibility
Process control	Clean room checklist	FO 00400203	Printed	Clean room	Shift foreman
Protocol	Quality test protocol	FO 00500201	Excel chart	Server	Quality tester

Types of records include process forms, test protocols with results, certificate of compliance (COC) accepted from suppliers, full questionnaires, quality records such as management reviews or internal audit reports, labels with production details such as serial numbers, validation forms, REACH registrations from suppliers, customer orders, records of machine maintenance, production tool status reports, job release approvals, and batch approvals.

It is recommended to maintain a table that specifies the records of the QMS along with different characteristics. The fields of the table will be:

- Identification number
- Description or name
- Relevant process/relevant department
- Responsible
- Media
- Location
- Internal/external
- Other characteristics such as public or classified

Example of Table 4.13.

Storage of Records

A storage location must be defined for each type of record: a closet, a designated folder, a computer folder, a file. The method shall allow each person in the organization who browses the records control procedure to trace back records according to their type. Storage definition shall refer to the archival of old documents as well.

There are two popular methods for managing records: design history file and design history record. In case you are managing and controlling the records with such methods, they will be mentioned in the procedure.

The design history file (DHF) is a file containing all the records related to the design and development of the medical device: design inputs, validation tests of design, verification and reviews of the design, and development activities. In practice the records in the file are collected during the design and development activities: reviewing and documenting customer's requirements, design of the medical device, development activities, prototype building, and testing. Such a file allows two things:

- Verification of the effectiveness. Control that the required results are achieved through the comparison between inputs and outputs.
- Change control. Tracing the changes and evolution of the medical device.

The design history record (DHR) is a file containing records concerning the realization processes of a specific model or version of a medical device. These are the records that prove the conformity to the requirements and specification, and demonstrate the effectiveness of the realization processes: certifications of materials, quality test reports, and delivery notices. The DHR method and content will be planned according to the characteristics of the medical device and its realization processes. Its objectives are to:

- control the procession of the medical device in processes
- ensure that all activities are conducted
- review the effectiveness of activities through the records

How? Through the provision of information concerning various properties of the medical device: dates of manufacture, quantities that were manufactured in each batch, registration and tracing serial numbers of medical devices, quantities that were delivered from each batch, and evidence of packaging and storage activities. You can maintain a checklist and place it in a folder and store all records or copies of them in the folder, or you can maintain a list of the records and refer to their location throughout the organization. I find this very effective.

Protection of Records

The records will be appropriately protected. For each record you need to identify the risks that records will be damaged or lost and apply appropriate methods of protection: organizing folders in the work stations, ensuring that records will reach the responsible parties and will not be lost, and ensuring no confusion when filing the records. The solution for protection shall extend to all areas and scopes of the organization.

Backup systems are one good example of how the organization protects its records. Such a system proves integrity of records as well as providing a solution in case of a disaster.

Each activity and method for protecting the records shall be documented in the procedure.

Authorization

The method will define an authorization management for access to the records, in order to protect the records from unauthorized entries. Some records will bear customer's property and include classified information and thus must be confidential.

Identification of Records

Each type of record (internal or external) must be identified. A record must have a name, catalogue number, or other means of identification: an element that identifies it and submits it to the method. Anyone in the organization that stumbles upon it will know where to assign it. The ISO 13485 Standard requires maintenance of a method for identification of records. I usually use the following method:

- FO-004-002-003: Clean room checklist.
- FO: Stands for form.
- 004: The first three digits represent the process related to this form.
- 002: The second three digits represent the subprocess related to this form.
- 003: Represents the third form related to this subprocess.
- Clean room checklist: The name of the form.

But the identification of a record does not end with its name and number. As stated before, a record is an evidence of performance. The question is not only which process but who performed the process. Each record must have the identity of the person that filled it or at least the function that is responsible for it. The classic way is the name, date, and a signature on the record. The identification of the person will be clear and understood. A digital signature counts as well. The method and manner for identifying the records shall be documented in the procedure.

Legible Records

The method shall ensure that the records will be legible for their entire retention time. When determining the method the organization shall consider the following issues:

- The deterioration of electronic or magnetic media on which the records are kept plays an important role. Media such as CDs or magnetic tapes do not last forever. In fact their lifetime is shorter than you think.
- Changing of technology used to save and access the records is a major aspect. You may find yourself one day not able to access a file because the properties of the operation system were changed or your system administrator removed the software from your computer.
- Conversion of analog records to digital formats will enable retrieval of 100% of the data and information on the records. If you decide to scan records to computer files, please ensure that the scanning is done appropriately and the information on record is readable and clear after the scan. I have already found myself kneeling on all fours, searching for old documents in cold cellars just because the scanning was hard and it was impossible to use these records.
- Filling forms will be done clearly and correctly. People with problematic handwriting will have to work harder and provide legible data and information on the record. I am not expecting you to include it in the training program but do pay attention and comment to people about this issue.

Errors on Records

When a mistake or error is made on a record, it is acceptable to correct it, but the wrong original entry will stay visible on the record. The person who corrected the error will be identified and the correction will be dated (similar to a correction made on a contract). The reason for the correction will be recorded. The activity and manner of correcting the error on the records shall be documented in the procedure.

Archiving Records

Activities for archiving records will be determined and documented in the procedure. It is required to define what should be done with old records, how they should be handled, how long they should be retained, and whether they are to be disposed of or archived. An authority will be appointed for disposing of or archiving the records. You are responsible for implementing awareness of the issue throughout the organization.

The storage of old records will be defined. The activities will define the location of the archiving, the retention time, and in which media. Once again I suggest managing a table that describes the archiving parameters for each type of record (Table 4.14).

Retention Time

The ISO 13485 Standard requires retaining records as long as the lifetime of the medical device and in any case not less than two years from the date the product was

TABLE 4.14
Where Records Are Archived

Type	Location	Media	Retention Time
Customer's complaint	I:\Public Quality\Quality Archive\Customer's Complaint (a computer file path)	Electronic	7 years
Test protocols	Archive	Paper	7 years
COC	Archive	Paper	7 years

delivered, or other period required by any applicable regulatory requirement. Once again I have prepared a visual example in order to explain it. Let us assume:

- The defined lifetime of the medical device is one year after it has been delivered.
- ISO 13485 Standard requirement: The organization is required to retain records referring to the medical device for at least two years after the delivery.
- Regulatory requirement: The organization is required to retain records referring to the medical device for at least four years after the delivery.

So, on one beautiful morning the organization delivers the medical device and the count begins. Refer to the timeline (Figure 4.6).

Let us analyze the various time indications:

a. The organization is not allowed to dispose of any records referring to the medical device—the medical device is still valid and functions.
b. The organization is not allowed to dispose of the records referring to the medical device—it has not been two years since the delivery date (standard requirement).
c. The organization is not allowed to dispose of the records referring to the medical device. True, the lifetime of the medical device has terminated, but it has not yet been two years and there is a regulatory requirement that demands records are kept for at least four years.
d. The organization is not allowed to dispose of the records referring to the medical device. It has been two years but there is a regulatory requirement that demands records are kept for at least four years.
e. The organization is allowed to dispose of the records.

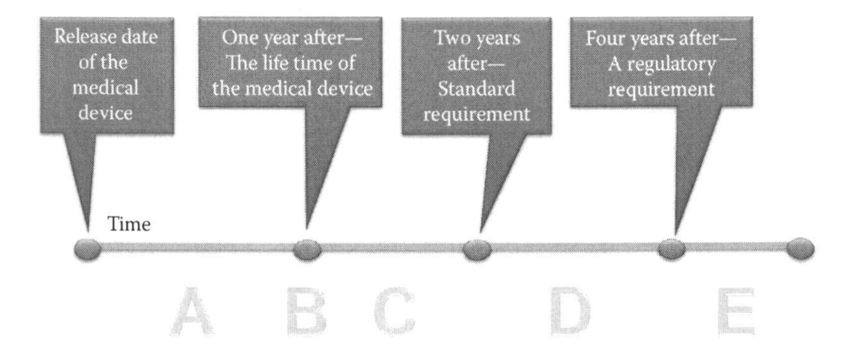

FIGURE 4.6 Retention time of records.

Risk Management

When determining the retention time, it is necessary to verify that the residual risks on the medical device do not demand a longer retention time. It may be that the retention time will have to be as long as the residual risk is valid. Check the risk file when determining the retention time.

TABLE 4.15
List of Standard Requirements for Records

Clause	Description	Document Type
5.6.1	Management review	Record
6.2.2 (e)	Competence, awareness, and training	Record
6.3	Maintenance	Record
7.1 (d)	Planning of product realization	Record
7.1	Risk management	Record
7.2.2	Review of requirements related to product	Record
7.3.2	Design and development inputs	Record
7.3.3	Design and development outputs	Record
7.3.4	Design and development review	Record
7.3.5	Design and development verification	Record
7.3.6	Design and development validation	Record
7.3.7	Control of design and development changes	Record
7.4.1	Supplier evaluations	Record
7.4.2	Purchasing information	Record
7.4.3	Verification of purchased product	Record
7.5.1.1	Batch records	Record
7.5.1.2.2	Installation activities	Record
7.5.1.2.3	Servicing activities	Record
7.5.1.3	Sterilization parameters	Record
7.5.2.1	Validation (process)	Record
7.5.2.2	Validation (sterilization)	Record
7.5.3.2.1	Product traceability	Record
7.5.3.2.2	Consignee name and address	Record
7.5.4	Customer property	Record
7.5.5	Preservation of product	Record
7.6	Calibration (as found)	Record
7.6	Calibration (corrected)	Record
8.2.2	Internal audits	Record
8.2.4.1	Product release	Record
8.2.4.2	Product inspection and testing	Record
8.3	Nonconformances (authorization)	Record
8.3	Nonconformances (nature)	Record
8.4	Analysis of data	Record
8.5.1	Customer complaints (investigations)	Record
8.5.1	Customer complaints (no action)	Record
8.5.2	Corrective action (including investigation)	Record
8.5.3	Preventive action (including investigation)	Record

Standard Requirements for Records

The ISO 13485 Standard requires maintenance of specific records in addition to those that prove conformity and effectiveness. These records will be submitted to the record control activities just like any other records. A list specifying all of the standard requirements for the records is as in Table 4.15.

A tip: When you browse the ISO 13485 Standard you will notice a note that is constantly repeated: see 4.2.4. This note actually directs you to subclause 4.2.4 of the standard: Control of Records. Still confused? Any clause or subclause that ends with that note means that you must maintain a record.

5 Management Responsibility

5.1 MANAGEMENT COMMITMENT REQUIREMENTS

As far as I can say, the success of a quality management system (QMS) depends on the top management. This is no secret. But how can one evaluate whether the management is truly devoted to the quality management system or just acts like it once a year when the external auditor pays a visit? Then all the special suits come out, everybody is smiling and saying how important the QMS is and blah blah blah… (Table 5.1).

This chapter (Management Responsibility) lays out the requirements of top management regarding the quality management system. Chapter 5.1 specifies the principle that will construct the commitment of top management. In this chapter the general requirements for top management regarding the quality management system are presented. Specific requirements appear in chapters 5.2–5.6. This chapter should be regarded as a basis for self-evaluation of your top management's status and its role

TABLE 5.1
Standard Requirements of Clause 5.1

ISO 13485	ISO 9001
Top management is required to prove with evidence its commitment to the implementation of a quality management system. The commitment will ensure maintenance of the effectiveness of the quality management system	Top management is required to prove with evidence its commitment to implementing a quality management system. The commitment will ensure continual improvement of the effectiveness of the quality management system
Top management shall convey and inform the organization of the importance of meeting customers' and regulatory requirements	Top management shall convey and inform the organization of the importance of meeting customers' and regulatory requirements
Top management shall determine and document a quality policy	Top management shall determine and document a quality policy
Top management shall see to it that quality objectives are defined and obtained	Top management shall see to it that quality objectives are defined and obtained
Top management shall conduct management reviews of the quality management system	Top management shall conduct management reviews of the quality management system
Top management shall allocate resources for the quality management system	Top management shall allocate resources for the quality management system
Statutory requirements refer to regulations concerning the safety and performance of the medical device only	

within the quality management system regarding its commitment. Here, the management is required to demonstrate, with actions and evidence, how it assures that the quality management system is effectively implemented. In order to prove its commitment, top management will supply evidence of its actions.

Ensuring the Effectiveness of the Quality Management System

The ISO 13485 Standard requires maintaining the effectiveness of the quality management system. It is clearly emphasized that top management is not only responsible for developing the quality management system but also implementing it and maintaining it effectively. Effectiveness will be achieved when carrying out the following fundamental activities:

- Establishing communication channels with the lower levels in the organization
- Defining a quality policy
- Implementing the quality policy throughout the organization using measurable quality objectives
- Fulfilling them by reviewing the QMS periodically and systematically
- Allocating the required resources

Communicating

One of the missions of top management is communicating to the organization the importance of meeting customers as well as statutory and regulatory requirements during the realization processes. The purpose here is to ensure that the management has defined means of communication to deliver and implement as well as receive information, data, and messages regarding the QMS objectives among the employees.

Defining a Quality Policy

Top management is required to define a quality policy or other statement demonstrating the commitment of top management and the organization to the implementation of a quality management system, and to the maintenance of its effectiveness (with reference to the requirements of clause 5.3 (Quality Policy)).

Quality Objectives

Top management will establish the quality objectives and will ensure that these objectives are achieved. This will be done by determining the objectives that are relevant to the quality policy and the nature of the organization. After determining the objectives, top management must collect and analyze data regarding these objectives and evaluate whether they have been met or not. The objectives will be determined with reference to the requirements of subclause 5.4.1 (Quality Objectives).

Management Review

Top management will conduct a systematic and periodical review of its QMS, in order to evaluate its effectiveness. The management review will be analyzed in more detail in chapter 5.6 (Management Review).

Allocation of Resources

Top management shall ensure allocation of all required resources in order to ensure the effective operation of the quality management system.

5.2 CUSTOMER FOCUS

The ISO 13485 sets requirements to ensure top management's commitment to the customers (Table 5.2). Chapter 5.2 (Customer Focus) sets the level of involvement of top management regarding its customers. There are two main goals:

- Understanding and implementing customers' and regulatory requirements
- Realizing a product that will meet the customers' and regulatory requirements

The standard refers us to two of its requirements: 7.2.1 and 8.2.1, because as far as the standard is concerned, these goals will be achieved once the top management will plan, implement, and control the two issues mentioned on these subclauses.

Determination of Requirements Related to the Product

Top management shall define a method for identifying and implementing customers' and regulatory requirements. The objective of the method is to identify the requirements and to introduce them to the realization processes. The method will cover all the necessary activities: which roles are involved, what their activities are, which information is to be maintained, frequencies and intervals, and data analysis actions. The method will be determined according to the standard requirements as specified in subclause 7.2.1 (Determination of Requirements Related to the Product). The methods shall include internal customers as well. After establishing the method, top management is responsible for examining its effectiveness:

- To verify whether the method was implemented as required
- To validate that the customers' and regulatory requirements are met

Implementing Feedback Activities

Top management shall define a method for monitoring the information regarding whether the product met customers' and regulatory requirements. The activities will be defined according to the standard requirements in subclause 8.2.1 (Feedback). The method shall indicate types of data, responsibilities, and activities. After establishing the method, top management is responsible for examining its effectiveness:

TABLE 5.2
Standard Requirements of Clause 5.2

ISO 13485	ISO 9001
Top management is responsible for ensuring all customer requirements are understood	Top management is responsible for ensuring all customer requirements are understood
Top management is responsible for ensuring all customer requirements are implemented and met	Top management is responsible for ensuring all customer requirements are implemented and met
	Customer satisfaction will be enhanced as a result

- To verify whether the method was implemented as required
- To validate that the information and data that were collected and analyzed are providing the appropriate situation report

Clause 5.2 ensures that top management or its representative will be fully involved in these quality activities.

5.3 QUALITY POLICY

The organization will define a quality policy that will express its quality intentions regarding various issues (Table 5.3).

Quality Policy: The Definition

A quality policy is the general guidelines, intentions, and goals of the organization referring to quality. The policy is defined and published by top management. The policy will be implementable, available, active, and communicated and will be documented as required in paragraph 4.2.1 (mainly in the quality manual).

The policy will demonstrate what quality means to the organization: the intention to provide your customers with quality products according to defined requirements using a controlled system of processes and procedures. The system will be effective and subject to constant improvement.

Association with the Organization

The quality policy shall define the areas, subjects, and scopes where the organization would like to implement its quality efforts. The quality policy will be planned and

TABLE 5.3
Standard Requirements of Clause 5.3

ISO 13485	ISO 9001
Top management will establish a quality documented policy	Top management will establish a quality documented policy
The quality policy must suit the organization's nature and type of activities	The quality policy must suit the organization's nature and type of activities
The quality policy shall demonstrate the organization's commitment to maintaining the effectiveness of the quality management system	The quality policy shall demonstrate the organization's commitment to continually improving the quality management system
The quality policy shall demonstrate the organization's commitment to meeting customer and regulatory requirements	The quality policy shall demonstrate the organization's commitment to meeting customer and regulatory requirements
The quality policy will define the basis for setting quality objectives	The quality policy will define the basis for setting quality objectives
Top management shall indicate the manner in which the quality policy is to be distributed and presented throughout the organization	Top management shall indicate the manner in which the quality policy is to be distributed and presented throughout the organization
The quality policy must be periodically reviewed in order to ensure its competence	The quality policy must be periodically reviewed in order to ensure its competence

designed in order to suit all the activities of the organization that are included under the quality management system: marketing, sales, finance, administration, production, development, and logistics.

Effectiveness of the Quality Management System

The policy shall demonstrate the intentions of the organization regarding the maintenance of the effectiveness of the quality management system; top management must initiate defined actions and intentions in order to maintain an effective quality management system.

Relation to Quality Objectives

The quality policy shall lay the foundations for the definition of quality objectives. This relation between the quality policy and the quality objective will turn it into a useful document rather than just a documented statement. Usually the policy includes strategic objectives that refer to more specific and measurable objectives. The quality policy defines areas and scopes in which the quality will be active and valid. The quality objectives will be derived from these areas and scopes. If the policy declares a desire to manufacture precision products to meet the most critical design requirements in a wide range of applications, the appropriate relevant objectives would be as follows:

- Promoting design and development in the organization
- Identifying new unfulfilled market needs

Setting objectives correlated to the policy will assist in maintaining an effective quality management system. But whatever the objectives are, there are two main goals that must be implemented regarding the quality objectives: meeting customer and regulatory requirements. The policy will include a clear reference to the issue.

Communication and Distribution

Top management shall determine a method to inform all employees related to the QMS about the policy:

- The employees do not have to learn the policy by heart but must be familiar with the main principles of the policy.
- The employees must understand their position in the quality management system and the impact of their activities on the product.
- Their work shall indicate that they carry the quality policy out through their activities.

This matter shall be documented in the quality manual.

Periodical Review

The quality policy will be reviewed periodically in order to ensure its competence. The review will ensure that changes that affect the QMS (internal and external) have been taken into account and when applicable the policy has been updated appropriately.

Example

An example is given here of a quality policy that covers what the chapter has discussed:

Our company is committed to the highest level of quality in the manufacture, marketing, service, and support of our products. Quality and compliance with all applicable regulatory and customer requirements shall underline all of our efforts. We are committed to monitoring, improving, and continuously maintaining our quality system and its effectiveness. Our success in meeting this objective is systematically measured by the performance of our processes. Our quality objectives are as follows:

- The company will act to provide its customers with the appropriate product according to their specifications and expectations.
- The company will act to effectively identify implement applicable regulatory requirements throughout all the realization processes.
- The company will promote its human resources and allocate all the required resources.
- The company will promote its infrastructures and work environment conditions and allocate all the required resources.
- The company regards suppliers as partners and will act to implement them fully in the quality management system.

5.4 PLANNING

5.4.1 Quality Objectives

The quality objectives are an integral part of the quality policy and maintain a close relation with it. The quality objectives are the manner in which the quality policy is implemented within the organization (Table 5.4).

The purpose of the quality objective is to carry out the quality policy practically and implement it in the quality management system. By planning and implementing quality objectives a meaningful, powerful, and impressive quality policy is integrated. The real proof for implementing the policy is its translation into a set of implementable clear objectives. The objectives will ensure all customers' as well as regulatory requirements are met. In order to obtain this, the relevant parameters for measurement must be identified. This is why a reference to chapter 7.1 (Planning

TABLE 5.4
Standard Requirements of Subclause 5.4.1

ISO 13485	ISO 9001
Top management shall determine appropriate quality objectives including objectives necessary for the achievement of realization planning	Top management shall determine appropriate quality objectives including objectives necessary for the achievement of realization planning
The quality objectives shall be documented	The quality objectives shall be documented
The objectives will be submitted to appropriate and relevant functions on different levels throughout the organization	The objectives will be submitted to appropriate and relevant functions on different levels throughout the organization
Quality objectives will be measurable and consistent with the quality policy	Quality objectives will be measurable and consistent with the quality policy

of Product Realization) where objectives for the planning of product realization are defined is added:

- Quality objectives for product realization
- Requirements for documented procedures and specifications
- Implementations of all controls, verifications, and validations
- Reference of the results to acceptance criteria
- Definition of the required records

Your quality objectives will strive to cover these issues.

Effectiveness of the QMS

The quality objectives will allow you to maintain the effectiveness of your quality management system through obtaining a systematic and continual improvement. This relationship between achieving objectives and effectiveness will be forwarded to the employees at all levels. It is important for them to understand the direct connection between the two. Understanding this point will motivate them in achieving their goals. They will know that their actions generate results and these results are collected, measured, and reviewed, but more importantly promote the organization in its planned course.

Measurable Objectives

The quality objectives will be subdivided into specific operative objectives that could be assigned to specific roles, functions, divisions, or departments in the organization and be measured using techniques. It is hard to measure a quality objective such as "Promotion of human resources." Such an objective must be developed into a practical plan (Table 5.5).

This is actually a training program but it reflects and carries out the organization's objective in promoting the human resource. Such plans can be measured. The resources required to achieve the objectives shall be allocated. If training for computer operations is determined the necessary means must be provided: a budget, a tutor, schedules, appropriate computers for use, and training materials.

The quality objective will be documented in a controlled document. Usually the quality manual includes the list of the strategic objectives and a reference to another document containing the specific operative objectives. This is an effective way because the specific objectives are submitted to frequent change and update. This document will be controlled under the documents control process in the organization as required in subclause 4.2.3 (Control of Documents).

TABLE 5.5
Practical List of Objectives

Schedule	Theme	Target Group
Jan 2010	Preparing for sterilization processes	Production employees
Feb 2010	Computer operation	Administration
Mar 2010	Quality procedures: refreshment	All departments

An essential and integral aspect of the quality objectives is the definition of the methods and techniques concerning the data: obtaining, collecting, recording, analyzing, and drawing conclusions. The analysis of the objectives indicates whether improvement and effectiveness are achieved.

5.4.2 Quality Management System Planning

The quality planning is a critical phase in the design of the quality system. During the planning the organization considers all the key elements and factors relevant to the quality system and identifies the activities needed for the realization of the medical device. While planning you must stay focused on your main goal: providing a safe and effective medical device that meets all the customers' and regulatory requirements. The outputs of the planning will generate the required methods, documentations, and records that will support these activities. The planning shall cover all the relevant aspects and areas in which the organization is active: design and development, manufacturing, logistics, sales, installation, service, and support (Table 5.6).

Quality planning is the definition of the operational resources, activities, and support necessary to fulfill quality objectives or elements of the quality policy. The output of the quality planning is the quality plan. The quality plan is a document specifying activities, their resources, their sequences, and the responsibilities necessary in order to achieve an objective or planned results. A quality plan can be derived directly from quality planning and may appear, for example, as a procedure (quality or realization).

Levels of Quality Planning

There are three levels of planning:

- Planning related to the strategic concept of the organization done and agreed on by top management: quality objectives, deciding upon marketing a new product, opening a new department, or a yearly business plan with objectives. Such planning may affect the lower levels of the organization and might demand them to plan or change their further activities.
- Planning related to the quality management system: results and conclusions of management reviews, an external audit with requirements for corrective actions, and a review by a regulatory body with requirements for new activities,

TABLE 5.6
Standard Requirements of Subclause 5.4.2

ISO 13485	ISO 9001
Top management will ensure planning of the quality management system with the aim of meeting all the requirements of chapter 4.1 and the quality objectives	Top management will ensure planning of the quality management system with the aim of meeting all the requirements of chapter 4.1 and the quality objectives
Any changes or updates of the quality management system will be controlled and its integrity will be ensured	Any changes or updates of the quality management system will be controlled and its integrity will be ensured

or corrective or preventive actions. This second level may affect both directions, up the organizational ladder or down to the operative levels.
- The third level of quality planning is the operative level: implementing work procedures or instructions, carrying out training, and implementing validation plans with acceptance criteria.

Principles of Planning

The standard refers to clause 4.1 (Quality Management System General Requirements). Your quality management system will be planned according to the principles mentioned there:

- Establishing an effective QMS and activities that will ensure its effectiveness
- Identifying the processes and activities necessary for the realization and defining the relations and interactions between them
- Defining methods for operating, controlling, and measuring the processes and activities
- Identifying the necessary resources for the operation

Elements of quality planning:

- Determining quality objectives
- Developing models for the management of product life cycles
- Defining activities
- Establishing documentation necessary for the realization
- Designing required records, information, and data for activities
- Defining realization plans
- Setting authorities and responsibilities as job descriptions
- Introducing and certifying human resources to the processes
- Identifying methods for product realization
- Identifying tools and infrastructures for realization
- Designing work environment for the realization
- Defining the relations and interactions between activities
- Determining methods for improvement using measuring, monitoring, and analyzing activities

Recruiting the Appropriate Personnel for the Task

Key roles and functions in the organization shall participate in the planning and will verify that all the important aspects are being considered. This includes not only the department managers and the chief engineer but also production employees or other parties that will operate the activities and will face everyday challenges during the realization processes. It is important to hear what they have to say. The participants will have a clear understanding of the activities, and the necessary documents and records. Such a review will ensure that the activities, plans, documentation, and records will be effective (achieve their planned results) and assist in achieving the quality objectives. The roles will review whether the plans enable the manufacturer in realizing a medical device that meets all the customers' and regulatory requirements.

Changes

When planning and designing the quality management system, one must consider and relate to how changes will be introduced to the system: defined, implanted, and controlled. The principle is quite simple. Each change in the quality management system shall be submitted to a controlled process. The control will ensure that it is reviewed, approved, and appropriately introduced to the relevant parties and parts of the organization. A good example is documents control. Documents are an essential element of the QMS and each change must be submitted to a controlled process. Because we are dealing here with the ISO 13485 Standard, changes are to be expected throughout regulatory and statutory requirements as well. Expected changes:

- Changes in customer's requirements or specifications
- Improving processes or activities
- Update of regulatory requirements
- Organizational changes or addition of functions or roles
- Changes occurring in processes

5.5 RESPONSIBILITY, AUTHORITY, AND COMMUNICATION

5.5.1 Responsibility and Authority

Implementing the standard requirements demands the definition of authorities and responsibilities of the quality management system and product realization. Defining the authorities and responsibilities has several important objectives concerning the quality management system (Table 5.7):

TABLE 5.7
Standard Requirements of Subclause 5.5.1

ISO 13485	ISO 9001
Top management must ensure the definition of authorities and responsibilities throughout the different organizational levels	Top management must ensure the definition of authorities and responsibilities throughout the different organizational levels
The definitions will be documented and communicated to all the relevant levels of the organization	The definitions will be documented and communicated to all the relevant levels of the organization
The independence and authority of functions and roles that review and verify activities and processes will be ensured	
Interrelations between the various functions and participants of the quality management system that have a direct affect on the medical device will be determined and documented	
Where regulations require specific personnel for activities related to the postproduction stage and reporting of adverse events (8.2.1, 8.5.1), the organization will nominate them	

- Determining the hierarchy of decision making in the organization in order to achieve the quality objectives
- Clearly allocating human resources to processes and activities
- Identifying training and qualifications needed for each function
- Allowing the orientation within processes regarding the realization of the product, data and information, and responsibilities
- Enabling a structural sharing of information between the different participants of the organization

Organizational Structure

The organizational structure is the definition of hierarchy in the organization and relates to the nature of the organization. The structure describes all the functions, roles, and relations in an organization and demonstrates who is subjected to whom and who reports to whom. Defining the structure is the first step in defining the authorities and responsibilities of the QMS: the authorities and responsibilities that will operate the processes and activities are to be mapped. An example of an organizational structure is given in chapter 4.2.2 (Quality Manual). Although there is no specific requirement regarding the documentation of the organizational structure, it is highly recommended to include an organizational chart in the quality manual.

Job Description

Every role defined in the organizational structure must have a job description describing its responsibilities and authorities. It is important to mention that all job descriptions must correspond to the list of processes included in the QMS. This will ensure effectiveness of process realization. The job description specifies what a function does daily and organizes the list of responsibilities and authorities of this specific function: development manager, secretary, production manager, or quality manager. The job description will cover the following issues:

- Identification of the function. The title of the role or function is important to identify every role: operational manager, lab technician, administrative secretary.
- Dependence. Which role is the function subject to or to whom must he report at the end of the day? The dependence will be determined according to the organizational structure.
- Responsibilities. The responsibilities are activities that combine the function's work and effect on the medical device. The responsibilities relate directly to the realization processes. Try to be as accurate as possible. At the end of the definition each realization activity must be related to a function.
- Authorities. The authorities are the points and events in a process where the function is authorized to make a decision that will determine the flow of the process or affect the quality of the medical device. For example, a production manager decides which machine will be allocated to a process. A quality manager decides whether a product conforms or not and therefore has control over the release of the process.
- External qualifications: The organization will decide which external qualifications are required for the role in order for it to operate the processes: machine

engineer, electrical technician, certified lab technician, certified account manager, forklift driving license.
- Internal qualification: The organization will decide which internal training and certifications are required for each function: working procedure training, ERP system training, machine maintenance. These may be the introductory conditions for an employee to perform a process.

For several review and auditing activities an independence from other subjects (like auditee) must be granted for the authority that performs these activities. A good example to demonstrate the importance of the independence is the internal audit processes: the auditor must have his own opinion on things and should not be influenced by the environment he is auditing. Design and development review is another example where the authority that evaluates the progress of the development must perform it independently without being influenced by subjective factors. What defines independence?

- Accessibility to data and information
- Collaboration with his work colleagues
- Acquisition of the relevant knowledge and qualifications

All employees at all levels of the organization will be aware of their responsibilities and authorities. The matter will be communicated to each role. I suggest integrating it into the training and certification process of each function.

Documenting the definitions is necessary for the verification of the job description at later-stage audits or reviews. The documentation of the job description may be carried out in several ways: work instructions, procedures, or designated documents stated as job descriptions (I personally recommend an independent document).

Interrelations

The interrelations between the authorities define how a process "flows" between the different authorities and between different areas in the organization. The interrelations are expressed through the activities. The characteristics of the interrelations are:

- Inputs and output of processes
- The transferring of data and information between entities
- Organizational relevance of an authority

The standard expects you to determine these points, events, and requirements where an interrelation between two functions is initiated. Most process activities are performed by personnel but there are activities where personnel interrelate to a nonhuman system or two nonhuman systems communicate between themselves (automatization of processes). When such activities may affect the product, the matter will be documented and controlled. The determination may appear on the relevant procedure or work instructions but may also be described on a designated flow chart diagram.

Regulatory Requirements

There are regulatory requirements that demand the appointment of specific personnel or functions for specific activities or processes. The regulations may demand certain qualifications to be nominated and certain activities to be carried out. When such requirements exist, top management shall ensure that these personnel are hired. In addition, the standard refers us to two subclauses: 8.2.1 (Feedback) and 8.5.1

(Improvement—General). Actually the ISO 13485 Standard expects that a specific authority and responsibility will be allocated to the following activities:

- The treatment of customer's complaints including the issue of gaining experience from postproduction phase activities
- The authorization and approval of complaints that were not followed by a corrective or preventive action
- The activities of reporting of adverse events to the local or national authorities

These three issues will be submitted to an authority within the organization. But either way, they must be verified with local, national, or international regulations.

Expected Documents

These activities of defining the authorities and responsibilities generate documentation:

- An organizational structure
- Job descriptions
- Identification of qualifications and training needs
- Definition of interrelations

Each of the documents mentioned above will be submitted to the process of documents control in the organization as required in subclause 4.2.3 (Control of Documents).

5.5.2 Management Representative

A part of the management's responsibility is to appoint an authority that will have the task of imparting the quality policy and expectations of top management to the organization on one hand, and to receive feedback regarding the status and performance of the QMS on the other hand (Table 5.8).

TABLE 5.8
Standard Requirements of Subclause 5.5.2

ISO 13485	ISO 9001
Top management shall appoint a representative that has authority and responsibility for the quality management system in the organization	Top management shall appoint a representative that has authority and responsibility for the quality management system in the organization
The representative will ensure the establishment, implementation, and control of processes and activities required for the quality management system	The representative will ensure the establishment, implementation, and control of processes and activities required for the quality management system
The representative will report to top management on the performances, competence, and implementation of the quality management system and the need for improvements	The representative will report to top management on the performances, competence, and implementation of the quality management system and the need for improvements
The representative will act to promote the awareness of customers' and regulatory requirements throughout the organization	The representative will act to promote the awareness of customers' requirements throughout the organization

The Representative

Although it is common, the representative must not be a quality manager. However, they must be a member of top management and shall have the authority to decide. Here are a few considerations when selecting and appointing a representative:

- In cases when the management representative is not the quality manager, it is required to define the interrelations and applications between the representative and the quality manager.
- The representative may be an external responsible body in which top management has confidence, for example a consulting firm.
- Delegation of assignments and tasks of the representative to other roles and parties in the organization is possible. But the responsibility to top management rests on one person's shoulders only.
- It is recommended that the representative has the appropriate background and knowledge relevant to the area, technologies, and nature of the medical devices.
- When appointing a role that performs or is involved in more activities in the organization related to the quality of the product, it is important to ensure that no conflicts arise due to its obligation to the quality management system.

There are a lot of possibilities to determine the representative, but it is important to document the issue. If it's a quality manager or another role in the organization, then document the fact that they are the representative on their job description. If it's an external party you must produce some sort of document that specifies its responsibilities to top management and the organization. An agreement is one option.

Examining and Reporting

The goals of the representative are to:

- Ensure that quality objectives are achieved
- See that all the required processes are established and maintained according to the specifications
- Inform of need for improvements

The main task of the representative is to examine and evaluate the status of the QMS and to report to the top management whether the main objectives of the quality management system are achieved and of the status of improvements. The examination will be done through the assessment of the processes that were identified as relevant to the QMS and were defined in the quality manual. There is no exact requirement regarding the reporting methods or intervals. They may occur as management reviews, as complaints reports, or as internal audits reports. The reporting may vary according to different areas and activities. Another issue is to define what will act as evidence and findings that will support the reporting. As a representative, aside from the management review and the internal audit I used to submit to my CEO weekly reports with different issues concerning the quality of the products. Whatever manner of reporting is decided upon, the reporting requirements, methods, and intervals must be defined and documented in the appropriate documentation.

Promotion of Awareness

Another role for the management representative is to promote the awareness of the employees of regulatory and customers' requirements. The representative will define the topics and issues that are relevant to the regulatory requirements and customers' requirements. I suggest they identify on each organizational level how customers' and regulatory requirements are expressed and verify that measures to promote awareness are being taken. They may be defined on a training plan for example. The ways to promote the issues will be planned according to the nature and activities of the organization: training, lectures, publications, certifications, distributing information, etc.

5.5.3 Internal Communication

In today's business environment, communication channels (internal as well as external) play one of the most important roles in an organization. Companies invest millions of dollars in order to implement effective communication channels. In the organization, the internal communication channels have some strategic objectives (Table 5.9). The channels:

- Boost the processes in the organization and contribute to their effectiveness
- Promote sharing of information between entities
- Promote and convey to employees the importance of meeting customers' and regulatory requirements
- Help identifying problems and opportunities for improvement

Effectiveness of Communication Channels

Effective communication channels are an important component of a healthy organization. They create transparency and allow the efficient flow of data and information. The effectiveness of communication channels is measured by the following:

- Verification that information reaches its destination at the right time
- Awareness and familiarity of employees with their relevant channels and knowledge of where to report and what information or data they must submit

The communication channels define the reporting methods and relationships in an organization and so will be planned in accordance with its organizational structure and flow of processes. Each employee, function, or role will know to whom

TABLE 5.9
Standard Requirements of Subclause 5.5.3

ISO 13485	ISO 9001
Top management shall provide means and resources for implementing active and effective internal communication channels	Top management shall provide means and resources for implementing active and effective internal communication channels
The communication channels will be used to transfer data and information regarding the effectiveness of the quality management system	The communication channels will be used to transfer data and information regarding the effectiveness of the quality management system

they must report or who reports to them, what is requested to be transferred or to be received, and in what manner. When a production manager needs raw material or components for a realization, communication channels with the warehouseman will be defined and established in an effective way; the request will arrive on time and through an appropriate method, the warehouse man will have all the necessary information and a defined way to return an answer to the production manager (information or materials). Communication channels can be used for the enhancement of human resources: training and sharing of knowledge (knowledge management processes).

So the characteristics of effective channels are:

- Encouraged
- Clear and understandable
- Bidirectional
- Active on all organizational levels

But why does the standard imply the responsibility of the communication channels belongs to top management? Because implementing communication channels is a strategic decision. Effective channels will promote processes and encourage parties to share information and knowledge, but they do require a lot of resources.

Choosing the Communication Channels

Examples of communication channels: ERP system, PLM system, BPM system, brochures, internal news mails or e-mails, periodic meetings, training, and lectures. For each channel it is necessary to define the frequencies of use and the types of data or information it will handle: job assignments, customer complaints, administrative messages, and decision and resolutions from the management review. But it can be planned using a different approach: review what the required information to be transferred is and then plan the channels appropriately. If it can be seen that the process of handling customer complaints in the organization is not effective and parties are neglecting their duties, a designated system may be implemented that will encourage the process.

I would like to review some strategic communication channels that meet all the objectives and might assist in enhancing the effectiveness of processes:

- The ERP (Enterprise Resource Planning) system is the classic example of a communication channel. The system binds all of the organization's activities and departments under one application and merges all processes to one level. The organizational entities communicate and share information through the system processes.
- The BPM (Business Process Management) system is a relatively new trend. It is based on the MRP principle but boosts its control and effectiveness by collecting data from defined organizational entities, analyzing it, and releasing information needed to support decisions. The system encourages the systematization and integration of management principles with the strategy of the company (quality policy for example) and thus optimizes the processes.
- The PLM (Product Life cycle Management) is a system that bundles under one application various areas and ranges that usually do not have direct contact between them (planning, production, and customer handling) and might use different tools for communication. The system supports and encourages each to share its information.

5.6 MANAGEMENT REVIEW

5.6.1 General

The management review is a management tool in the hands of top management needed to keep up with the quality management system. It is one method (among others) dictated by the standard for monitoring the quality management system and evaluating its performances and effectiveness (Table 5.10).

Management Review

The management review is an activity usually performed as a meeting where representatives of top management are presented with data and information regarding the performances of the QMS. The objective of the review is to give top management a chance to periodically evaluate the quality management system.

The review must cover all the topics that are mentioned in the ISO 13485 Standard through a review of the activities: review of activities related to quality, documentation, human resources, work environment, and infrastructure, quality planning of the product, development, purchasing, realization of the product, and so on. The data and information presented to top management are reviewed on various levels:

- The conformance, suitability, and adequacy of the activities to the quality policy
- The achievement of quality objectives and the fulfillment of customers' and regulatory requirements
- The need for improvement and changes throughout the quality management system
- The need for resources in order to maintain an effective quality management system

TABLE 5.10
Standard Requirements of Subclause 5.6.1

ISO 13485	ISO 9001
Top management shall survey the quality management system at defined intervals	Top management shall survey the quality management system at defined intervals
The review shall verify the consecutive suitability, adequacy, and effectiveness of the quality management system	The review shall verify the consecutive suitability, adequacy, and effectiveness of the quality management system
The review shall evaluate opportunities for improvement and required changes throughout the quality management system	The review shall evaluate opportunities for improvement and required changes throughout the quality management system
The review shall evaluate competence of the quality policy and the status of achieving quality objectives	The review shall evaluate competence of the quality policy and the status of achieving quality objectives
The results and conclusions of the review shall be documented and the records shall be submitted to the records control process as required in subclause 4.2.4 (Control of Records)	The results and conclusions of the review shall be documented and the records shall be submitted to the records control process as required in subclause 4.2.4 (Control of Records)

Quality Objectives

One of the most important purposes of the management review (in my opinion) is the examination of quality objectives. Quality objectives are an efficient tool for achieving an effective QMS. The control and review of the management play an important key role in this mechanism. And what better opportunity for a close checkup than the management review (when top management is already "in the mood")? The examination will focus on two areas:

- The achievement and fulfillment of quality objectives like quality plans, objectives of performances, marketing objectives, customer-related objectives (for example, complaint or feedback related), or quality objectives (for example, audit or training related).
- The compliance of the objective and their level of effectiveness concerning the quality management system. This examination will determine whether the objectives are truly suited to the nature of the organization.

Changes and Improvements

Another objective of the review is the assessment of changes and improvements:

- Changes and improvements that were implemented will be reviewed for their effectiveness and suitability to the QMS.
- Potential changes and improvements will be reviewed and discussed concerning their applicability to the QMS and to plan required resources and execution.

Intervals and Participants

The review shall be performed at least once a year. It is important that delegates and representatives of top management attend the review. The organization shall determine the frequency and participants according to its nature and complexity of activities but at least once a year with justified participation of top management is necessary. Once a year is not often enough in my opinion. In our business environment a year is a long period of time when many things happen and some important decisions regarding the QMS are to be taken. Therefore I have defined (as a member of top management) that the QMS will be reviewed by me and other delegates from the different organizational levels (that are not considered as top management) once a week as a quality circle. The meeting will cover all the topics that are dictated by the standard and will provide all the required outputs in a frame of one year. In addition, top management will review the status of the QMS twice a year. In cases and situations where a higher decision or intervention is needed, an extraordinary meeting with the rest of top management will be summoned. I have documented this matter in a procedure: management review.

Records

Outputs and records of the review activities are to be documented. The standard does not specify any particular method for documenting the review, but bear in mind that this is the beginning of a long-term review process, with inputs and outputs of the process. It should be documented in a way that allows follow-up and comparison at later stages: a report, form, or a presentation. I suggest designing and maintaining a designated form for the matter that will document:

- The date and location where the review took place
- The participants

- The issues that were discussed
- Evidence or reference to the evidence
- Decisions, schedules, and responsibilities for execution

The form itself will be submitted to the process of document control as in subclause 4.2.3 and the records of the review will be submitted to the process of record control in the quality management system as required in subclause 4.2.4 (Control of Records).

5.6.2 Review Input

The management review is a strategic tool for examining and evaluating specific issues through the use of certain data and information. The principle is simple: compare the performance against the objectives and come to a conclusion about whether the organization followed its processes. This list of inputs reflects the quality management system and involves aspects of control, consulting, and taking decisions. The topics are reviewed in Table 5.11.

As you might have noticed, the information and data required to be reviewed are pretty much explicit. You need only to identify the sources of data and the responsible parties in the organization that can provide the data, collect it in an orderly manner, and present in an acceptable way. The data and information will be presented as documented evidence that will support top management in discussing and taking decisions: results of surveys, reviews, and audits, summary reports, presentations, and statistical charts.

At this point I would like to make a remark: always point out where you succeed in achieving the specifications and objectives as well as failures. The objective is to learn from successes and duplicate them in other events, cases, products,

TABLE 5.11
Standard Requirements of Subclause 5.6.2

ISO 13485	ISO 9001
Audit results: internal, external, and customer audits	Audit results: internal, external, and customer audits
Customer feedback: may include customer complaints as well	Customer feedback: may include customer's complaints as well
Process conformance and product conformity: including data on the processes, quality of products, and nonconformities regarding the process and the product	Process conformance and product conformity: including data about the processes, quality of products, and nonconformities regarding the process and the product
Status of CAPA	Status of CAPA
Follow-ups from previous reviews	Follow-ups from previous reviews
Any change that might affect the quality management system	Any change that might affect the quality management system
Recommendation for improvements	Recommendation for improvements
Any new or revised applicable regulatory requirements needed to be implemented	

or processes and to analyze failures in order to avoid them in other events, cases, products, or processes.

Result of Audits

Evidence of whether the organization's activities and processes conform to planned arrangements and are effectively implemented and maintained will be presented through audit results. This includes results from internal, external, supplier and customer audits. The review shall refer to the findings, the rejections, required actions, and recommendations for improvements.

Customer Feedback

Information and results of customer feedback activities will be presented and will enable top management to evaluate whether it has met customer requirements. The information shall relate to different issues and aspects: user surveys, aspects of products, customer requirements and contract information, regulatory compliance, and service. It may include passive feedback data that was received in the organization like customer complaints, and active feedback that the organization initiated such as customer feedback surveys or analysis of data gathered during service activities.

Process Performance and Product Conformance

Evidence that demonstrates the ability of realization processes to achieve planned results and the conformity of products (process outputs) to the acceptance criteria will be presented. The information will include data from statistical analyses of product characteristics and process performances. In other words, allow top management to evaluate the processes and products in comparison with the criteria. Try to reflect successes and failures of certain cases onto other cases.

Status of Corrective and Preventive Actions

Status of actions taken to eliminate the causes of nonconformities or potential nonconformities will be discussed. The corrective and preventive actions that were initiated throughout the organization are to be analyzed. In particular, relate to the effectiveness and the extent of objective achievement of the actions. Again, try to analyze and reflect successes and failures.

Follow-Up Actions from Previous Management Reviews

Decisions for actions determined in previous reviews will be discussed: what was decided, what was carried out, and what was turned down, rejected, or postponed. The review will not only examine whether they were applied and implemented, but also whether the actions were effective and achieved their objectives. At this point some people may try to bury themselves in their chairs…

Changes Affecting the QMS

Changes implemented in the quality management system that might have affected the quality management system or the medical device will be reviewed for their effectiveness and suitability to the QMS. That means all events that occurred since the last management review and were not referred by top management. This is their chance to be informed. What is considered as a change?

- Changes in customer specifications
- Organizational changes
- Changes in the production installation
- Changes in work procedures
- Changes concerning human resources

Improvements

Improvements that were initiated and implemented in the QMS and may affect the medical device will be reviewed. Top management must review the implementation and effectiveness of improvements in the organization: the consistency in the implementation of manners or methods, promotion of awareness among employees, and achieving planned results. Improvements may occur as:

- Improvements recommended by audits
- Changes in processes for better efficiency
- Decisions of previous reviews

Regulatory Requirements

Top management will review changes in current applicable regulatory requirements and the demand for the implementation of new or revised regulatory requirements. The review shall relate to all areas and activities of the manufacturer: design, development, purchasing, realization, storage, sales and marketing, delivery, installation, maintenance, and service. The review is led by two parameters:

- The location where the medical device is marketed
- The location where the medical device is developed

5.6.3 Review Output

The objective of the review output is to document top management's evaluation of the QMS concerning the effectiveness of processes and the achievement of the quality objectives. The outputs will demonstrate the satisfaction (or dissatisfaction) of top management with the quality system and its ambition or expectations for the initiation of improvements, changes, or corrections. In other words: what is top management's opinion of the quality system. This statement will be expressed through decisions, both strategic and operative (Table 5.12).

Taking Decisions

The outputs of the management review process are decisions. The decisions are to be documented and communicated to all relevant parties in the organization:

- For the purpose of information within the organization
- For the purpose of performing, executing, and controlling tasks and assignments

By the way, a decision such as: the management is satisfied with the current situation of the production and chooses to take no further actions, is a legitimate decision that will be respected by all auditors, but it will need to be documented and justified with evidence that the results were satisfying.

TABLE 5.12
Standard Requirements of Subclause 5.6.3

ISO 13485	ISO 9001
The outputs of the management review will include decisions and actions covering the following issues:	The outputs of the management review will include decisions and actions covering the following issues:
Improvements and changes necessary for maintenance of the effectiveness of the quality management system and its processes	Improvements and changes necessary for the effectiveness of the quality management system and its processes
Improving and changing of product related to customer's requirements	Improving and changing of product related to customer's requirements
Description of resources needed for the implementation and execution of the decisions	Description of resources needed for the implementation and execution of the decisions

Decisions will be followed up in order to verify their accomplishment. And just like the ISO Standard, each (operative) decision will be characterized with the following factors:

- The content and description of the decision.
- The decisions can be classified according to the review issues: improvement on products or processes, changes and improvements in the QMS, compliance to regulatory requirement, corrective or preventive actions or other issues referred to during the review.
- The implications of the decision for the quality management system will be evaluated: which system elements, entities, processes, and products are involved or will be influenced by the decision.
- The relevant party or function in the organization that will be responsible for carrying out the decision will be submitted.
- Objectives will be set in order to examine the effectiveness of the decision or action.
- Target dates will be scheduled in order to frame it.
- The required resources for the accomplishment will be addressed.
- The decision will include reference to the appropriate documentation in the QMS (if applicable).

If a decision related to training of production employees was taken, the relevant functions or roles will be informed about the decision, and its objectives and target dates. In the next management review the decisions will be followed up regarding performance and results.

Effectiveness of Processes

The outputs of the review shall serve the effectiveness of the QMS and its processes. So whenever suggestions are made—changes in processes, corrective actions, or improvements—their consequences for the quality system and the processes will be weighed. Let us review an example, where a change in the realization processes was decided in order to increase process effectiveness:

- Effectiveness of process. In order to reduce the risk of product contamination, the transportation in the production hall must be shortened.
- Decision. The top management decides to reorganize the layout of the packaging production line.

Another example of effectiveness is the reference to decisions of the last management review. When decisions of the last review were accomplished, their execution and results will be referred, with a justification and when needed a corrective actions.

Quality Policy and Objectives

When quality objectives are updated, changed, or added, the relevant quality system elements and documentation are updated as well:

- If the change in the objectives was strategic, an update on the quality policy will be considered.
- If the change in the objectives was quantitative, the relevant objective control will be updated.

However, it is important to submit and communicate the decisions regarding the quality objectives to the lower levels of the organization for awareness and execution.

Customers and Regulatory Requirements

The decisions of the review shall increase the competence of the medical devices and promote the ability of the manufacturer to meet customers' and regulatory requirements. The suggestions and decisions are to be oriented to this matter: safety, performance, functionality, and intended use of the medical device. For example:

- An analysis of last year's complaints showed a reoccurrence of a certain complaint: The user manual does not cover a specific area related to the use of the medical device.
- The short-term corrective action: An annex was added to the user manual.
- Top management decided in the review: A new and revised user manual will be designed, produced, and distributed to all customers or distributors.

Allocation of Resources

Resources necessary to obtain the improvements to or changes in processes and products, and the achievement of quality objectives will be mentioned. No one expects budgeting and calculation of the expenses during the review. But top management are obliged to allocate the required resources. If you insist on including numbers in the review, you are welcome to do so.

Another issue that will be accounted is the allocation of resources needed to implement, perform and complete effective Risk Management processes and their appraisal.

The ISO 14971—Application of risk management to medical devices (which the ISO 13485 refers to as guidance for effective risk management) requires management review as well, where you need to discuss the policy regarding risk Management and the allocation of appropriate resources. This is a good opportunity to combine the management review of both standards or at least display outputs of the risk management review that may affect the QMS, because I can assure you the decisions that will be taken regarding the implementation of one standard will affect elements by the second.

Documentation, Approval, and Distribution

The outputs of the management review will be documented. The documentation may appear on a designated form, a meeting summary, or a special report—whatever suits the organization. If a form is being designed for this, it must be submitted to the documents control process. However the outputs of the review are to be approved by top management and communicated to lower levels in the organization. The approval may occur as a signature on the form or just a statement. The records of the review (containing the outputs) will be submitted to the process of records control, as required in subclause 4.2.4 (Control of Records).

6 Resource Management

Resources—one of the foundation stones of the quality management system. The standard requires us to define, manage, and control our resources. The standard relate to three kinds of resources: human resources, infrastructures, and work environment. These are responsible for critical areas and scopes of the realization processes, especially when it comes to medical devices. Therefore the appropriate definitions and controls are expected.

6.1 PROVISION OF RESOURCES

The resources required for the establishment of a quality management system and the maintenance of its effectiveness are to be determined. The standard considers the allocation of appropriate resources as a key factor in realizing an effective quality system. The manufacturer is expected to analyze its needs for resource while considering certain organizational aspects. In other words, to sit, think, and examine what its resources needs are in Table 6.1.

Clause 6.1 (Provision of Resources) is regarded as clarification of the requirements regarding the provision of resources. In order to determine effective resources that will support the manufacturer and promote the achievement of its requirements and specifications (and there certainly are a lot of these), the standard presents us with guidelines for the determination:

- Quality policy. A correlation between the resources and the quality policy is essential. In the quality policy the nature of the organization and its processes is determined, there is a commitment to meet customers' as well as regulatory requirements, quality objectives (or principles for their determination) are set, and scope of activity is determined. Now it is time to identify the necessary resources.

TABLE 6.1
Standard Requirements of Clause 6.1

ISO 13485	ISO 9001
Resources needed for the implementation and maintenance of an effective quality management system are to be determined	Resources needed for the implementation and the continual improvement of the quality management system are to be determined
Resources needed for the achievement of customers' requirements as well as regulatory requirements will be determined	Resources needed for the achievement of customers' requirements and the enhancement of customers' satisfaction will be determined

- Quality objectives. The defined resources that will support the manufacturer in achieving its quality objectives.
- Realization processes. The processes are a crucial constituent in the definition and the amount, extent, and complexity of the processes will determine the required resources.
- Requirements. The resources are to support the manufacturer in meeting customers' and regulatory requirements.
- Effectiveness. The resources are to support the activities necessary to achieve the above-mentioned: quality objectives, realization processes, and customers' and regulatory requirements.

All of the above are the expectations of the quality management system. The standard requires specification of what resources are needed to assist and support in achieving these strategic aspects and to reach the appropriate determination of the resources: human resources, infrastructures, work environment, tools and equipment, information systems, suppliers and partners, natural resources, and financial resources.

A tip: There is an old debate regarding the documentation of the issue. The standard does require documentation but the conservatives (and I am a part conservative) claim that the documentation is needed in order to answer other standard requirements (which is true). But if you stop and think for a second, the quality management documentation is full of definitions and determinations of resources: SOPs, work instructions, test instructions, user manuals, forms, and maintenance plans, where you mention and refer to resources. I suggest you include, in your quality manual, a clause referring to the provision of resources, stating the commitment of the management to identify resources needs and to provide them. In that clause define all the resource types in your organization: human resources, infrastructures, tools and equipment, machines, and budgets. In addition, insert a remark that specific resources are specified in the proper documents.

Reference to Risk Management

The provision of resources applies to the allocation of adequate resources necessary for the risk management activities. The main objective is to ensure that appropriate resources will be allocated for the effectiveness of processes and activities related to the risk management:

- Employees with appropriate qualifications
- Responsibilities and authorities for the activities
- Tool and equipment

6.2 HUMAN RESOURCE

6.2.1 General

Human resource has a significant weight and effect on the realization processes. Everybody is aware of that. But the question is whether everybody assimilates it. In order to verify and validate the fact that human resources are suitably addressed

TABLE 6.2
Standard Requirements of Subclause 6.2.1

ISO 13485	ISO 9001
The organization shall ensure that personnel and employees performing activities, tasks, and work that affect the quality and conformity of the product will be competent and acquire the adequate skills	The organization shall ensure that personnel and employees performing activities, tasks, and work that affect the quality and conformity of the product will be competent and acquire the adequate skills
The effect on the conformity of the product may be direct or indirect	The effect on the conformity of the product may be direct or indirect
Competence and adequate skills include education, qualification, training, and experience	Competence and adequate skills include education, qualification, training, and experience

when planning a quality management system, the ISO 13485 Standard presents us (in stages) with how to analyze, plan, and determine the human resources (Table 6.2).

Subclause 6.2.1 is a general introduction to chapter 6.2 where specific requirements appear. The main principle of the chapter is as follows: the organization shall verify the allocation of appropriate personnel for the realization of the medical device. In order to verify this, it is required first to define:

- What are the qualification requirements for each role of function?
- What evidence is necessary?

These two questions will be discussed in detail in chapter 6.2.2 (Competence, Awareness, and Training). But I would like to briefly discuss the importance of and relationship between qualifying personnel, the implementation of a quality management system, and maintenance of its effectiveness. The main objective of enhancing your human resource is to provide your employees with the ability to perform their job and activities as planned. Your personnel are responsible for the realization of the medical devices and meeting customer and regulatory requirements; they operate machines, assemble products, sit in front of computers, or contact your customers. It is no secret that industries and services today are evolving on a daily basis, products are becoming more complex, the global environment challenges you more and more, and thus knowledge becomes an essential element. You must give your employees the tools and instruments to deal with this new reality. In other words, training today is an integral part of your product. The organization must combine the two together: the human resources and the knowledge. Such integration will enhance the effectiveness of the QMS.

6.2.2 Competence, Awareness, and Training

While planning the human resources for the realization processes, the organization shall refer to the issues in Table 6.3.

TABLE 6.3
Standard Requirements of Subclause 6.2.2

ISO 13485	ISO 9001
For each function or role that performs an activity that may affect the quality of the product or its conformity to the requirements, the organization shall determine necessary qualifications, training, and certifications needed for the work	For each function or role that performs an activity that may affect the quality of the product or its conformity to the requirements, the organization shall determine necessary qualifications, training and certifications needed for the work
Where applicable, the organization shall plan and implement training and certification activities, in order to enhance the personnel to the required qualification level	Where applicable, the organization shall plan and implement training and certification activities, in order to enhance the personnel to the required qualification level
Effectiveness of actions regarding training and certifications will be evaluated	Effectiveness of actions regarding training and certifications will be evaluated
The organization shall ensure the awareness of personnel regarding the effect and importance of their actions and activities on the quality of the product and the conformity to the requirements	The organization shall ensure the awareness of personnel regarding the effect and importance of their actions and activities to the quality of the product and the conformity to the requirements
The organization shall ensure the awareness of personnel of the relevance of their actions and activities to the achievement of the quality objectives	The organization shall ensure the awareness of personnel of the relevance of their actions and activities to the achievement of the quality objectives
Records and evidence of training and other actions will be maintained and submitted to the records control process as required in subclause 4.2.4	Records and evidence of training and other actions will be maintained and submitted to the records control process as required in subclause 4.2.4
Where regulatory requirements require the establishment and maintenance of documented procedures or methods for identifying training needs, such procedures will be maintained	

Identifying the Training Needs

The first step in establishing an effective training and certification process is the identification and location of the training needs. The training and the certification of employees in a work place are a process with the purpose of assisting the members of the organization in fulfilling their activities and tasks better and more effectively by introducing them to skills, knowledge, and professional and organizational approaches. Training and certifications may be needed in the following cases:

- Hiring and introducing new personnel
- Improvement of knowledge and skills
- Introduction of innovations in the organization
- Supporting organizational processes

By initiating actions the organization promotes its personnel in achieving work objectives. The qualifications, skills, and knowledge required for the fulfillment of the product objectives need to be defined and determined according to the characters of the medical device and the nature of the activities:

- Customer requirements
- The characters and features of the medical devices
- The raw materials or components it is made of
- The processes that operate the medical device and constitute its functionality
- The processes that realize the medical device

In the organization, in each organizational structure (production, logistics, development, purchase, marketing), different workers perform different tasks and activities that promote one shared goal: realization of the medical device. For each level in each organizational structure it is necessary to define the level of qualifications and skills that the worker needs to perform their tasks. Usually the issue is managed by the function responsible for human resources. But as far as the ISO 13485 Standard is concerned, some elements and job characteristics must be defined and documented:

- Education: The level of knowledge and education required for a role will be determined: engineer, technician, programmer, biologist, certified logistician. Some roles may not require an education or external certification at all. These definitions will be the preconditions for the hiring of personnel for specific roles.
- Regulatory requirements: When a regulatory requirement requires a certain certification according to a law or a standard, it will be mentioned as a precondition for hiring a person to the job. The matter will be verified with evidence prior to the hiring.
- Experience: The extent of experience and background in parameters of time as well as areas and scopes of activities will be defined.
- Certification: The manufacturer will define a certification plan or process needed to introduce a person to a specific role: training about processes, procedures, work instructions, or activities related to the job. The plan shall cover both operational tasks related to the realization of the medical device as well as administrative and quality tasks.
- Training: The training (external as well as internal) for the role will be planned. It is necessary to identify the critical points or events in a process, which may affect the product and its integrity and to plan the trainings in accordance.

All of the above will be defined and documented. The end objective is to define a certification character for an employee and to ensure that only certified personnel perform a certain job and task. The documentation will be submitted to the documents control process in the organization as required in subclause 4.2.3 (Control of Documents). Let us assume that the manufacturer employs personnel for sales and marketing activities, production processes, and logistics processes. For each role in each department the manufacturer shall:

- Define the required education, experience, and skill
- Define the certification process for the job
- Define a training plan

The activities of training and certifying employees for tasks will be recorded. The records will serve as quality records and will be submitted to the process of records control as required in subclause 4.2.4 (Control of Records).

Certification Plan

Each employee that is recruited to the organization and will participate in the realization of the medical device is obliged to go through a planned and documented process of introducing him to the organization and the relevant processes. The plan will cover specific areas and topics in the organization such as:

- Introduction to the organization
- Administrative issues, for example, registration by accounting
- Introduction to different people and functions throughout the organization, for example, work colleagues
- Introduction to the different zones and areas in the organization: canteens, parking, toilets, offices
- General processes: working hours, vacations, terms of use, social conditions
- Designated realization and quality processes

The plan will be documented and controlled. Records indicating the performance of the plan shall be maintained as quality records.

Training Plan

The training and certification needs are the objectives and requirements of human resources for qualifications and skills. Now, after the definition, the organization is required to plan training or other activities in order to satisfy these training needs. The objective of the training plan is to fill in and complete the gaps between the training needs and objectives and the current situation of your human resources (regarding qualifications and skills). The matter can be completed in four stages:

1. The determination of target groups in the organization: departments, workers, divisions, roles, or functions
2. The review and evaluation of the status with a defined method
3. The identification and mapping of the gaps in the organization
4. The development of the training plan according to the results

Training is a broad and complex issue. Whole libraries have been written on the subject. But there are some elements required by the standard that the plan must include:

- The plan will be based on the nature of the processes and of the organization and the training activities will be oriented to support the realization processes.
- Each function, role, area, department, or field in your organization that is related to the realization of the medical device or may affect its quality will have a designated training plan that will relate to their field of activities. In the plan, the subjects of the training—the audience or target groups—will be defined.
- The plan will be periodical: monthly, quarterly, or yearly, and will include dates and schedules (you are not required to provide specific dates—periods of the year are sufficient). The period will be set according to the type of the training and the target group. For example, refreshing work procedures may occur once a year. But customer complaints and nonconformities must be introduced to employees almost immediately.
- A minimal specification of the topics of the training will be included.
- The plan shall define the methods for the training. The matter will be discussed in detail in this chapter.
- The plan will define the tutor: is it an internal tutor (an employee training another employee) or is it an external tutor.
- The plan will cover quality aspects such as quality procedures and quality controls implemented throughout the quality management system. For example, each employee must know how to identify nonconformity and how to react. But

the matter will be different for a production employee and a logistics employee. Therefore for each target a designated plan is needed.
- The plan will relate to customers' and regulatory requirements. The plan may cover specific requirements and will indicate to employees of how he or she may access these requirements during the performance of its tasks and activities: training of the structure and content of the device master record (DMR), or referring employees to the regulatory requirements or procedures that cover them.
- The training shall be correlated with the quality policy and objectives. The matter will be discussed in details in this chapter.
- The plan shall relate to training requirements derived from the risk management. The objective is to ensure workers whose activities or tasks that may pose a danger to the medical device are appropriately identified and trained. It may include specific qualifications or certifications for particular processes or products. Please refer to the risk management plan and derive from their the targets groups (authorities and responsibilities) and their qualification requirements.
- The plan will be evaluated for performance and results.

The plan will define specific organizational events where training is necessary:

- Refreshing work instructions and work procedures
- Quality or work procedures
- Training related to structural changes; transfer of employees between departments or roles (structural changes) within the organization
- Transfer of employees between processes or products (within a department)
- Introduction of innovations within the organization; new products or projects
- Introduction of new technologies or new developments in the industry
- Introduction of new infrastructures, machines, or tools
- Training required by regulations or applicable standards
- Introduction of new regulations or refreshment of old ones
- Special, specific events that may affect the quality of the product (special projects, or special visits at various sites)
- Coaching employees (very popular at the moment)
- Training required by your customers
- Training provided to your suppliers
- Customers' complaints, nonconformities, or feedback results

One objective of training is to enhance the human resources. It is recommended to consider expanding the training in a way that will include the development of skills and provision of knowledge in the area of product realization. The technology, area, and market where the medical device is active will be periodically reviewed in order to identify new training areas. It may be integrated with feedback activities as mentioned in chapter 8.2.1.

In order to create effective training—training that will assist your employees and provide them with tools and knowledge for their everyday work—I personally recommend that someone with a background in a specific field will plan the training for each field or area of activity in the organization, for example, a department manager or a technical manager. It should be someone who is aware of problems, special events or situations, and particular cases that your employees will face during the daily tasks or activities, and the plan will cover these and indicate to the employee how they should react. The plan must not be inflexible; on the contrary, you may update it at any time. It is possible to define further parameters within the training plan, such as:

- The location of the training: meeting rooms, auditorium
- Required resources: computers, software, projector
- The length of the training
- Who is the tutor

Types of Training

There is no requirement to perform the training in the traditional way as frontal courses, lectures, or personal training. You may define training as self-learning or online tutoring, for example. The purpose remains the same however; only the method needs to be defined. Here are some examples of types of training:

- Frontal training
- External courses
- A visit to exhibitions, conferences, or conventions
- A visit to suppliers' facilities
- A supplier training about his products (very important, especially in commerce)
- E-learning courses
- Purchasing literature or special training software

So in case your employees or work colleagues paid a visit to a supplier, or participated in a conference, the matter may be considered as training as long as it is related to the realization of the medical device.

Evaluating the Effectiveness of the Training

Before I start, please allow me to remind you that effectiveness is the extent to which planned activities are realized and planned results achieved. In terms of training, it is measured by whether the training has achieved its goal and to what extent.

Training has objectives and goals. Specific training has its objectives, which support and promote the whole of the organization's objectives. The ISO 13485 Standard is aware of that and thus requires a systematical evaluation of training. The standard relates to certain aspects of training:

- The evaluation will determine whether the training was effective or not. It is necessary to define methods for the evaluation of the effectiveness of the training: reviewing processes, counting defective parts, measuring personal performances (qualitative as well as quantitative), production analysis, and inquiry of employees.
- The evaluation will be done periodically and will include physical examinations: health and infections are important factors in the medical device industry.
- Each employee (on a personal scale rather than functional) will be evaluated for their competence for the training needs: required qualifications against current status of qualifications.

The evaluation of training will be done based on several parameters:

- Evaluation of the relevancy of the training to the medical device and its field of activity. For this reason the training is to be planned by professionals who have background, knowledge, skills, and experience in the field of activity. This is exactly where their added value is required.
- Evaluation of the employees. Check whether the employees have assimilated the training, skills, and knowledge that were assigned to them and implanted it in the realization processes. You can check this by conducting an exam at

the end of the training or analyzing processes in a defined period of time. It is always recommended to examine the results of the related processes rather than gathering information from the employees themselves. An employee can always claim that they have implemented what they have learned, but the question is what is happening during the realization processes. Inspect for yourself what is going on.

- Evaluate the tutor or trainer. Do they really know what they are talking about? Do they have the required qualifications and skills? How are their training skills? Can they really perform the training effectively?
- Evaluate whether the training is updated. In our modern world changes occur on a daily basis. What was relevant a year ago could be totally irrelevant today. Perhaps the organization has implemented new processes or technologies but the training refers to the old ones.
- Regulatory requirements. Regulatory requirements tend to change and be updated. In any case, it is required to update documentation regarding regulatory requirements regularly. This should also be done for training.

The most important evaluation is whether the training has achieved its goal. If the training is related to a certain customer complaint, it must be reviewed to ensure that complaint will not be repeated. If the training is related to work instructions, the processes must be sampled and it must be verified that they are being done as specified. Such an examination will be planned in advance.

Awareness and Motivation of Employees

The quality management system includes the quality policy and the quality objectives. Training is one means of implementing the policy and achieving these objectives. Quality objectives are divided into subobjectives that are obtained through operative objectives. The issue filters down to the level of the single process: each process has its objective—the expected output. The employees must be aware of this hierarchy and understand the relevancy, relation, and effect of their actions and activities on achieving the quality objectives. Employees must be aware that their activities and the expected output promote the quality objectives of the organization. Such awareness will create the identification of employees with the quality objectives and initiate the motivation to meet them. The employees must understand that they are bearing the operative responsibility of achieving the objectives. How? By demonstrating, during the training, the relation between the results of their actions and the quality objectives. The basic principle states that each employee must be familiar with the policy and objectives and therefore they are to be an integral subject of the training plan. If one of the quality objectives is to meet all the regulatory and international standard requirements, employees must understand how their actions contribute to these objectives; during the installation processes, an employee must follow the instructions as given by the applicable regulatory requirements that the organization is obligated to. If one of the quality objectives is to provide a device that meets all customer requirements, the employee must understand that devices that leave the factory must conform.

Evaluation of Employees

Another required evaluation of performance, effectiveness, and competence of the human resource is the periodical assessment of employees. This evaluation has several goals:

- Assessing for each employee the competence and the quality of the work according to predefined parameters
- Identifying needs and suggesting measures for the promotion of the employee in the organization
- Initiation of a dialogue between the employee and their superior regarding their mutual expectations, satisfaction, and further actions

Parameters related to quality issues for evaluation:

- Professional competence of the employee: Does the employee have the necessary practical or theoretical knowledge and the technical experience and background to perform their tasks?
- Capacity for teamwork or ability to work in a team: Does the employee's approach contribute to or motivate other team members? Does he or she creates a good working climate? Does he or she support his or her work colleagues?
- Attitude for dealing with and solving problems. Does the employee recognize problems and suggest solutions? Does the employee constantly seek and suggest improvements and optimizations?
- Approach to the company: Does the employee display a high level of commitment to his or her work place? Is he or she proactive and reliable?
- Performance and approach to the company's objectives: Are the performances of the employee satisfying? Is the employee committed to the goals of the company and achieving his or her personal goals?
- Approach to the work environment, tools, and equipment: Does the employee treat and behave in the work environment according to the firm's values and code of ethics or conduct? Does he or she utilize the working tools and equipment with responsibility and according to the specifications?

Such an evaluation will place the employee with regard to their qualifications and training objectives. The next stage is to assess the results and to determine whether further measures are required. A reference of the supervisor or employer is obligatory. Such evaluation can appear as a checklist or a form, with a qualitative or quantitative assessment. The results of the evaluation will serve as quality records.

Example:

See Table 6.4.

Employee's satisfaction:

☐ Very satisfied ☐ Satisfied ☐ Not satisfied

Necessary training or qualifications for the employee:

____

____

Regulatory Requirements for Identification of Training Needs

Where regulatory requirements require the establishment and maintenance of documented procedures or methods for identifying training needs, such procedures will

TABLE 6.4
Evaluation of Employees

Features	Assessment 1	2	3	4	5	6	Remarks
Professional competence of the employee	☐	☐	☐	☐	☐	☐	
Capacity for teamwork or ability to work in a team	☐	☐	☐	☐	☐	☐	
Performances and approach to the company's objectives	☐	☐	☐	☐	☐	☐	

be maintained. The ISO 13485 prepares us for the possibility that national or regional regulations might require us to plan and establish a procedure for the identification of training needs. The intention here is to toe the line with other applicable regulations regarding the identification of training needs. The most common example is the FDA's 21 CFR part 820.25, which specifically states that the manufacturer will establish a procedure for the identification of training needs in order to ensure that personnel are appropriately trained for the tasks. When such regulatory requirements are applicable, the manufacturer will:

- Determine and document a method for the identification of training needs.
- Implement the method for determining, while planning the qualifications of the human resources.

An example of such an SOP (very briefly):

1. For each job the manufacturer will analyze the processes that are related to the job.
2. For each job the manufacturer will analyze the activities that are related to the job.
3. For each job the manufacturer will analyze the outputs that are related to the job.
4. Clauses 1–3 relate to the identification of the needs. Now we move on the planning stage.
5. According to the results of the analyses, the manufacturer will determine the required education, background and experience, and skills for the job.
6. According to the results of the analyses, the manufacturer will determine the required certification process and training for the job.
7. The results of the analyses will be kept on the appropriate records.
8. The definitions of paragraphs 4–5 will be kept in the appropriate documents.

This procedure will be submitted to the documents control process in the organization as required in subclause 4.2.3 (Control of Documents).

Expected Documentation and Records

As you have probably noticed, the issue of planning and managing human resources demands the establishment of certain documentations and the maintenance of records. For documentation, the following is required:

- Training needs. Definitions of qualifications and training needs according to a role of function. I personally used to include these definitions in the job descriptions. There is a direct relation between the list of activities and the required qualifications to perform it.
- Certification plan. A list of activities and training required to introduce a person to a specific job or function. It may appear as a form, a checklist, or a procedure.
- Training plan. Although there is no requirement to document the plan, please do so. It will assist in following the implementation of training activities and may save answering some tricky questions during the audits.
- Evaluation of employees. A plan that specifies the parameters for assessing and evaluating employees and proposes topics for discussion between the employee and his supervisor.

The documentation will be submitted to the documents control process in the organization as required in subclause 4.2.3 (Control of Documents). In case you are planning and maintaining a set of forms for the training records, these forms will be submitted to the control of documents as well.

Within records it is required to maintain:

- External evidence that proves the competence of an employee according to the training and qualification needs: diplomas, certification of education, regulatory certifications, or licenses. For each employee a correlation is required between evidence of education and the definition of the job.
- Records and evidence of the certification activities for an employee (certification plan). The records will identify the employee that participated with detail, dates and activities that were initiated in order to introduce him to the job.
- Documented internal certification of employees that allows them to perform certain activities or relates to specific roles or functions. This may appear as an approval on a copy of the certification plan or on a designated from. It is important to mention that the certification will be personal.
- Records and evidence that prove training activities have been carried out. The records will include details such as dates, tutor or trainer, participants, and topics of training.
- Evaluation of the effectiveness of the training actions taken. This may appear on the same records of the training or on a designated record.
- Records of employees' evaluations of performance, effectiveness, and competence. These records may include records of physical examinations necessary for the realization processes.
- Any other records required by regulatory requirements.

These records will serve as quality records and will be submitted to the process of record control as required in subclause 4.2.4 (Control of Records). A good way to manage it is to maintain for person a designated file with his or hers relevant quality records.

6.3 INFRASTRUCTURE

Infrastructures are the stock of the basic facilities and equipment needed for the operation of a process or the maintenance, storage, or distribution of a product. It provides the suitable conditions and accessories to perform the appropriate business tasks and functions and assist in achieving the desired conformity of product and service requirements. Thus, it is strongly related to the product and has a direct effect on the quality of the medical devices (Table 6.5).

The requirements of the ISO 13485 Standard are to ensure the availability of appropriate infrastructures throughout the realization processes. But beside the provision of the infrastructures, the manufacturer is required to maintain and take care of them in order to eliminate the probability of failure. The maintenance of the infrastructures is a necessary precondition for the preservation of processes' long-term capability, ensures reproducibility of processes, and guarantees the achievement of the product requirements. And what is a better way to reach such quality management goals than to identify, plan, document, control, and record. The control over the infrastructures shall reach all levels of process support. According to this basic rule, even equipment whose failure might not harm and affect the medical device, but will affect the organization' ability to supply the medical device on schedule, must be controlled and maintained.

TABLE 6.5
Standard Requirements of Clause 6.3

ISO 13485	ISO 9001
Infrastructures necessary for the realization of the product to ensure that it will meet its requirements shall be defined and determined	Infrastructures necessary for the realization of the product to ensure that it will meet its requirements shall be defined and determined
The organization shall provide and maintain the appropriate infrastructures necessary to answer and meet these determinations	The organization shall provide and maintain the appropriate infrastructures necessary to answer and meet these determinations
Infrastructures include applicable buildings, workspaces, tools, equipment, machinery, and associated utilities necessary for the realization of processes	Infrastructures include applicable buildings, workspaces, tools, equipment, machinery, and associated utilities necessary for the realization of processes
The provision of infrastructures shall include the resources and the necessary services needed to support and operate them: transport, communication, and information systems	The provision of infrastructures shall include the resources and the necessary services needed to support and operate them: transport, communication, and information systems
Requirements for the maintenance and care of the infrastructures will be defined and documented referring to activities as well as intervals	
Records and evidence of maintenance activities shall be maintained and submitted to the records control process as required in subclause 4.2.4	

Identification of Infrastructures as Process Equipment

The basic goal of the organization is to ensure the provision and availability of infrastructures. Within infrastructures we include all the means, applications, interfaces, and facilities necessary for the realization of the medical device from the design stages until its delivery. According to the ISO Standard the infrastructures include software (the collection of functions and programs that provide instructions for a unit for the operation of activities) as well as hardware (the physical layout of components or parts of a system). In other words the standard needed to make it clear that both areas are included under the definition of infrastructures, the spiritual as well as the material. The definition includes services that support software and hardware and assist them in meeting the specifications.

The first step in initiating the control will be to identify the infrastructures. The objective is to focus only on what is relevant to the realization of the medical device. The most effective way to do this is to:

- Review all the processes that are related to the realization and are included under the QMS: capture of customer requirements, operation of raw materials and parts, transportation through various phases of the material flow, production, assembly, and delivery activities
- To map and list all the infrastructures that are being used
- To analyze the relation between the processes and the infrastructures
- To indicate which parameters may affect the processes and quality of the product

Importance is given to the effect of an infrastructure on a given process and this is measured on various levels: process parameters, elements of infrastructure, operators and responsibilities, and stage of process.

The next stage is to list all the infrastructures that were identified. Customers, as well as national or regional regulations that may set requirements for infrastructures, will be included. The identification is a long and detailed process but will be done only once (not including updates of processes or installation of new infrastructures of course). During the review various types of infrastructure may be encountered:

- Buildings, structures, work spaces, halls
- Basic infrastructures like water supply, air systems, and electricity
- Design and development tools
- Storage facilities
- Working tools, equipment, accessories, and monitoring and measuring devices
- Production facilities and machinery
- Computers, information systems, record-keeping systems and servers, and process automation and management systems
- Means of transportation and distribution
- Communication channels
- Security and safety means

IT, ERP systems, and other information systems are regarded as infrastructures. This results from the perception that today's IT systems are integral elements of the realization process. Any system that processes information, data, process characters, or parameters related to the realization of the medical devices is included under the infrastructures. At the end of the review you will have a list of the infrastructures to be controlled. This list is very important to the later planning of the maintenance activities and prevention measures. The list will be documented, controlled, and submitted to the documents control process.

Examples for infrastructures: ovens, sterilizers, computer systems, ERP systems, CRM systems, labs, clean room controllers, CAD systems, operators and phone systems, HVAC, printers and copiers, air compressors, industrial vehicles, normal vehicles, forklifts, aisle pickers, lifts, motorized pallet jacks, trucks, cranes, security and alarm systems, and filters.

Buildings and Structures

Buildings and structures are regarded as infrastructures; these are facilities that support processes and are necessary for the realization of a product. Characters of buildings and structures, and layouts of work spaces will be planned and implemented according to the needs of the processes that they are supporting: realization processes and activities, and conditions of storage. These will facilitate:

- Provision of proper conditions for performing the working processes in an effective manner
- Planning of plant layouts and process flow, in order to eliminate the risk of mixing products with different status
- Optimization of plant layouts for safety of personnel and devices, and agronomical parameters
- Consideration of interfacing with other infrastructures such as the supply of electricity, air or water, or transportation

Thus, a multidisciplinary approach involving different roles and different aspects of the realization is recommended for the evaluation of whether work spaces and structures indeed support the processes. The output of the review will determine and define which controls are required for the maintenance of these structures and buildings and for the prevention of failures. The control will include aspects such as installation, periodical controls, cleaning, maintenance and services, repairs, licenses, and other necessary operations.

Customer and Regulatory Requirements

Customer and regulatory requirements may determine requirements for infrastructures, and thus their characteristics and their need the maintenance. For example,

- Customers may deliver to the organization tools or machines necessary for the realization of the medical device. Such equipment is to be considered as infrastructures.
- Customer requirements may demand the storage of the medical devices in certain conditions. Such conditions require the manufacturer to install the appropriate control systems. These systems will be included in the list of the infrastructures.
- Several international standards or regulations relate to the maintenance of storage and production areas and require specific measures to be implemented. The regulations shall be identified and such infrastructures will be counted and included in the list as well.

The manufacturer must identify such external requirements for infrastructures and include them in the maintenance activities, but, importantly, ensure their availability.

Supporting Services

The list of infrastructures will include the services which support the infrastructures and ensure that all elements of infrastructure remain in safe, effective, and operational condition:

transportation services, communication services, and resources services (gas, oil, electricity). These are regarded as integral parts of the infrastructure. The services may occur as:

- Services needed for the operation of the infrastructures: water and electricity, phone and mobile phone services, IT services, transportation or freight services, provision of gas, oil, electricity, environmental, heating, and air conditioning
- Services that are required for the maintenance of the infrastructures: IT services, machine and tool maintenance services and repairs supplied by the manufacturer, information backup services, and pest control

Please note that IT services appear twice. This is because there are cases where IT services are required in order to operate machines and production processes, and require operation of an IT employee aside from the periodical maintenance and update of the computer systems and servers. The services may be provided internally or externally. When the service is provided by a supplier, the necessary service activities will be defined and documented.

Evaluation of Infrastructures

The suitability of the infrastructures to the quality objectives and quality planning will be evaluated. This is the first step in determining the requirements for maintenance activities. The goals of the evaluation are:

- To ensure that the infrastructures are intact, sustainable, and stable
- To ensure that the infrastructures will support the manufacturer in achieving quality targets and plans
- To verify that the infrastructures will not disturb the achievement of objectives or reduce the capability of processes
- To identify areas and ranges for control
- To determine which controls are needed
- When needed, to implement improvements or to update the infrastructures

Effective evaluation may occur with the help of acceptance criteria: checklists that assure specifications, allowable tolerances of equipment and machine performances, and user or supplier's instructions. If certain infrastructures require no maintenance activities, mention it on the evaluation: such infrastructures were identified and evaluated, and it was determined that no maintenance is necessary. The evaluation may be internally planned by you with a form or a checklist: something like a gap analysis between the requirements and the state of the infrastructures. Another option is to order an external evaluation that assesses your infrastructures. For example, a company that assesses the electrical network in the production halls. This is preferable because it will be an objective evaluation. The auditor would definitely appreciate it. The output of this activity will be the controls that are to be implemented in your infrastructure referring to required activities, responsibilities, and required tools, equipment, and intervals.

Integration of Risk Management Outputs and Safety Measures

The use of the infrastructures throughout the realization processes may pose risks to the users as well as to the products themselves. Such risks will be identified and discussed. Risks may appear as

- Process failures
- Risks to human resources
- Harm to the product

When such risks are identified, the proper controls and prevention measures will be applied. For example, the use of materials and pressurizing activities during the sterilization processes may generate corrosion in the chamber. Risks like this must be identified and the appropriate controls are to be implemented at the appropriate process stages. Risks to human resources are to be referred to as well. A classic example which almost cost me a rejection of external audit is the common ladder; during one of my external audits, the auditor demanded to see records indicating that a ladder was safe for use (!?!). To tell the truth it never crossed my mind to examine the ladder. But in fact this ladder was used daily and required semiyearly maintenance according to the manufacturer's specifications. Imagine that. But a ladder is a simple system. What about machines, electro systems, cranes, conveyor belts, forklifts, etc.? Each type of infrastructure shall be reviewed for the risks related to it and the necessary control and preventions will be integrated into the maintenance activities. A risk management output may serve as a reference to the review.

A documented plan for a solution of a problem related to the infrastructures will be implemented in the organization. The purpose of the plan is to define for the relevant parties or employees in different areas or departments what is to be done in case of a quality problem or failure concerning the infrastructures. The plan will refer to different aspects of the realization: production, quality, storage, and distribution, and will provide details and instructions according to the case. Figure 6.1 shows a basic example.

Such a plan will be available at the work stations to the appropriate employees.

Documented Requirements for a Maintenance Plan

Any type of infrastructure with a risk of failure that may affect the integrity and quality of the medical device as well as customer and regulatory requirements must be submitted systematically for maintenance and prevention. The ISO 13485 Standard specifically requires the documentation of requirements for activities. There is no requirement for a standard operating procedure but for documented

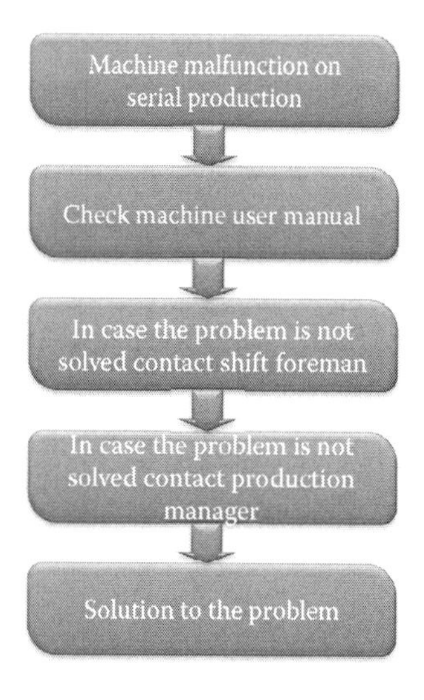

FIGURE 6.1 A problem–solution plan.

specifications, activities, and tasks. In other words the standard expects to see a plan including the definitions of responsibilities, maintenance activities and prevention measures concerning the infrastructures. The plan will cover the following issues:

- The infrastructures required for control and maintenance will be identified and documented: machines, tools, systems, computers, servers, forklifts, cranes. An identification method will be planned in order to identify infrastructures in a unique way: a number or a tag. The identification shall be visible on the tools or equipment and will allow the responsible party to identify it during use and operation.
- Determination of maintenance activities and tasks including the definitions of intervals according to the specifications of the infrastructures will be determined as a plan. The requirements and activities shall ensure stability of the infrastructure and the reproducibility of its processes over the long term. If water is supplied to the process, periodical inspection of the water system is required to be planned (not the quality of water but the system that is delivering it).
- Assignment of responsibilities of appropriate functions and roles for actions and tasks will be determined.
- The plan shall refer to the allocation of necessary resources: services, spare parts, special tools and equipment, materials such oils or lubricants, and external maintenance services.
- Necessary documents such as user manuals, technical instructions, technical schemes, or drawings shall be indicated including their location and availability.
- Inspections, controls, and examinations of the infrastructures will be planned and documented. These controls will verify that the activities are performed, and validate (when needed) the results. When applicable, acceptance criteria will be defined. For example, specifications of machine or equipment provided by manufacturer may serve as acceptance criteria for the comparison with the test results.
- The plan will initiate prevention measures through the identification of risks and the application of the appropriate controls.
- When repair is required, it will be documented and revalidated.
- Required records and evidence indicating that maintenance activities and preventions that were performed and controlled will be defined.

Once again, regarding risks, you may review the risk management plan and draw inputs from there. You may as well include the records of the prevention measures in the risk management file.

As mentioned above, a suitable function or responsibility for maintenance and control will be assigned to each infrastructure. The documented requirements shall identify which department is responsible for which infrastructure elements (at either the corporate or site level):

- The IT department is responsible for all computers, IT networks, databases (including backup services and computer security), e-mail servers, program licenses and updates, antivirus software, user applications and passwords, etc.
- Maintenance is responsible for water infrastructures, forklifts, fire control equipment, electrical infrastructures, natural gas, transportation, HVAC, landscaping, grounds maintenance, pest control, disposal of waste, recycling.

- Environmental health and safety (EHS) is responsible for environmental issues and safety equipment related to the different areas in the organization.
- When the responsibility lies with a supplier, the activities will be defined and documented, a responsible party will be appointed in order to evaluate the supplier's activities, and the supplier is obligated to provide you with the necessary recorded evidence.
- When distributors are required to maintain certain infrastructures or conditions, they will provide the manufacturer with the appropriate evidence for these conditions.

The matter shall not be limited to the appointment of a maintenance person, electrician, or IT department but will spread down to the level of employees using the infrastructures. For example, it is required to define for production employees how they shall safely use the infrastructures and what is required to be done at the end of each working day or each job: turning off systems, cleaning instructions, daily maintenance, etc. The matter shall be integrated in the training program.

Documented requirements may appear on a procedure (although this is not required), a form, a table, or a designated maintenance plan—whatever suits your organization and the nature of its infrastructures. The documents will be submitted to the documents control process in your quality management system as required in subclause 4.2.3 (Control of Documents). A very basic table appears above that may serve a maintenance plan for machines in a factory (Table 6.6).

But today there are qualified information systems that provide you with the required planning of activities and follow-ups. Most of today's ERP systems provide such a maintenance module. It may be that your supplier has already planned a maintenance plan and provides it. Make some calls and find it out.

Records Records Records

For each defined activity, the required records and evidence will be planned, indicating that maintenance activities and prevention measures were performed and controlled.

TABLE 6.6
Suggested Maintenance Plan for a Machine

Internal machine nr.:	10	20	30
Manufacturer:	Xxx	yyy	zzz
Type of machine:	aaa-bbb	aaa-bbb	aaa-ccc
Daily Inspection and Maintenance			
Hydraulic power unit	X	x	x
Safety devices	X	x	
Pneumatic facilities	X	x	x
Automatic central lubrication	X		x
Lamps and signals	X		x
Order and cleanliness	X	x	x
Weekly Inspection and Maintenance			
Programming unit	X	x	x
Fan filter	X	x	x

TABLE 6.7
Suggested List of Maintenance Activities

Daily Inspection and Maintenance

Internal machine nr.:	10			
Manufacturer:	xxx			
Type of machine:	aaa-bbb			
	Date	Name	Signature	Remarks
1. Hydraulic power unit				
2. Safety devices				
3. Pneumatic facilities				
4. Automatic central lubrication				
5. Lamps and signals				
6. Order and cleanliness				

The records will specify the activities that were done and prove the infrastructures' compliance to the specifications. The detail will include description of the activity, the date of the activity, and the identity of the performer. The records will serve as quality records and will be submitted to the process of records control in your organization as required in subclause 4.2.4 (Control of Records).

In relation to the table above, I have prepared here a short example of a concomitant record (Table 6.7).

6.4 WORK ENVIRONMENT

The work environment consists of the premises and other sites and locations where employees are engaged in work-related activities. The working environment is supposed to provide the manufacturer with the optimal conditions for the realization processes and thus has a direct effect on the medical devices. The work environment includes not only the physical locations, but also the influence equipment and materials used during the realization processes.

The goal of controlling the work environment is to determine, define, direct, monitor, regulate, document, and coordinate the conditions of the work environment by introducing them to predefined activities and controls. The activities cover specific areas and the parameters are confined to specified limits or definitions. The determination of work environment condition influences the characterization of tools, infrastructures, equipment, and human resources related to the realization processes. These elements are required to be synchronized in order to provide optimal qualifications to the work environment (Table 6.8).

The work environment is a collection of conditions (environmental, physical, ambient, and psychological) under which work and processes are carried out and includes all the spaces and halls that serve the organization for operation and realization of a product. These conditions are divided into various categories: physical elements of work spaces, factors that may influence the processes and activities, and resources

TABLE 6.8
Standard Requirements of Clause 6.4

ISO 13485	ISO 9001
The organization shall define and maintain the required work environment and its conditions in order to meet the product's requirements	The organization shall define and maintain the required work environment and its conditions in order to meet the product's requirements
Documented requirements for the control of health, cleanliness, clothing, conduct and behavior of personnel in and around work environments that may have an adverse effect on the device shall be established and maintained. Requirements of subclause 7.5.1.2.1 are to be referred to	
Documented requirements, such as procedures or work instructions, for the monitoring and control of the work environment and its conditions will be established and maintained, when these may affect the product or its quality or may have an adverse effect on the device. Requirements of subclause 7.5.1.2.1 are to be referred to	
Temporary employees and personnel working under special environment conditions shall be appropriately trained, certified, and supervised for working in such work conditions. Special training arrangements shall be planned and evidence of their compatibility will be maintained. Requirements of subclause 6.2.2b are to be referred to	
The organization shall plan, implement, and maintain a documented procedure describing activities ensuring that returned medical devices are identified and distinguished from other products. The purpose is to prevent any contamination of products, work environment, and personnel. Identification method as required in subclause 7.5.3.1 shall be considered	

that are invested in the processes or operate the activities in the work spaces. These three may influence the medical device on four levels:

- The ability of activities and actions and their outputs to achieve the product requirements
- The safety of the medical devices or the users
- The safety of the resources (personnel, tools, equipment, and materials)
- The quality of the medical device

Before we plunge into the specific requirements, I would like to distinguish between infrastructure and the working environment.

Working Environment vs. Infrastructure

When infrastructures include machines, the working environment is the area around the machine that is needed to realize the medical device: a place for the worker to operate the machine, lighting that the worker needs to perform a process, the noise around the work stations that may affect the worker, and the area where the process outputs are stored. Maintaining and controlling the infrastructure (the machine for example) would require a periodic control plan—in our example a maintenance plan for the machine. Maintaining and controlling the work environment would need a periodic inspection around the machine: cleanliness of the work space, sufficient lightning, and appropriate storage conditions. When the infrastructures refer to storage halls, the working environment includes the conditions in which the medical device is stored in these halls: temperature, humidity, safety, etc. Maintaining and controlling the storage halls as infrastructure will require building maintenance or electrical maintenance activities. Maintaining and controlling the storage halls as a work environment and its condition would require an environmental control system of temperature and humidity as well as an alarm system for the provision of safety. Examples of work environments and spaces include laboratories, logistic centers, clean rooms, production halls, stores, loading areas, meeting rooms, dressing rooms, and offices.

Definition and Determination of Working Environment

The work environment conditions and controls encompass all the different areas and scopes of the realization: storage of raw materials, parts, and components; transportation between departments and areas; production and assembly activities; storage of finished products, transportation to the customer; and storage at the distributor's premises. In order to reach and identify all the elements of the work environment that may affect the product, personnel, or processes, it is necessary to conduct a complete review, examination, and assessment of all realization activities and processes. The objective of the review is to understand the relationship between the product, personnel, and the work environment. This review includes the questioning and observation of employees' activities and the analysis of their work, tasks, and behavior around the work places and work stations, in order to understand how these may affect the conditions. Next stage will be to define the controls of the work environment. Another important task is the sampling of products in the process in order to study their status and to examine which conditions may affect them and how they are integrated into or influence the work environment. The sampling will occur at various locations and stages of the realization. Pay attention. Although the ISO 13485 Standard does not require this review to be documented, other standards that may be applicable do (the ISO 17665, for example).

Cleanliness Requirements of the Work Environment

In clause 6.4, the standard initiates the linkage between the cleanliness requirements and the work environment and refers to two main issues: control of the human resources and control of the work surroundings. The standard refers us to subclause 7.5.1.2.1 (Cleanliness of Product and Contamination Control). The objective of cleanliness processes is to remove any substances or process agents from the medical device prior to preceding processes or prior to the delivery, depending on the nature and use of the medical device. The principles are:

- Identification of sources of contaminants
- Removal of process agents
- Defining levels of cleanliness required for the medical device
- Planning tests and controls to prove these levels
- Documentation of the requirements and provision of records

The cleanliness processes define certain levels of cleanliness for the product that must be maintained and the activities with which they will be achieved. The controls of the work place and human resources will be planned in correlation with these requirements and will support the achievement of the cleanliness objectives. The objective is to relate the work environment to the cleaning processes. So when a cleaning activity of a product is planned and implemented, the influence of the work environment shall be considered. The next will be to plan the appropriate control of the work environment that will support the cleaning process.

Integration of Risk Management

Outputs of the risk management and risk evaluation shall be integrated in the planning and control of the work environment. The assumption opines that the environment may cause a failure in the product when the required conditions are not maintained. It is necessary to identify and control the risks related to the work environment that may affect the product. Such evaluation and mapping of the risks is a part of the risk management process. The output is the risk management file that specifies risks related to the medical device in general and in our case the risks related to the work environment. These risks will serve as inputs to the planning of the controls of the work environment. The most effective way is to identify the relation between risks and work environment elements including human resources, and to define which parameters are related to the surroundings and conditions of the workplace. Figure 6.2 demonstrates the flow.

The risk management will relate to different elements and activities and the relation between them:

- The identification of work environment conditions that may harm or endanger the medical device, its components, parts, or materials
- Reference to factors on the medical device that might influence or contaminate the work environment such as emissions of toxic materials or the effects of products with an expiration date on the environment
- Reference to the effects and results of disposal of the medical device on the environment
- Reference to the influence of the work environment on the package of the medical device and its integrity

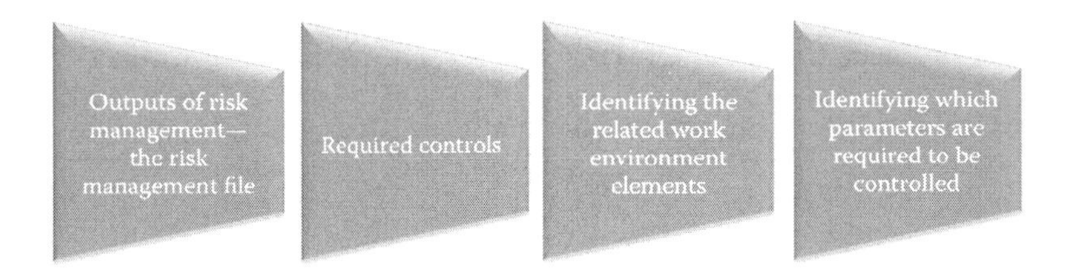

FIGURE 6.2 Integration of risk management in the control of the work environment.

- Reference to the influence that other equipment and tools have on the medical device such as electric or magnetic fields
- Identification of risks related to the human resources and the need to train and certify them for activities and jobs

Examples may be the review of magnetic parameters that may affect processes of the medical device and thus its intended use or the storage of the medical device near substances that may contaminate them.

Regulatory Requirements

Local, national, or international regulatory requirements may demand the establishment and maintenance of specific controls of your work environment. For example,

- ISO 11135 requires a documented assessment of the potential effect of sterilization processes on the work environment.
- ISO 17665 requires the implementation of various controls of the work environment.

When these are applicable and required, they are to be included in the planning of the controls; there is a good chance that such work environment requirements from different standards or regulations are applicable to your processes and products. I suggest a complete review of all these regulations and a listing of all the requirements according to type of process or product.

Human Resources Health

Regarding human resources the main risk is the contamination of the work environment by the spread of both microorganisms and particles. Such contamination may have adverse effect on the medical device. Situations and processes where the health of employees is critical may be sterilization and cleanliness activities. For example, validation of cleanliness of areas relies on bioburden control levels. Unhealthy employees may affect these areas and the level of cleanliness. In order to promote employee awareness of the issue, the organization may initiate a health policy with health indicators that define healthy situations. The policy shall establish a reporting system to communicate to employees the importance of this issue and wherewith the worker may report his or her health condition.

Authorization and Access

The manufacturer is required to define authorizations and access permissions to different areas, sites and locations: who is authorized and who is restricted to access the working environment. The matter applies to external visitors as well as internal. External visitors may be customers, suppliers, auditors, or even employees from other departments. For example, regarding manufacturing halls, the manufacturer shall define who is authorized to go into the halls and who is not! Otherwise you may find unwelcome guests... And when unwelcome guests are found, it should be defined what is to be done in order to verify that conditions were not changed and contaminations were not applied. Types of persons who could be moving around the facilities include the following:

- Internal: Manufacturing personnel, supervisors and productions managers, material handlers, storage workers, design engineers, quality control or assurance, management, service and maintenance personnel

- External: Suppliers, service providers, subcontractors, visitors, auditors, customers

In order to manage authorization and access effectively, it is required to define and implement a method. An authorization system that is implanted in the premises of the organization allowing access to areas to only certain personnel is such a method. Such a system defines and implements the requirements. In case such a system does not exist in the organization, you are required to determine and document who is authorized in the various areas in the organization. This document will be submitted to the records control.

Conduct and Behavior of Personnel around the Work Environment

One of the most critical elements that affect the conditions of the work environment is the conduct and behavior of human resources. In order to identify the activities and actions that may affect the conditions, the manufacturer is required to identify all the roles and functions that have contact with the work environment on two levels: contact with the product and operation of realization processes, and contact with the work environment elements that may affect its conditions. Functions and roles from all the realization processes are required to be reviewed: production, transportation, storage, quality, service, maintenance, and cleaning. For each role or function that was identified the following points will be addressed:

- The required level of health will be defined.
- A suitable dress code with the appropriate accessories will be assigned: gloves, hats, gowns.
- The work activities will be analyzed in order to verify that they are not creating a situation where the work environment is at risk.
- A set of activities and actions will be planned and defined to ensure that workers conduct is appropriate around the work stations and its conditions are maintained.
- The appropriate documentation and instructions will be established: instructions for behavior in the work environment, dress code, cleaning instructions, and identification of nonconformities or potential situations that may create nonconformities.

Regarding manufacturing processes, it is required to define how one shall handle the manufacturing surroundings around the machines during and after any processes, for example material handling, cleaning requirements, and order requirements.

After the identification of all relevant roles and functions it is necessary to define for each the training needs regarding the work environment. These needs will be integrated in the job description and the certification process of an employee, and will be included in the training plan according to the specifications of subclause 6.2.2.

The next reference to human resources regards the employment and integration of temporary personnel in the designated work environment. Here the requirements are clear:

- Temporary personnel shall be trained and certified to work in a special work environment under special conditions.
- The integration and work of such personnel will be supervised by a trained person.
- The organization shall develop and implement special training methods for temporary employees and the matter shall be incorporated in the training methods of the organization as required in subclause 6.2.2b.
- Records and evidence proving their relevant competence shall be maintained.

Sometimes the standard cannot be clearer. The emphasis here is on the requirement to identify the training needs (according to the requirements of 6.2.2b) and to develop training methods or at least to refer to the issue of conduct and behavior in the work environment while receiving and certifying temporary personnel. All the requirements of 6.2.2 apply to this matter: planning the training, setting programs, performing, and evaluating.

Control over the Work Environment

So, what has been achieved until now?

- We have distinguished the work environment from the infrastructures.
- We have identified the elements of the work place that are to be controlled.
- We have identified and discussed the integration of all the work environment requirement inputs (risk management, regulations, cleanliness, and employees' health).
- We have set the requirements for the human resources.

Now all that is left is to discuss the work environment itself, what are the crucial conditions, which parameters are to be controlled, and how.

Environmental conditions are the definitions of several parameters creating a situation or a status in a certain location to which the devices and the workers are exposed. The devices can be subjected to various conditional stresses during processes and activities, such as vacuum and pressure changes, radical temperatures, and changes in humidity. The conditions may be in forms such as air pressure, gases, aerosols, or particles. The conditions may consist also of physical factors that might affect the product.

The start point is the evaluation of the required work environment conditions and the potential effect that these conditions have on the environment and on the medical device's characteristics. These conditions are supposed to preserve the medical device properties, functionality, and safety, and eliminate failures that may result in an adverse effect on the product. These conditions are derived directly from the character and type of the medical device and will be controlled and verified through parameters that affect them. The evaluation will cover the entire supply chain from the storage activities of raw materials and parts until the storage of finished goods. The evaluation shall detect extreme conditions that the products may be exposed to. Examples of environmental conditions include air quality, temperature and humidity, magnetic fields, external electrical influences, electrostatic discharge, acoustic conditions, clinical conditions, work space layouts, storage requirements, dust and particles, and ESD (for electronic components). An effective analysis:

- Reviews all the environmental inputs and requirements such as product, cleanliness, human resource, and risk management
- Reviews all the related processes and activities
- Examines the flaws of the material throughout the realization processes
- Inspects all the outputs of the processes
- Involves all the participants of the processes in order to cover all aspects and information
- Determines at each phase what the required conditions for the work environment are
- Plans the required records and evidence that prove the achievement of the conditions
- Enables the manufacturer to identify the sources when problems with the product arise

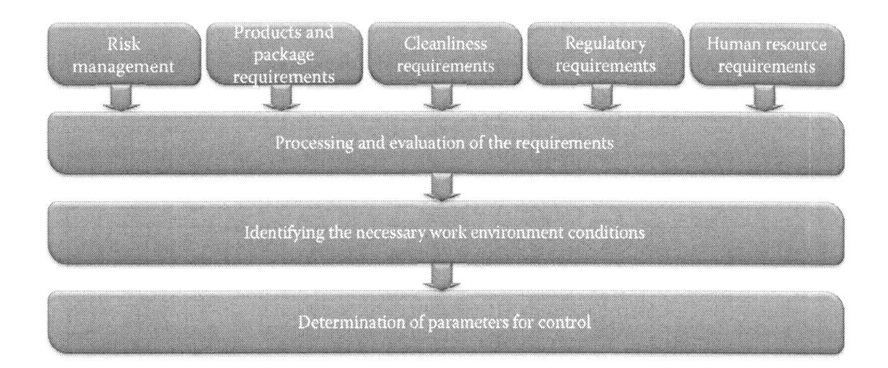

FIGURE 6.3 Evaluation of work environment conditions and parameters.

Figure 6.3 demonstrates the evaluation.

The result is a list of parameters that should be controlled around your work environment. For example:

- Surrounding conditions in the production halls: temperature, relative humidity (RH), pressure, emission of gases
- Air quality: circulation of air, concentration of airborne particles
- Acoustic conditions: level of decibels
- Mechanic or kinetic conditions: level of vibration
- Sterility: SAL

Determination of the conditions allows the manufacturer to detect in advance which activities or lack of activities may create unwanted conditions and reduce the functionality of the medical device, for example, increase unwanted or unaccepted levels of bioburden in the work environment. Another example, for some parts or components high levels of temperature and humidity are crucial for their integrity and functionality. On the other hand, for electronic components such levels are harmful and in addition for such components it is highly important to provide an environment free of electrostatic discharge. For each of these parameters you need to plan the suitable control.

- In some cases you may need to define acceptance criteria for effective control, for example, by the control of measurable conditions such as temperature or humidity. The criteria will relate to the fluctuations of these parameters, and to limits and tolerances.
- In some cases it will be necessary to integrate the controls of the parameters in the validations of the product's provision (as required in subclause 7.5.2), in order to prove that the work environment's conditions were as required during processes. For example, in sterilization and cleaning processes, it is necessary to ensure that environmental conditions at the manufacturing site achieved predefined criteria. This is one of the process validations. Through the control of these parameters is the guarantee that these products were produced and packaged in a qualified, controlled environment. More examples of environmental parameters, indicators, and controls: cleanliness of work surfaces, air filtration, pressure, and airflow.
- Psychological effects play an important role in the work environment. Agronomic and psychological factors may affect the human resources and

prevent them from operating the process as expected. For example, long-term exposure to noise may result in distractions and disturbances, and certain shades of light create an undesired reaction in certain people. Such distractions may lead to inattention to the process. If preventions or accessories for these matters and issues are determined, the controls will verify their availability.

- Work environment conditions that may affect the packaging are to be taken into account. There are conditions that may affect the packages and the packaging activities as well as storage conditions that may affect the integrity and quality of the package. For example, high temperatures may affect the material the package is made of and harm it.
- The use of tools and equipment necessary for the controls shall be specified. The specification shall relate to safety measures of the environment as well as the personnel that operate it.
- When controls of the work environment are required by distributors of the medical device, the requirements shall be communicated to them and they will implement them.

The next stage is determining the means and tools that will deliver you the required controls over these parameters:

- Control devices: monitoring tools, sensors, particle counters, devices to measure temperature and humidity, gas filters
- Instructions: work instructions, procedures, checklists, forms, environmental review instructions
- Tests: the verifications and validations that the level of parameters were measured according to the definitions and that the required conditions were achieved through demonstration of results

The controls will be planned in order to support and provide appropriate data regarding the conditions and the appropriate sample rate devices shall be addressed. For example, when selecting and installing a device to control particles, the shape, volume, and aerodynamics of these shall be taken into account. When selecting a gauge to measure temperature, it is necessary to ensure its scope supports the criteria. Examples of work environment controls:

- Access control to areas and work stations for humans: controlled work areas and access, segregation of work areas, traffic controls
- Control of areas of the material flaw: decontamination areas, sterilization rooms, clinical areas
- Environmental controls: particle counts, humidity, temperature, noise measurements, and vibrations
- Facilities and necessary accessories that support the work environment conditions: hand wash facilities, work surfaces, cleaning solutions, racks, bins, baskets, special tissue papers, shoes, overcoats, gloves, and hangers
- Procedures and defined activities for conduct and behavior around the work environment: hand-washing instructions, cleaning instructions, dress code
- External services that control the work environment

The controls will be implemented throughout the working processes and activities. Tools and equipment and control devices shall be submitted to the requirements of chapter 7.6: Control of monitoring and measuring devices. These conditions, processes, parameters, control tools, and equipment as well as activities, actions, criteria, and the requested results will be documented. These are the documentation requirements that the ISO 13485 Standard expects to find. Documented requirements may appear on SOPs, work instructions, forms, checklists, etc. This matter will be elaborated upon in the appropriate paragraph of this chapter.

Control against Contamination

Contaminated or potentially contaminated products may risk the work environment. The ISO 13485 Standard requires establishing, documenting, and maintaining requirements for special arrangements, activities, and measures for the control of returned, contaminated, or potentially contaminated products. The objective is to eliminate the contamination of the work environment or personnel. Returned medical devices may contaminate, pollute, infect, or trigger another illness that may affect the work environment or personnel. The requirements shall indicate activities such as accepting the returned medical devices, identifying them, separating them, segregating them, distinguishing them, and storing them in the designated areas. The manufacturer is required to set and document specific activities and arrangements where the objective is to protect the work environment, other medical devices, and the personnel. The activities and arrangement shall refer to issues such as:

- The identification of the products. The identification is one of the controls that the manufacturer is to implement in order to distinguish contaminated products. The standard refers us to subclause 7.5.3.1 (Identification), where identification requirements for the returned medical devices are specified and in particular the requirements for documented procedure regarding the identification activities and arrangement of contaminated or potentially contaminated products. Now do not get confused. On this matter a documented procedure is required to rather than documented requirements. You may integrate the issue with the procedure of the identification activities of other types of products (you are required to establish a procedure anyway) or you may establish an independent procedure. The procedure will be submitted to the control of documents as required in subclause 4.2.3.
- Revalidation of products. Returned medical devices that are designated for resale are to be revalidated and reverified that they are in the same condition as a new product, before being submitted to the work environment; they are intact and unharmed, and the package is sealed and complete. The objective is to ensure that the status of these products is acceptable and that there is no danger of contaminating the work environment, personnel, or other products. The matter shall include the processes of submitting medical devices to rework.
- Handling the products. The manufacturer shall plan and document activities for handling contaminated or potentially contaminated products: receiving, accepting, cleaning, segregating, and decontaminating procedures. Materials, parts, components, products, or finished goods that were detected as defective or with nonconformity are to be segregated and controlled until their repair, rework, or disposal. Can the issue be integrated with the "Control of nonconforming product" procedure? Yes. According to subclause 4.2.1 a single document may include requirements of one or more procedures. But bear in mind that there are activities that are not related to the control of nonconforming products that are also related. Evidence and records proving activities are according to the planned requirements shall be provided.

TABLE 6.9
Principles of Documentation with Reference to Instruction for a Clean Room

Principle of Documentation	Example of Clean Room Instructions
Definitions of the objective and purposes	Defining implementation and control of the cleanliness and sanitation levels in controlled environments
Identification of the responsibilities and authorities, and reference to the required training and certification needs	The shift manager will monitor and ensure that cleaning and sanitation activities are documented and will sign and approve the monthly cleaning checklist
	It is the responsibility of operators of processes to clean their work stations at the beginning and end of each shift. It is also their responsibility to report leaks, oil spills, etc. to the department supervisor
	Only certified employees are authorized to perform activities in the clean area. The certification will appear documented in the employee's personal file
Specification of the areas that are to be controlled	Production halls A, B, and C
Reference to the appropriate documentation	SOP-011: Personnel Training
	WI-01: Gowning and Health and Cleanliness
	FO-32: Clean Room Cleaning Checklist
Identification of tools and equipment, dressing accessories, and other accessories necessary for the control activities	Equipment is to be cleaned prior to entry into a clean area. No brushes, brooms, feather dusters, aerosols, dry mops, or steel wool are allowed in the clean room. A list of chemicals approved for use in the clean area appears in Appendix A.
	Approved equipment for cleaning activities:
	HEPA-filtered vacuum
	Lint-free cleaning mops
	Lint-free wipes
	Stainless steel or plastic buckets
Determination of activities and controls including reference to responsibilities and interval	Direct contact without protection with product is not allowed
	It is required to wear powder-free gloves when performing cleaning tasks
	When using disinfectants it is necessary to allow them to remain on the surface for a period of 10–20 minutes
	Opening a vacuum cleaner in the clean room to change filters and bags or to perform other maintenance is prohibited
	HEPA filters are to be cleaned once a week and only when face guards are installed
Reference to the required records for collecting data concerning the conditions of the work environment and evidence proving the execution of expected activities	Documentation and evidence of activities will be recorded on the appropriate cleaning checklist. Full identification is required

- Service and maintenance. Medical devices that are returned for service and repair shall be segregated from other medical devices. Receiving activities of devices for service and maintenance shall be planned in order to eliminate the mixing of devices with different status or the access of unauthorized devices to certain areas. The matter shall refer to relevant working tools and equipment when the transfer of these between products with different status may contaminate the product or the work environment.

The activities shall be planned according to the nature of the product, the processes that the product performs, and the type of use. If the medical device has contact with human tissues, naturally special segregation and decontamination activities will be planned.

Documentation

Throughout clause 6.4 the standard demands the establishment of documented requirements necessary for the implementation and maintenance of work environment conditions. True, the standard does not indicate a documented procedure, but there is a "trap":

- Reference to other standard requirements which do demand the establishment and maintenance of SOPs.
- The fact that due to the nature of controls and requirements, only documented procedures may be effective.
- Applicable regulatory and standard requirements demand the maintenance of documented procedures.

For example, the FDA CFR 21 SEC 820.150 requires specifically an SOP to describe the controls over storage conditions. Other designated ISO Standards such as the ISO 11137 or the ISO 17665 require specifically documented procedures for the control of the work environments related to their scope of activities.

The documented requirements shall specify to a user how it is required to operate elements in the work environment and what is required to control in the work environments. Basic instructions for a clean room are given with reference to the principles (Table 6.9).

Expected Records

The objective of the records is to prove that the conditions were according to the definitions and to supply historical data regarding levels of environmental contamination or levels of risks during the realization processes. Records may appear as:

- Outputs and printouts of control systems, tools, or devices: printed reports, screens, files
- Definitions of authorization and accesses to areas and sites
- Records of environmental reviews regarding the conditions: forms, checklists, tables, or charts with data
- Process verifications and validations regarding the conditions of the work environment
- Evidence of human resource compatibility: records of training and certifications
- Records and evidence required by regulatory requirements

7 Product Realization

7.1 PLANNING OF PRODUCT REALIZATION

Chapter 7.1 (Planning of Product Realization) initiates the master planning of the realization of the medical device and refers for the first time to the term "quality plan." Planning of this will cover the entire life cycle of the medical device (including the design and development activities). The objective of the quality plan is to lead, guide, and instruct all the participants on the different functions and roles that are involved in the realization of a device; how to manage the design and development of a device; how to prepare for the realization; which resources are required; which activities are needed; what are the controls to be applied; and what evidence is expected. A quality plan provides the organization with the means of integrating the quality management principles throughout the realization processes—for a product, a project, or a service (Table 7.1).

Quality Plan

A quality plan is a list of specifications or activities for the organization to follow, meet, or maintain in order to realize a product according to requirements (customer's or regulatory). The objective is to carry out the requirements given earlier in clause 4.1 (Quality Management System: General Requirements):

1. Identifying all the required processes for product realization
2. Defining the relations between the various processes
3. Defining the required resources
4. Defining the acceptance (or rejection) criteria
5. Defining the validation and verification of products and processes (control and monitoring processes)
6. Evaluation of effectiveness

These are the principles with which the manufacturer shall plan its realization activities. Quality planning integrates the relevant requirements for resources and information concerning the realization of a product and makes them available to any involved party. It may also be viewed as a guideline for the product's realization processes; it consists of all the necessary information that would assist the participants to produce a product that meets its requirements.

Reference of the Quality Plan to the Quality Objectives

In clause 5.4.1 (Quality Objectives), the standards refers us to clause 7.1, which requires that top management ensures the implementation of quality objectives related to the realization. On the quality manual, describe the quality objectives and targets that would be achieved when implementing a quality management system, and would assist the realization of a product that meets the requirements. Now is the time and the place to refer to those objectives regarding the product realization. For example, let us

TABLE 7.1
Standard Requirements of Clause 7.1

ISO 13485	ISO 9001
Processes needed for the realization of the product shall be developed, planned, and implemented	Processes needed for the realization of the product shall be developed, planned, and implemented
The planning of the realization processes shall relate to the principles and concepts of the quality requirements and processes as required in clause 4.1	The planning of the realization processes shall relate to the principles and concepts of the quality requirements and processes as required in clause 4.1
The quality objectives and quality requirements of the product shall be clearly defined and shall be controlled throughout the product realization	The quality objectives and quality requirements of the product shall be clearly defined and shall be controlled throughout the product realization
The organization shall determine the processes, methods, and activities needed for the realization of the product. Documentation and resources necessary to support these activities shall be planned, allocated, and implemented	The organization shall determine the processes, methods, and activities needed for the realization of the product. Documentations and resources necessary to support these activities shall be planned, allocated, and implemented
The organization shall determine the activities required for verification, validation, monitoring, and measurement of processes and products. The appropriate criteria (acceptance or rejection) for these activities shall be determined	The organization shall determine the activities required for verification, validation, monitoring, and measurement of processes and products. The appropriate criteria (acceptance or rejection) for these activities shall be determined
The organization shall determine the records providing evidence that the realization processes are performed according to the quality plan, at the right sequences, and that outputs of processes meet the product's requirements. These records must be kept and included under the records control process, as required in subclause 4.2.4 (Control of Records)	The organization shall determine the records providing evidence that the realization processes are performed according to the quality plan, at the right sequences, and that outputs of processes meet the product's requirements. These records must be kept and included under the records control process as required in subclause 4.2.4 (Control of Records)
The planned activities and methods must be suitable to the nature of the organization's processes and operations, and to the nature of the product	The planned activities and methods must be suitable to the nature of the organization's processes and operations, and to the nature of the product
Note: The organization may refer to the outputs of design and development activities, as specified in clause 7.3 of this standard, when planning the realization processes	Note: The organization may refer to the outputs of design and development activities, as specified in clause 7.3 of this standard, when planning the realization processes
Risk management activities shall be planned, and the requirements shall be documented and incorporated throughout the realization of the product.	
Records of risk management shall be included under the records control process as required in subclause 4.2.4 (Control of Records)	
Note: The planning of risk management shall refer to the ISO 14971 Standard for guidance on risk management	

TABLE 7.1 (Continued)
Standard Requirements of Clause 7.1

ISO 13485	ISO 9001
Note: The organization may maintain a document specifying all the requirements and quality, as well as realization processes, referring to the resources and documentations involved. The document may be considered as a quality plan. Such a document may be assigned to a product, project, or a contract	Note: The organization may maintain a document specifying all the requirements and quality, as well as realization processes, referring to the resources and documentations involved. The document may be considered as a quality plan. Such a document may be assigned to a product, project, or a contract

assume that the organization declared on its quality manual that it would like to reduce the number of customer complaints. After a review of last year's complaints, it was discovered that most of these relate to the packaging of the product and, in particular, the packaging processes. As a result of this discovery, the organization must review the exact definitions and controls regarding the packaging processes and consider redefining them in order to reduce the number of complaints. In other words, when planning the realization processes and establishing the quality plan, the organization shall refer to the relevant quality objectives—reducing complaints—and plan the required controls in order to achieve these objectives. A great deal of the planning of the realization and the determination of the product's objectives take place during the design and development stages of the product, such as:

- The definitions of the product and its characteristics
- The definitions of the required resources and functions
- The definitions of the necessary activities and their sequence

The planning of the realization processes shall use, or at least refer to, the outputs of the design and development plan.

Processes

Defining the processes is the first step in defining a quality plan. The quality plan shall describe the processes with which the manufacturer realizes the product. The objective is to provide a reference for the verification of process outputs and to allow you to test whether the product has progressed according to plan. The definitions shall relate to the methods, activities, techniques, practices, responsibilities, documentations, and specific records that would provide evidence for these processes. These will be documented. The plan may include or refer to documented realization requirements—procedures, flow charts, diagrams, routing charts, checklists, work instructions, test instructions, or forms of any kind. You may define generic procedures or plan specific procedures using a high level of detail. For example, a work instruction is a part of the quality plan that assists the manufacture in achieving one part of the realization process. It is a list of planned activities for operating a process, reference to the appropriate documentations, and a specification of the records. The issue is well addressed in chapter 4.2 (Documentation Requirements). Another important aspect to be considered when planning the processes is the integration of quality principles and processes that are required by this standard: control of documents and records (planning, review, approval, release, and control of changes); the implementation of processes to handle a product according to its status; analyses for improvements; the handling of nonconforming products and so on.

Regulatory Requirements

During the planning of your product realization, regulatory requirements have an essential role in the designing stage. Thus, the quality plan will refer to the appropriate regulations regarding various aspects of the medical device. The manufacturer will review the applicable local, national, or international regulation directives or standards that apply to its medical devices and will review whether there are specific requirements regarding the planning of the realization. Requirements may be for verification or validation activities, packaging and labeling, clinical evaluations, examination, and quality assurance. These are all critical aspects in the planning of product realization. When there are such demands they will be naturally implemented. This is one aspect of the harmonization that ISO 13485 aspires to. Examples for standards that may be applicable include:

- EN 980 (labeling)
- EN 10993 (biological compatibility)
- EN 11607 (packaging)
- EN 14155 (clinical evaluation)
- ISO 14971 (risk management)
- EN 60601 (medical electrical equipment)

Another example is the IVDD 98/79/EC (in vitro diagnostic directive). The directive characterizes the framework of regulations regarding in vitro medical devices, discusses issues such as the design stages and establishment of a technical file, and dictates particular requirements. These requirements are to be considered planned and implemented in the realization processes. Advisories and safety warnings related to the medical device shall be referred and defined. When an advisory or a warning are required to be posted or labeled on the medical device, the quality plan shall indicate or refer to a documented specification where these warnings or advisories shall be assigned, and by whom. If it is required by a regulation to publish the presence of some material or component (in the medical device) due to certain considerations (health or danger) you shall refer to it on the quality plan. If a regulation demands that employees acquire a qualification or a certification in order to realize the medical device, as mentioned in subclause 6.2.2, then this would have to be mentioned on the quality plan, the relevant regulation, and the implication on human resources.

Production Requirements and Resources

The organization shall define the required production resources related to the product realization: raw material, required machinery, required production means (molds, tools, safety equipment), production parameters, work instructions, necessary work environment, storage requirements, and human resources—including training and certification needs. Regarding human resources, the organization shall define those necessary to the product realization: employees required; necessary qualifications, training, or certifications. When it is necessary to employ workers that have specific training in order to realize the product, this should be defined and documented; that is, give the name of the product or process along with the qualification needed for its realization. This may seem somewhat confusing as it may be considered that such a definition has already been given during implementation of the requirements in Chapter 6 (Resource Management). This is partly correct, as there is some congruence; the difference, however, is that here you define the needs, while in Chapter 6 you plan the management and controls.

Verification of Product

Verification is the confirmation, through the provision of objective evidence, that product requirements have been fulfilled. Verification is achieved through the review activities such as calculations, quality tests, and a review of process outputs and records. The quality plan defines which verification is needed throughout the processes; which parts, components, activities, or scopes on the medical device are to be verified; and the acceptance criteria. When the plan does not include the description of the verifications, it shall refer to documentations and specifications related to them. The best example is the quality test instructions and the quality protocols. The test instructions describe what the required product verifications are, and the protocols provide the evidence. The difference between a test instruction and the work instruction is that the test instruction specifies the inspection tasks and indicates the criteria for the output; big, small, long, or short. As a manufacturer, you must compare the accepted results of a process with the expected results documented on the test instruction. Another example is a customer's order. Let us assume that a customer's order should not be transferred for production without a set of defined documentation in order to ensure that the relevant inputs are at the right place and time: a copy of the order, design history file (DHF), updated product diagram, incoming material quality tests, product portfolio, certification of training, and routing cards. The manufacturer must verify that the requirements were fulfilled and define how they shall be ensured; a check list, a status management on the information system, which requires signatures. The verification of products and processes would be planned according to the standard's specific requirements, as shown in clauses 8.2.3 (Monitoring and Measurement of Processes), and 8.2.4.1 (Monitoring and Measurement of Product).

Validation of Product

Validation is an approval, through the provision of objective evidence, that the requirements for a specific intended use or application have been fulfilled. The organization is required to define the activities that would evaluate the compatibility of the product and what are the acceptance criteria. Compatibility is the extent to which the realized medical device achieved the predefined specification—functionality, performance, safety, and intended use through the demonstrations of process parameters. Issues to be concerned with include:

- The plan shall indicate the production stages and activities that are required throughout the realization processes and validation of products or processes.
- Planning of validation activities shall indicate who is to perform these activities on products or processes.
- The plan shall refer to the appropriate specification and documentation—such as work instructions, test specifications and instructions, list of equipment for monitoring and measurement, integration tests, scientific criteria, and research.
- Planning of the validation processes shall refer to the resources required in order to validate a process, and shall specify the monitoring and measuring devices that are needed to perform these activities. Usually the definition would

appear on test instructions. This is also the place to mention any special equipment that is required for validation.
- A plan shall include the acceptance or rejection criteria for products or processes, or provide a reference to documentation that includes tolerances and limits.

Labeling and Identifying Products

The quality plan shall define the labeling and identification requirements for products throughout the realization processes. The plan shall indicate:

- The data and information to be placed on the labels.
- The stages of the production in which the products are to be labeled.
- The parts or components that are to be labeled.
- The responsibilities for the labeling activities.
- A reference to the appropriate forms and records.

The contents of the label depend on the type of medical device and its nature—contents of the medical device, warnings, safety instructions, or advisory notices.

Traceability and Status Management

The quality plan shall refer to the instructions and procedures related to the traceability and status management requirements. The ISO 13485 requires defining a method for managing traceability throughout the whole realization process and maintaining documented procedures. At the same time, the quality plan relates to the status management of materials, parts, components, and finished goods; and will describe the tools and techniques with which the status will be managed throughout all the realization processes. Specific requirements will be discussed on subclause 7.5.3 (Identification and Traceability).

Customer Requirements

Customer requirements and references to their technical, functional, or performance specifications shall be included in the planning of product realization. The reference to customer requirements may influence various aspects of the plan—additional verifications or validations, specific identification or labeling requirements. A good example could be a contract or a project where the organization is delivering a tailored product to the customer; aside from the regular production requirements, there are also exceptional specifications to be fulfilled. These specifications must be documented. When such requirements are the case, the quality plan should be designed in accordance with them.

Risk Management

The ISO 13485 Standard requires the planning of risk management processes and activities and the integration of them into the quality management system. Successful implementation of the risk management system would obtain for the organization a systematic method for identifying risks, evaluating and controlling them, and—where needed (and defined in advance)—eliminating or reducing them. Since risk management relates to the realization processes and shall cover the entire life cycle of the product, a reference shall be included on the quality plan. The issue is regarded as any other realization activity: storage, packaging, or transportation. The standard expects that you include on the quality plan how are you going to implement risk management evaluations and controls throughout the realization processes. The requirements for activities related to risk management will be documented and shall be submitted to the documents control process as required in subclause 4.2.3 (Control of Documents).

Risk controls may be executed in various ways: warning or advisory notices on the product, altering work procedures, adding safety measures, changing components or features of the product—activities that are derived from the risk management outputs. The issue is applicable to all stages of the life cycle of a medical device:

- The planning stage of the medical device
- Purchasing of material
- Production of the medical device
- Marketing
- Delivery
- Installation
- Service maintenance
- Disposal

Clause 7.1 (Planning of Product Realization) initiates the harmonization of two management systems—the integration of risk management systems and processes in your quality management system. The quality plan shall refer to the critical elements of the risk management system—such as the risk management plan, the risk management file, the risk management report, and the integration of their outputs in the work processes.

I will review here the relation between the risk management plan and the planning of the product realization. The activities of the risk management system are defined and documented in the risk management plan (given the fact that a risk management system is implemented in the organization). The plan includes:

- Identification of the relevant products or components
- Identification of any requirements for the risk management: standards, technical, safety, customer, and, most important, regulatory requirements
- Definition of criteria for risk acceptability
- The required verifications of validations of risk controls
- Definitions of the different stages of the realization in which the risk management activities are to be applied and control implemented
- Reference to the responsibilities and authorities

The quality plan reviews the various stages of the product realization; and just as it refers to the quality tests of a part or to the packaging activities of a product, it will relate to the risk management requirements mentioned on the risk management plan on the appropriate stages of realization. Regarding the records, the ISO 13485 Standard is clear and expects to find records and evidence of the risk management activities. These records shall be submitted to the control of records in your quality management system. If you are implementing the ISO 14971 Standard, note that for every medical device being submitted to the risk management process, you will be required to administer a risk management file containing records and evidence produced by the risk management process. The objective is to establish one location in the organization where all documents and records related to risk management shall be kept and maintained.

The ISO 13485 Standard refers us to the ISO 14971 Standard for guidance of developing, planning, and implementing a risk management system. The basic purpose of the ISO 14971 Standard is to propose a process to identify the hazards related to medical devices—including in vitro diagnostic (IVD) medical devices—in order to evaluate and control the risks and to monitor the effectiveness of the controls that are implemented: in other words, to systemize the risk management process and to boost control (a typical ISO organization requirement). The main objective is to establish a standard for a risk management process and to toe the line among various industries and geographic regions. The term, "risk management," is to be considered in the medical device industry as more than just a nice management term. It is considered essential, both by ISO and the FDA, for ensuring the safety and reliability of medical devices. The ISO 14971 Standard is a risk management standard that is specifically designed and developed for the medical device industry. The standard suggests an effective risk management system model and uses principles for the development, production, and maintenance of medical devices. It was also designed in a way that it could be relatively easily integrated with other quality or environmental management systems. It is not required that you implement the ISO 14971 Standard but it is suggested that you consult it as a guide on how to plan risk management activities, and how to integrate and implement an effective risk management system. The standard is acknowledged in medical device industries and market regions around the world. The FDA recognizes and accepts the model for risk management as suggested by the ISO 14971 Standard. The European Union declared it as mandatory for obtaining the CE mark although recently objections were raised regarding the standard's coverage of essential requirements of the applicable medical device directives related to the realization of the medical device. It means that you will have to make further investigations and clarifications regarding the applicability of the ISO 14971 to your type of medical device or relevant applicable regulatory requirements.

Practical Quality Plan

There is no requirement for a procedure describing the quality plan; however, it is highly recommended to define and draw an independent document bearing the title "quality plan," or a set of documents specifying the different stages of the realization processes as a quality plan: requirements, processes, resources, verifications and validations, activities, and records. The document may appear on a procedure, a table, or a form. Table 7.2 is an example for a list serving as a quality plan.

Notes:

- The table shall include reference to the appropriate documentations (procedures, instructions, forms).
- QM—quality manager.
- PM—production manager.
- DDM—design and development manager.
- ITM—IT maintenance.

Such specification may be known as DMR (device master record) or as technical documentation and design dossier. However, the principle must be made clear—specifications of the controls over different realization processes should include: the requirement, the documentation, the responsible party, and the location availability. For example, were you an employee in this plant, you should be able follow the plan and find yourself around the realization process and the related details. If a problem occurs, you then would have access to the necessary information in order to investigate the matter.

TABLE 7.2
Example of a Documented Quality Plan

Requirement	Required Documentation	Responsible	Location
Procedures	Controlling purchased product	Store man	Company's server
	Cleanliness procedure	PM	Company's server
	Validation procedure for software	PM ITM	Company's server
	Identification and traceability	PM QM	Company's server
	Work instructions		Company's server DMR, machines
	Assembly instructions		Company's server DMR, machines
	Quality test instructions		Company's server DMR, machines
Customer's Requirements	Copy of customer's order	Salesman	ERP system
	Product's specifications, design testing reports, risk controls, design reviews, product's diagram, design verification, validation reports, specifications for raw materials, product labeling and packaging, design changes	DDM QM	DHF
	QS example part	QM	Examples Room
Risk Management	Risk management plan	QM DDM	Company's server
	Risk management report	DDM PM QM	
	Risk management file	QM DDM	
Material	Raw material quality report (COC)	Store man	ERP system (scanned)
	Purchase order report	Store man	ERP system
	Delivery notice	Store man	ERP system (scanned)
Production Requirements	IQ specifications, protocols, and records	QM PM	DHR
	OQ specifications, protocols, and records		DHR
	PQ specifications, protocols, and records		DHR
	List of monitoring and measurement equipment		DHR
	Production order	PM	DHR
	Batch records	PM	DHR
	Cleanliness records	PM	DHR

(*continued*)

TABLE 7.2 (Continued)
Example of a Documented Quality Plan

Requirement	Required Documentation	Responsible	Location
	Identification barcodes	PM	DHR
Human Resources Requirements	Scheduled working shifts	Shift foreman	Notice board
	Instruction for worker		Training folder
	Training form		Training folder

Reference to Chapter 7.3

The standard suggests applying the planning principles mentioned in chapter 7.3 (Design and Development) while planning the realization processes. The principles are:

- The establishment of a documented plan that describes the stages and milestones of the realization.
- The determination of the required inputs to the realization processes—the inputs shall consist of product specifications as well as instructions, including reference to risk management requirements.
- The determination of the expected outputs—the outputs shall consist of process outputs as well as records and evidence.
- Definitions of review activities for the control of the progress of the plan.
- Definitions of verification activities.
- Definitions of validation activities.
- Definitions of controls over changes.

Records

As part of the planning of the realization of a product (processes, activities, required resources, and documentation), the manufacturer will decide and determine the records and evidence needed as proof for the compatibility of the product to its specifications. Each activity that takes place during the realization of the medical device must produce evidence that:

- The activity was conducted on the appropriate stage and sequence, and by the appropriate responsibility.
- The results of the process meet their predefined requirements.

For example, when the quality plan indicates that a certain qualification is necessary for conducting an activity, you would be required to provide documented evidence that employees on a certain production session (tracked with an identifier in order to achieve traceability) obtain this qualification. If preparation for a sterilization load requires obtaining and documenting evidence that equipment has been provided and installed in accordance to predefined specifications, you would be required to provide this evidence. The quality plan shall indicate or refer to the appropriate instructions concerning which documents are expected, and where the records are stored. The ISO 13485 Standard refers us to subclause 4.2.4 (Control of Records) and requires that these records shall be part of your quality management system and be submitted to the records control process.

7.2 CUSTOMER-RELATED PROCESSES

7.2.1 Determination of Requirements Related to the Product

Product requirements are a collection of inputs to set criteria for its validation; but what are the product's requirements? In order to accurately identify these, the organization needs to develop a method to collect and review these inputs (Table 7.3).

When determining the requirements related to the product, the organization must first verify the feasibility of supplying the product according to the customer's expectations and specifications. Thus, it is required to review all requirements from various inputs and conditions—customer, regulatory, safety, and organizational. Another objective is the guarantee that all the requirements are clear, documented, and distributed. Through the development of a systematic method for the identification of all the inputs that shape and determine the product, the organization may determine exactly what the product specifications are, and evaluate whether it has the ability to meet these specifications. This type of evaluation requires cooperation with other organizational parties, such as design and development, production, and logistics. The method shall cover stages such as:

- Communicating with the customer (this will be defined under the requirements of subclause 7.2.3—Customer Communication)
- Accepting and collecting the customer requirements related to the product
- Collecting other products' requirements, such as the regulation or risk management outputs
- Translating and processing requirements into the required realization activities

TABLE 7.3
Standard Requirements of Subclause 7.2.1

ISO 13485	ISO 9001
The organization shall determine product requirements as defined by the customer. The determination shall refer to delivery and postdelivery activities too	The organization shall determine product requirements defined by the customer. The determination shall refer to delivery and postdelivery activities too
The organization shall determine product requirements that are not expressed or forwarded by the customer, but are required for obtaining the intended use of the product	The organization shall determine product's requirements that are not expressed or forwarded by the customer, but are required for obtaining the intended use of the product
The organization shall identify and implement regulatory requirements applicable to the product	The organization shall identify and implement regulatory requirements applicable to the product
The organization shall determine additional requirements necessary for realization of the product	The organization shall determine additional requirements necessary for realization of the product

- Evaluating whether the organization can provide the customer with an adequate product
- Distributing the requirements among the different relevant organizational units

The standard is aware that achieving all of customers' requirements is almost impossible. However, there are some areas and product scopes—such as regulatory and safety requirements—that do not leave much room for compromise. For example, in the medical device industry a significance weight is given to the apprehension of customer safety as well as intended use requirements. The organization is to present a method for:

- Capturing all the inputs that may serve as requirements
- Fully apprehending these requirements
- Assurance that all relevant documents are provided
- Distributing all the requirements to the appropriate organizational units

There is no standard demand to document the method; however, during an audit, you will have to prove that this method is defined and implemented. Thus, you must plan and introduce key tools into your organization that will assist it in meeting the necessary requirements. These include:

- Customer files
- Checklists
- Order forms
- Management systems
- A summary report of research
- A document characterization

The standards introduce us to several main types of requirements that need to be reviewed when accepting or collecting requirements related to the product. Reviewing these will bring you closer to an accurate determination of the demands.

Customer Requirements

Product requirements define the customer's expectations of the product; the customer formally communicates their needs through defined communication channels (see chapter 7.2.3) and transfer product specifications, including performance requirements. Possible types of customer requirements include:

- Product-related requirements such as functionality, quality, performance, safety, intended use
- Technical specifications of materials, parts, components, processes, the use of certain equipments, and the qualifications of personnel
- Packaging and identification
- Transport and delivery specifications and schedules
- Storage and protection
- Certifications for standards

- Prices and conditions of payment
- Service and maintenance
- Guarantee

In order to ensure a systematic means of capturing and reviewing the customer's requirements, the organization is expected to develop a method for receiving these requirements, which may be transferred in various ways. This is a critical contact point with your customer regarding the capturing and understanding of all his/her needs. Requirements can be delivered through the following:

- Documentation (of an order, contract, or agreement)
- Technical specifications
- Diagrams and drawings
- Request for proposal (RFP)
- Tenders
- Markets surveys
- Clinical research

Records of orders or contracts will be dealt with in subclause 7.2.2.

Additional Requirements not Stated by the Customer

While determining the requirements related to the product, some areas that were not considered or taken in account by the customer may include:

- The operating environment: The manufacturer shall verify that the operating environment in which the medical device must operate is clear and understood. If the medical device is to operate under a controlled temperature, it must be reviewed and mentioned to the customer. This requirement is valid, for example, when software must be installed and there are technical specifications for the installation.
- Interfacing with other products or equipment: It must be made clear whether the product is to interface with other devices and what the implications of the interface will be. This has a direct relation to the risk management process outputs.
- Transportability: The organization must verify that it has the ability to perform delivery and transportation activities while preserving the product. In some cases it will be a controlled transportation; in others it may be the installment of medical devices. The review shall ensure that the customer is aware of such requirements.
- Service and maintenance: When service and maintenance are part of the product and need to be delivered regularly, they must be reviewed and determined. The organization must evaluate whether it has the abilities to perform these activities and the customer must be made aware of the matter.

Additional Requirements

The organization shall evaluate other realization requirements that are not of the customer's concern but are nonetheless crucial to the realization processes. Such requirements must be verified for their availability. They include:

- Qualifications, skills, or knowledge
- Special equipment, tools, and accessories (such as clothing or software)
- Material or components
- Workshops, workstations, and production resources

- Necessary processes
- Required standards
- Activities for the disposal of materials

Regulatory Requirements

The identification of relevant regulatory requirements is critical when determining requirements related to the product. These contain provisions for product safety, product characteristics, and functions; and they may affect or set the product's requirements—design and development, production, assembly, storage and transportation, handling, recycling, and the disposal of materials or products. The logic behind the requirement claims is that a lack of compliance with regulations regarding the use and safety of the medical device may have a negative implication on the user or operator. The organization shall define a method for the identification of the relevant regulatory requirements. The goal here is to develop a method to ensure that regulations are available and understood when product requirements are being considered and planned. The method will ensure that any changes or updates in the regulatory requirements are identified, seized, and accounted for. This is how you may ensure that the relevant product requirements will be up to date with regard to the regulations. Availability of the regulations is not measured only by their physical presence, but also by employees' awareness of the regulations and their influence and affect on the product's realization.

The regulatory requirements may include applicable government, safety, and environmental regulations. They may apply to the acquisition, storage, handling, recycling, elimination, or disposal of materials or products. One of the first stages of identifying the applicable regulations is the classification of the medical device according to its characters, functionality, type, and level of risk that it may pose to the user or operator.

Note: In subclause 5.6.2 (Review Input) top management reviews new or revised regulatory requirements. This point can be covered during the management review; you may indicate that the regulatory requirements and changes related to the customer requirements review are assessed during the management review.

Also, updates on regulatory requirements changes may be obtained through newsletter registration, a periodical review of information sources (such as websites), or a periodical application to the authorities for inquiries on whether changes were issued.

Reference to Risk Management

The risk management outputs will serve as inputs for the determination of product requirements. Risk analysis, along with its results, presents controls that will act as product requirements which must be referred or implemented. The importance of reference to the product is similar to the regulatory requirements.

Clarity of Requirements

Product requirements shall be clear and unambiguous in a way that would allow effective product validation during later phases of product's life cycle. In other words, the organization shall undertake measures to eliminate misunderstandings or gaps between the product requirements and their interpretation by the organization. There is always an element of risk in the difference between the perspectives of the organization regarding the product requirement. Here are some practical measures to eliminate these gaps:

- Appointing a designated authority or function for receiving and understanding customer requirements will reduce the number of opinions and interpretations.

- Identifying and contacting functions and roles by the customer or local authorities relevant to specific topics. Such functions may assist and support the manufacturer in understanding the requirements: quality control, purchase, design, and development.
- Ensuring that technical or professional terms and abbreviations are understood, well interpreted, and explained.
- When the requirements are in a foreign language, the organization shall ensure that it has the capacity to have these translated.
- Creating a communication channel designed to receive specific inputs will ensure the submission of definite inputs. A good example is to install by the customer a terminal of your system for submitting orders.
- Accepting the approval from the customer or the local authorities is one of the most effective ways of eliminating misunderstandings.

7.2.2 Review of Requirements Related to the Product Requirements

The specifications of a product are the sum of all the customer's expectation of the medical device. These specifications contain requirements for functionality, performance, safety, regulations, quality, packaging installation, service warranty, and standards. The ISO 13485 Standard approach reflects the dependency of the organization on its customers. Thus, the organization is required to develop a method to identify its customers requirements and capture and review their needs, along with a system that will to manage relations with the customer and preserve its loyalty (Table 7.4).

Accepting a Request from the Customer

A review of requirements related to the product essentially means the development of a method that is necessary to understand the needs and demands related to the medical device, and to coordinate them with the your organization. The objectives of the review are:

- Understanding the needs and requirements of the customer
- Translating the needs to organizational terms—product specifications, functionality, risk management, and regulations
- Reviewing and approving the ability of the organization to produce and deliver the product

These will be conducted before the submission of a commitment to the customer. The goal of the review is to clarify and interpret the customer's requirements, translate them into organizational terms, and ensure that the organization can meet them. The requirements may be divided into set, planned, programmed, or fixed product properties, as well as variable or specific customer requirements. Among the requirements are: schedules, quantities, technical specifications, quality requirements, regulatory requirements, risk management, packaging, delivery, installation, service, and warranty. Objectives are to be achieved through these basic principles:

- Accepting a request for a proposal or identifying a need
- Reviewing the needs
- Delivering a proposal to the customer
- Accepting a confirmation, an order, or a contract

TABLE 7.4
Standard Requirements of Subclause 7.2.1

ISO 13485	ISO 9001
The organization must examine and survey the requirements related to the product	The organization must examine and survey the requirements related to the product
The examination of the requirements shall be performed initially to engagement of the organization to provide the product to the customer through the submission of tenders, acceptance of contracts, orders, or changes to contracts or orders	The examination of the requirements shall be performed initially to engagement of the organization to provide the product to the customer through the submission of tenders, acceptance of contracts, orders, or changes to contracts or orders
The organization shall ensure that product's requirements are defined, documented, and are clear and understood, including the delivery requirements and the postdelivery requirements	The organization shall ensure that product's requirements are defined, and are clear and understood, including the delivery requirements and the postdelivery requirements
The organization shall ensure that differences between the request from the customer and the actual requirements submitted to the customer are settled	The organization shall ensure that differences between the request from the customer and the actual requirements submitted to the customer are settled
The organization must ensure and confirm that it has the ability to supply the product as required	The organization must ensure and confirm that it has the ability to supply the product as required
Records of the review shall be maintained and included under the records control procedure as required in subclause 4.2.4 (Control of Records)	Records of the review shall be maintained and included under the records control procedure as required in subclause 4.2.4 (Control of Records)
A documented approval or verification from the customer is required prior to the agreement, when the customer did not deliver documented product requirements or specifications	A documented approval or verification from the customer is required prior to the agreement, when the customer did not deliver documented product requirements or specifications
Changes of customer requirements are to be documented, updated on the relevant documentation, and distributed to the appropriate organizational parties	Changes of customer requirements are to be documented, updated on the relevant documentation, and distributed to the appropriate organizational parties
Note: when the customer requirements are based on a constant fixed list which represents all the product characteristics, a formal review is not required. A review of the information and detail on the list is required.	Note: when the customer requirements are based on a constant fixed list which represents all the product characteristics, a formal review is not required. A review of the information and detail on the list is required.

In practice, the organization shall develop and plan a method that defines:

- The interface between the organization and the customer to receive, exchange, and transfer information related to the product
- The definition of the information required from the customer
- The identification of all accessories and facilities that the customer must provide
- The different organizational responsibilities in the review, with the distribution of the requirements among them—marketing, design and development, production, and logistics

- The documented requirements
- The records and evidence of the review

The method for identifying customer needs and expectations shall begin with defining the organizations communication channels with customers:

- It may be that the requirements of the product would be delivered by the customer in the classic manner of request for a proposal, a price quote, an order, a tender, or a contract.
- The organization may determine the requirements based solely on surveys, market evaluations, or research.
- It may be a joint venture between the customer and the organization.
- The requirements may derive from postmarketing activities such as customer complaints, advisory notices or service feedback.

This stage must not be documented (these requirements shall be documented once you review them) unless the organization determine that the details sent by the customer serve as the records. However, I recommend maintaining records that the customer has submitted, since the next stages (the review and the answer to the customer) must be documented—though this also depends on the nature of the organization. For example, documenting requests for offers along with various parameters in commerce organizations may serve as a statistical database for later research.

Regulatory Requirements

The identification of relevant regulatory requirements related to the customer is crucial to the review. The logic behind such claims is that there is a possibility that different regulations apply to different customers due to different geographical locations or markets. The manufacturer must bear the responsibility here. The method shall identify the relevant regulations, directives, standards, or any other legal or statutory conditions. These will be available and understood when product requirements are being reviewed. These may refer to the different aspects of the medical device: functionality, safety, labeling, package, delivery, distribution, service and maintenance, advisory notice, and recall. And thus may display the customer's requirements in a whole different light.

Risks Review

The review of customer requirements shall include a review of risks related to the provision and delivery of the medical device. The objective of this risk review is to evaluate where the manufacturer might fail to deliver the medical device as required and how this may be avoided. The risks are to be analyzed on three levels:

- Providing a medical device according to the customer's need and quality requirements
- Providing a medical device that meets all the regulatory requirements (according to the geographical location of the customer)
- Providing a medical device that meets all the risk management requirements

Such a review is necessary when there is a chance that the organization could fail to provide the product due to various reasons or aspects, including:

- Provision—the ability to supply the product on schedule.
- Geographical constraints—where the medical devices are required to be delivered to distant geographical regions in which the organization has not yet delivered, or has not yet provided support (service and maintenance).

- Security issues—above all the issue of handling confidential health data or customer property.
- Availability of realization resources—the liability of production, time, and human resources to supply the product.
- Qualifications—when the customer requires personnel of certain qualifications, these shall be ensured.
- Subcontracting, purchasing, or outsourcing—when such are needed, the organization shall evaluate their availability, integrity, and compatibility.
- Technological aspects—does the organization govern the technological skills, qualifications, tools, methods, and innovation that it is necessary to provide?

Let us review some examples of how such review of risks may proceed. When the organization is obliged to deliver the medical device in a special package, it must verify that such a package is available and a process supports it. Another example is when the manufacturer is compelled to deliver the medical device according to specific schedules, and must thus perform some kind of availability check, and verify that it can deliver it on time. If the medical device is to be installed in a specific environment with specific conditions, the manufacturer must verify that all the conditions are available to them. This kind of review is to be documented and the records maintained. The records of such a review depend on the nature and type of the product.

Resolving Differences between the Manufacturer and the Customer

One of the objectives of the review is the confirmation that the manufacturer can deliver a product to the customer according to their needs—though this may have a side effect. After the review, when the organization knows what the customer wants, and what it must deliver, differences, obscurities, or disagreements may arise; the customer wants something that the manufacturer can deliver, but not entirely. This is natural. For example, differences may appear as price disparities, functionality, attributes, or delivery schedules. These differences must be resolved before the customer approves the offer. In other words, according to the standard, a customer's order should not be submitted for realization before all disagreements or differences between the customer and the manufacturer are resolved. Such differences can be resolved by accepting an approval from the customer of the terms for supplying the product. When it is a mass-produced product, and the customer has submitted an order, most organizations would check whether they can supply the product according to the request, and will return a document stating their terms to the customer for approval. An approval may come in the form of a signature or a message. In other cases, when the product is more complex, it may be resolved with documented specifications agreed by both sides (for example, in an agreement, a contract, or a meeting summary). However, some contracts or agreements may not contain all the requirements. They may contain products, models, delivery methods, and prices—but not schedules. It would therefore be required to gain customers' approval for these variables. When the organization is performing sittings and conferences with the customer regarding their requirements and specifications, and the outputs of these sittings act as the customer's specifications, it is necessary to define the method. It is also possible to define each realization stage, where a customer's approval is obtained. For example, in a contract a manufacturer may obtain general approval, but on an order they may obtain specific approval. In other situations manufacturers may submit the product for approval after each production stage. The question is what reflects you nature of organization?

When an organization knows that it cannot deliver a product according to the needs of the customer, it must notify them before the customer's order submission. When a certain operating environment is required for the medical device, or it is known that the customer will operate or use the medical device in an environment which may harm or disqualify the product, the manufacturer must raise the issue and draw it to the attention of the customer.

Control and Review of Changes in Customer Requirements

The organization must control changes in customer requirements. The ISO 13485 Standard is aware that customers may change their minds and needs. This is why manufacturers must maintain control over the actualization and validity of the requirements. Changes required by the customer must be reviewed on several perspectives that may affect the medical device. The review shall determine whether the manufacturer is capable of providing the necessary changes:

- Product characteristics or technical specifications
- Implications of risk controls
- Compatibility with regulatory requirements
- Technical abilities
- Availability of resources

The first stage in the process is accepting a request for a change. Here the organization is required to integrate the request for change into the method. The matter must not be documented in a procedure, but documented requirements shall be planned and provided; for example, forms or information system, for example. The documented requirement shall include a responsibility, which may be documented on the job description. The next step is to identify the type and extent of the change. This has several implications:

- Identification of the product and the extent of the change
- Identification of the relevant organizational parties

The matter can then be submitted for review. At this stage the manufacturer should determine:

- Who is responsible for the evaluation
- What is to be evaluated
- Which documentation is it necessary to review and update (diagrams, specifications, instructions)
- To whom must the changes be distributed
- Who approves the changes

As said before, the issue will be structured in a method, and records of the review shall be maintained. When changes on the product are initiated by the organization—such as changes in materials, packages, processes, human resources, transportation, or any other conditions that were agreed with the customer and to which the organization is committed—the organization shall receive approval from the customer.

The classic example is updating an order form on an information system and submitting its status. Say, for instance, that the customer has made an order, and after a few days they decide add or subtract some items from that order, or to change the delivery dates. The sales person simply updates the order, performs an availability check with the relevant parties, and submits it. The issue becomes complicated when the product is more complex and more parameters must be evaluated, or where the product is a specially tailored one. In this case you may need to update a whole set of documentation and to inform various department or functions. The approval of the change is critical. Take, for example, a product that involves technical plans or diagrams, and the customer wants to make a change to the technical specifications. This means that plans and diagrams should also be changed or updated. The approval of the change would ensure that all relevant technical documentation was updated according to the change, and that all relevant parties were informed. I recommend appointing a function to such review and approval. The method could be integrated with the method for records control as presented in chapter 4.2.4.

Records

The records of the review have two main objectives. The first is for the maintenance of product requirements needed for later verification and validation. The second is for evidence of the review, and as a proof of the ability of the organization to supply the product according to the requirements. Thus, the records are divided into two types:

- Documented product requirements: RFP, request for price quote, product specifications, customer's order (external document), customer approval, approved technical specifications, internal order, contract or agreements, quality, and package and delivery specifications
- Records of the review: production plans with reference to orders, records of stocks or inventory, records of consignation, and contracts agreements

The ISO 13485 Standard refers us to subclause 4.2.4 (Control of Records) and requires that records related to the review shall be part of your quality management system and would be submitted to the records control process.

7.2.3 Customer Communication

One of the most common business activities in an organization is the communication with customers; the customer wants and needs the attention, and, in most cases, also pays for this attention. The ways to communicate with your customer may vary according to the type of medical device, or the type of the agreement that an organization has with its customers. The scope of a contract, for example, may determine different communication channels or manners regarding the provision, operation, or maintenance of the medical device. There are cases and scenarios where communication will be dictated and controlled by third parties. All these affairs will be structured in planned arrangements for communicating with the customers (Table 7.5).

The main objective of clause 7.2.3 is to initiate effective communication channels with the customers, whether they are internal or external. The effectiveness would be obtained by answering the following questions:

- Is the method for accepting customer requirements properly defined and maintained in the organization?
- Does the customer receive all the information and data that they need and that answer their enquiries?
- Does the organization maintain an effective way to receive complaints from the customer and provide them with answers?

TABLE 7.5
Standard Requirements of Subclause 7.2.3

ISO 13485	ISO 9001
The organization will develop a method for communicating with the customer on various topics related to the product, its delivery or postdelivery activities	The organization will develop a method for communicating with the customer on various topics related to the product, its delivery or postdelivery activities
The communication will include sharing information with the customer regarding the product	The communication will include sharing information with the customer regarding the product
The organization will exchange information with customer regarding enquiries, orders, and contracts, including changes and updates relevant to the product	The organization will exchange information with customer regarding enquiries, orders, and contracts, including changes and updates relevant to the product
The organization must determine a method for handling customer complaints and feedbacks as specified in subclause 8.2.1.	The organization must determine a method for handling customer complaints and feedbacks
The organization must determine the method for communicating advisory notices to the customers (subclause 8.5.1)	

- Are the communication and information transferred to the customer planned and maintained according to regulatory requirements?
- Does the organization maintain an effective communication channel when it needs to transfer advisory notices or perform recalls?

Try to understand the philosophical aspect behind this requirement—the customer and their needs stand in the center of your attention. When the customer has needs they initiate communication with the manufacturer through defined channels. The manufacturer is obliged to answer and fulfill these needs, which are divided into several themes and subjects, and may take place at different phases of the realization processes: marketing, design and development, production, delivery, installation, warranty, service and maintenance, and advisory notice and recalls. For each need or type of interaction, you must define the right response and reaction: channel, responsibility, and information to be handled. Thus, plan your responses using the organizational structure and processes according to the needs of the customer.

Information Regarding the Product or the Service

Planning communication channels with your customers may be affected by the information related to the product or service, which will be exchanged with the customer—either transferred or received. The definition shall relate to information regarding the product and its attributes:

- The description of the medical device
- The use of the medical device

- Training instructions or warnings regarding the use and operation of the medical device
- Previous editions or versions of the medical device
- The medical device materials, components, and characteristics
- Processes and realization activities of the medical device (sterilization, storage, and delivery)
- Warnings and advisory notices regarding the medical device

Information regarding the product including changes and updates to the medical device:

- Changes that may affect the characteristics of the medical device
- Improvements in the medical device
- Problems regarding the medical device that the customer must not know about

Changes, updates, and improvements must be brought to the attention of the customer. According to the standard, "changes" is understood as meaning any alterations made to the product's features or to the attributes of a contemporary or future model that was ordered and agreed with the customer. The same applies to improvements (which are a kind of change). The organization is to define the suitable media and form of communication—e-mails, telephone calls, written correspondence, or meetings.

Information for processes that depend on interaction with the customer and their submission of inputs:

- Development or design plans
- Results of acceptance testing
- Requirements for inputs such as customer specifications
- Demonstrations and presentations of products, prototypes, or results of tests

The ISO 13485 Standard requires the determination of communication means with the customer through the implementation of effective arrangements. The objective is to reassure that all the necessary inputs have been accepted or transferred.

Investigations, Applications or Inquiries Regarding Orders or Contracts

The standard requires a definition of a system and an organizational function that handles all applications from the customers regarding the business collaboration between the manufacturer and the customer (orders or contracts). The objective is to allow for the customer's access to information regarding subjects that may be of interest to them. When defining the method, the manufacturer must take into consideration what information will be transferred to customers:

- Orders or contracts—the processes of submission orders or contracts, as well as inquiries or investigations
- Status of orders—inquiries or investigations concerning production activities or the realization of the medical device, delivery dates, transportation, installation, and warranty
- Technical support—how the support will be organized and the means of communication with the customer
- Service and maintenance
- Progress of activities that are under the responsibility of the customer
- Reporting over present or future changes

A Defined System

After the necessary information to be exchanged with the customer has been defined, the organization shall define the method to handle each type of information. The method will be based on three simple principles:

1. How—the means or manner in which the information will be accepted or delivered: printed media, interaction center, service center, e-mail, fax, online via website or a designated program. The definition will be bi-directional—client to business and business to client.
2. Where—the format and means where the information will saved and kept: handbooks, user manuals, internet sites, forms, records on the information system, e-mail, or client portfolios. This requirement refers indirectly to chapter 4.2.4 (Control of Records). These records are an integral part of the quality management system. Some of them are required to be maintained (see chapter 4.2.4 for the specific list). Include them under the process of controlling the quality records. This will ensure that they would be kept in the desired manner and under the required control.
3. To whom—the distribution of the data to the relevant parties: marketing, design and development, production, logistics, and technical service.

Authorities and Responsibilities for Customer Communication

In order to maintain effective communication channels, the manufacturer shall appoint designated roles for each type of customer communication. Each role will be responsible for managing the communication channel according to the definition related to the specific case (marketing, production, or logistics). For example, a sales representative is responsible for delivering price quotes, and to input orders to the marketing and sales information system. When developing a specific product with the customer, a project manager will be designated for the tasks of communicating with the customer, receiving and documenting product specifications and requirements, conducting meetings with the customer, conducting meetings with the internal functions to realize the product, and so on. The objective is to appoint a person or a function that will bear the responsibility of operating the communication with the customer and exchanging the required information. The documentation may appear on the job description, the role definition, or on a work instruction. Strong emphasis is given to the treatment of complaints and the handling of customer feedback. These will be covered in more details later.

Time Frames

The objective here is to specify the exact time frame for a response—that is, over what period of time must the requested information be transferred to the customer. Normally this depends on the nature of the notice. In principle it is necessary that every type of communication defines the required response time. For example:

- An offer—a request for an offer would be normally handled within 24 hours.
- A complaint—an immediate answer would be delivered to the customer stating that the complaint is under review and that a full answer will be delivered to the customer within four business days.
- Changes in the medical device—the response time would be determined according to the nature of the change.

Although documentation is not required, the control report is. Such parameters are related to the business development and usually appear on a business or a project plan. The manufacturer may refer to these plans, and can draw the definitions from such documents and implement them on the relevant control system; in an interaction center they may generate control reports to analyze time responses, and in a sales department they may review the time responses for leads.

Verification

The organization must verify the effectiveness of the communication channels. In other words verification that the information reached its designated target is required. This aspect is critical for achieving customer satisfaction. It is also a matter of great importance because the organization may distribute the medical device through dealers or distributors, and therefore might not have any direct contact with the end users. This means that a manufacturer might not have control over the contact they have with their customers. It is therefore critical to verify the mechanism of the communication. However, bear in mind that the distributor's and dealer's interests may differ from those of the manufacturer.

The practical approach toward maintaining this involves defining the verification for each communication process. If a customer needs to approve an order, it would be necessary to obtain their approval document. Send the customer a copy of the order and request to have it returned with their signature. When using e-mail as a communication channel, verify that the recipient received the message by defining an automatic respond notice; this acts as a sort of verification. If a distributor is to communicate for the manufacturer (you), request that they deliver sufficient evidence. A registered letter may also provide verification. When a meeting is being conducted with the customer and agreements or understandings have been concluded, produce a meeting summary and send it to the relevant parties. This verification will serve the manufacturer in case of advisory notices or recalls.

Customer Records

Customer records shall be kept according to the nature of the communication. The purpose is to define the needed inputs for communicating with the customer. At first, the organization shall define which records are required in order to maintain effective communication with the customer—that is, name, contact person, telephone number, e-mail address, postal address, activity hours, bank account details, credit card numbers, particular notices and remarks, examples of products, types of documents (order, delivery notes, invoices), or technical specifications—anything that would be necessary for communication with the customer. If the customer maintains a designated system for correspondence, then the relevant parties should receive training with instructions on how to use the relevant system. For example, if the customer installs a system terminal in the organization for maintaining the business relationships, performing orders, or exchanging documents, then the required records on this case are list of responsible and authorities for maintaining the system and the relevant instructions. The documentation could take place on the job description and the guidance could appear on a work instruction. The verification will be on a training form or the certification of an employee.

The next stage is to define where customer's records will be kept, along with how they will be kept, or in which format, referring to realization phases (when) and responsible functions (who). By "when" and "who" I refer to the different stages during the

TABLE 7.6
Process Examples and Related Customer's Records

Process	Customer Records
Marketing lead	The name and telephone number of the customer, plus a completed lead survey for the sales representative to communicate with a potential customer
Sales order	Full customer details, including account details
Development	The name of a contact person by the customer related to the production of the medical device
Production	The details and communication means with the quality control
Delivery	Address for delivery and a contact person in the logistics clause
Accounting	Details for debit

business process. Each stage demands a different type of information that forms the communication with the customer. In other words, define the records that are related to a process and a function. For each stage define which customer records are required, and verify that the information is well distributed. Review the process examples and the customer's records requirement (Table 7.6).

The ISO 13485 Standard suggests a CRM process; the manufacturer must find an effective way to implement it. Mostly, these requirements are already implemented, though they need to be identified throughout the processes so that it is made certain that they are carried out. One effective way is to use the management information system. I refer here to the Enterprise resource Planning (ERP) or Customer relation Management (CRM) systems—a system that manages processes in the organization:

1. The system defines the records that must be gathered and used for communication with the customer.
2. The system verifies that these records are really gathered for the customer and processes.
3. The system ensures that the records are distributed to the appropriate functions.

Customer Feedback

The ISO 13485 Standard requires monitoring customers' feedback. We will discuss the reason for this in chapter 8.2.1 (Feedback). The main principle to bear in mind is that customers' satisfaction may be submitted to subjective opinion while feedback provides an objective point of view on whether the organization supplied the medical device according to the requirements. The main issue of this process is to provide an early warning about potential quality problems. This process effectively generates the inputs for improvement, and initiates the necessary corrective and preventive actions. Feedback evaluation is maintained through the following:

- Customer complaints—the organization must monitor customer complaints regarding to the performance and functionality of the medical device.
- User surveys—the manufacturer may conduct surveys regarding the functionality, characteristics, and performances of the medical device.
- Reviews—the manufacturer may order or initiate a review regarding their medical device.

- Journal reviews—to research sector and industry tendencies.
- Periodic postproduction preview phase—activities conducted after the product's design is completed and the product had been manufactured.

Handling complaints is dealt with in detail in the following paragraph. For each of the aforementioned actions, it is necessary to define a communication channel—if you are using a product review for receiving feedback regarding the medical device, you must determine how this review will be conducted. The method of the review will be dealt with in chapter 8.2.1. The means with which you will communicate the customers will include conferences, personal interviews, focus groups or e-mails. Since clause 8.2.1 requires a documented procedure for the feedback activities, the topic of communication will be documented there.

Complaint Handling

The ISO 13485 Standard regards the issue of complaints as being highly significant. An important aspect on this issue is the facility with which a customer can communicate with the organization and convey a complaint. No less important is the organization's delivery of a satisfactory response to the complaint. The first concern of the organization is to define the application process of the complaint. The handling of a complaint should be managed using a tested method. The method should deal with various aspect of the process:

- Communication: The method shall describe to the customer how they may reach the organization to file a complaint. The method could be incorporated with other types of inquiries (such as information or the ordering of products). However, the organization must notify its customers of the ways that they can deliver complaints—a specific or free-phone number, an online form, a designated e-mail address, an interaction center—such options for filing a complaint must be made known to the customer. Contact details can be printed on a brochure, the contract, the firm's website, or on the product itself.
- Details: The method shall define the required information and details that must be recorded during a complaint. The details should be sufficient in details and information in order to ensure effective treatment. The manufacturer must document the information to ensure effective investigation into the nature and cause of the complaint. The matter is discussed further in chapters 8.5.1 (Improvement—General) and 8.5.2 (Corrective Action). The details of the complaint are the inputs to these quality processes and activities. If the complaint refers to a product, then the following information must be specified—the model, batch number and production details, contact person, delivery date, and any other detail that would identify the product and support the investigation. If the complaint refers to a service, then specify when the service was given, by whom, and the service identifier. The best way to ensure that such details are provided is to design a form (manually or electronically), and verify that all fields are completed. You may encounter such methods when filling a form on the web with fields that are marked with a star suggesting that certain fields are mandatory.
- Distribution: The method for handling a complaint shall define to the communication of the complaint to the appropriate role or function in the organization through the definition of the interface between the organizational unit that receives the complaint and the one the shall handle and investigate it; an e-mail, form, or designated system.

- Responsibilities: The function that would be in charge of the process of accepting the complaints must be defined (e.g., an operator, an interaction center agent, a customer relationship manager, or an account manager). As well as defining the function responsible for accepting the complaint, the function responsible for handling the complaint must also be defined. Some complaints may need to be passed on to a designated person in order for them to be appropriately handled. This person should be clearly appointed.
- Time frame: It is necessary to determine the exact time frame for the response and the treatment. The customer should not be left waiting for an answer. Especially in the medical device sector where it can be matter of life and death. If the answer is taking too long, the customer should be notified and assured that their complaint is under investigation. Another aspect related to time frames is local or national regulations; where regulations require that you submit an action in a defined period of time, the organization must apply these requirements and implement them in its processes.

  A sample response to a complaint would include the following steps: send the customer a message apologizing for the inconvenience caused, and notify them that the complaint is being processed. Ask them to allow X number of working days before an answer is submitted. The message will be signed by the person handling the complaint. Attach a copy of a complaint form (to gain trust), with contact details included.
- Answer: After accepting, processing, and handling the complaint, it is necessary to inform and communicate the results to the customer or to the regulatory authorities. The method shall define the means and details. You cannot ensure that each complaint is closed to the satisfaction of the customer, but you can verify that the results were transferred and the customer received them.

Advisory Notices

As for advisory notices, the organization is required to determine and document a process for communicating with the customers, notifying them of any cases where a malfunction or deterioration in the characteristics of the medical device have occurred or may potentially occur. For example, if the manufacturer discovers that the product may, under certain conditions, present a risk to the user, the organization must notify the customer through informing local authorities, using the media, posting messages, notifying the distributors, or tracking down batches with customer records. This topic is dealt with in greater depth in clause 8.5.1. The ISO Standards also refer us to this clause. Clause 7.2.3 requires that you define the communication aspect and determine how the advisory notice shall be communicated to customers. Since clause 8.5.1 demands a procedure, the communication requirements of clause 7.2.3 would be defined and documented there. When defining the communication aspect, you must refer to the following issues:

- The target group to receive the notice—customers, distributors, local authorities.
- Key roles that are responsible for communicating with the customer—quality manager, head of development, public relations.
- The information that will be delivered—details of the medical device, model, batch number, production date, applicable references.
- The documentation that must be delivered—a notice of information, a malfunction advisory, a designated report.
- The method through which the information will be delivered—e-mails, fax, post, telephone.

- Regulatory reporting—in certain locations the manufacturer will be subjected to specific reporting regulations according to certain cases, event, or incidents. In each area of operation, manufacturers are required to identify the suitable regulatory body and to find out when, and in what manner, it is required that they report. It may be that certain countries require certain reports to several legal bodies.

A good way to define and present the communication regarding advisory notices is to design a flow chart that specifies the interaction between the organization and the relevant target groups, supported by the necessary documentation.

Regulatory Requirements

Although the standard does not relate to regulatory requirements in subclause 7.2.3 directly, they will be discussed here. As mentioned before, in many regions manufacturers will be subjected to specific regulations. These may require that they communicate with their customers on various topics other than complaints or advisory notices. It might be necessary to collect specific data or to design specific processes or documentation in order to respond to these needs. This is why manufacturers are requested to identify any national or regional regulations, or to review any changes at the beginning of the certification process (clauses 4.2.3 and 5.6.2). If there are changes regarding communication with the customer, the manufacturer must implement them. This fact may influence the entire communication process with the customer.

7.3 DESIGN AND DEVELOPMENT

7.3.1 Design and Development Planning

The ISO 13485 Standard requires that you plan and control the design and development of products. While doing so, the organization must refer to the following issues (Table 7.7).

The ISO 13485 Standard's (as well as that of the ISO 9001 Standard) bottom line regarding design and development planning is: determine a method for development and follow it through. The main goal is to reduce dependence on the verification and validation processes, and implement quality controls over the development processes. When it comes to the early identification of problems or difficulties, such an approach will assist the organization. The planning of the design and development has several objectives:

- To identify major design and development tasks
- To divide the design and development into phases
- To eliminate potential quality problems as much as possible
- To allow compliance with regulatory and customer requirements

The tactic is to examine whether the development advances within measured steps according to prior planning. It is important to update the plan as the development advances, and to change the plan according to what is required. This means that it is possible to change the plan during the development (if required), but do not forget to update the relevant documentation.

TABLE 7.7
Standard Requirements of Subclause 7.3.1

ISO 13485	ISO 9001
The organization is required to establish and maintain a documented procedure describing the process for controlling the design and development process. The procedure shall be submitted to the documents control method in your organization as required in subclause 4.2.3. The introduction must include updating documentation when it is appropriate	The organization is required to establish and maintain a process for controlling the design and development process
Milestones during the development process shall be defined	Milestones during the development process shall be defined
Responsibilities and authorities related to the design and development shall be defined and allocated	Responsibilities and authorities related to the design and development shall be defined and allocated
The method shall indicate where time frames, schedules, objectives, and resources are decided and documented	The method shall indicate where time frames, schedules, objectives, and resources are decided and documented
The method must allow identification of any requirements for the development: standards' requirements, market or customer requirements, or regulatory requirements	The method must allow identification of any requirements for the development: standards' requirements, market or customer requirements, or regulatory requirements
The method shall define effective reviews, verifications, and validations during the design and development process for every stage, as needed	The method shall define effective reviews, verifications, and validations during the design and development process for every stage, as needed
Transfer activities between the various design and development stages shall ensure that all development outputs are appropriate for production before termination of processes	
The planning of the development shall be reviewed in order to ensure its validation	
The organization must introduce the design and development outputs to the records control process within the organization as required in subclause 4.2.4 (Control of Records)	The organization must submit the design and development outputs to the records control process within the organization as required in subclause 4.2.4 (Control of Records)
The method shall ensure effective communication and information sharing between different parties involved in the development by managing and controlling the interface between them	The method shall ensure effective communication and information sharing between different parties involved in the development by managing and controlling the interface between them
The method shall ensure that the planning outputs are updated as the development proceeds. The control over the update shall be submitted to the documents control method in your organization as required in subclause 4.2.3	The method shall ensure that the planning outputs are updated as the development proceeds

In the following paragraphs I will review the issues to be considered when determining the design development plan.

A Documented Procedure

The first distinguished difference between the ISO 13485 Standard and the older ISO 9001 Standard is the requirement for a documented procedure describing the design and the development processes. The procedure must cover all the requirements mentioned in the table above. As expected, the procedure will be submitted to the control of documents process as required in clause 4.2.3 (Control of Documents), and will be included in the appropriate procedure. A form or a chart describing milestones or the development stages is not sufficient here. Another procedure is required.

Control over Related Documents

Any document that is related to design and development will be submitted to the control of documents process as well. To put it another way: set up the design and development plan and the related documentation according to the method of document control. Updating documents during the design and the development is crucial. Given this fact, any documents related to design and development must answer all the requirements of chapter 4.2.3—that is, they must be reviewed and approved, updated when needed, be of relevance, and so on. This is applicable to all kind and types of forms—flow chart diagrams, instructions, programs, templates, and computer software—all the documentation platforms of the design and the development.

Milestones

Milestones describing the development process must be defined. When an activity is considered to be a stage of design and development, contributes to the progress, and generates outputs, it should be counted as a "milestone." Milestones represent the stages that the organization must follow and complete while designing and developing, such as:

- Marketing reviews
- Brainstorming
- Gathering relevant information
- Research from prior developments
- Delegation of tasks
- Scheduling
- Risk management
- Design and development planning
- Design inputs
- Design outputs
- Design reviews
- Design verifications
- Design validations
- Design transfers
- Design changes
- Design history files
- Communication with authorities
- Obtaining approvals
- Training

The objective is to describe what activities are essential, and what is expected at the end of each activity—the outputs.

Responsibilities and Authorities

Each development and design activity must have the responsible roles for controlling allocated to them. It is very similar to organizational definitions—each participant in the design and development stage must have a clearly defined understanding of their responsibilities and the activities they are required to perform, how they are integrated into the development cycle, to whom they must report, and the outputs expected of them. When required, the definition shall include a development team structure (like an organizational structure) with the interrelationships between the participants outlined. One way to document this would be to describe it in the job description. I recommend, however, including the authorities and responsibilities in a structured procedure.

It is important to clearly define the responsible party for conducting the design and the development reviews. It may be an individual or a team. Part of their responsibility would be to assess the process according to predefined criteria. The question here is not what it is required to assess, but who. A reference will be given to the manner: meeting, review of data or results, interviews.

Time Frames

The method shall indicate where time frames, schedules, and time objectives with resources are determined and documented. The specifications must also refer to purchasing activities. The objective is to establish control over the development process in terms of time frames. Timing charts, Pert, or Gantt charts could be used for the purpose. The time control will relate to:

- The milestone of the design and the development—when an activity shall start and end; for example, approving data, ordering materials, creating prototypes.
- The allocation of different resources to the development processes—you may define time frames for the allocation.
- The applications between the different developing units—when the interrelations may take place.
- The validation and verification activities—determining when the validation and verification activities occur.

The easiest way to describe it would be setting time objectives for each activity, or allocating to each activity a required time frame for realization; for example, a "time budget" that should not be exceeded. It is important to define the control tool to be used for time management: various MS Applications, a self-planned schedule—something that may provide the manufacturer with the means of controlling the advance of a project in terms of time. In today's market there are countless systems and types of software for the purpose. It is important to find the most suitable to your own needs.

Validation and Verification

The plan shall provide effective controls over the design and development activities, and define for each activity the required verification and validation (when required). In other words, the manufacturer should describe how one will examine whether the development was conducted according to the plan, and whether the outputs of the processes achieved the required results. In some cases you may determine this in cooperation with your customer. The design and development activities must be:

- Verified—the examination that ensures that the development processes are advancing as planned
- Validated—the assurance that results and outputs of the development processes meet the objectives; the test will be with predefined criteria

The validation and verification requirements of the design and development will be reviewed in detail in subclauses 7.3.5–7.3.6. An important aspect in the validation of the design and development is the identification of the appropriate measurement devices and equipment monitoring tools. These must be able to provide you with the appropriate and reliable data in order to validate processes. When a tool or piece of equipment is required for the validation, it is required to define what it is, and to verify that it is available.

Say, for example, that you are using a certain material during the development and are required to monitor its behavior in certain conditions. First, you need to check how the data will be obtained. Second, you need to define which monitoring equipment will obtain the necessary data. Next, you must see whether the equipment is available and ensure that it will provide you with the desired data. You may simulate the process in order find to out exactly what is needed in to monitor it.

Advice: In order to be able to verify effectively the progress of the development process, you may want to consider describing the process in a table, using fields such as: development phase, activity, responsibility, time frame, risks, required output, recipients, validation activity, and verification activity. Framing the development process in such a document would help to maintain the required level of control.

Transfer Activities

Another goal of the verification is to ensure that the design and development activities are suitable, and are verified before submitting, releasing, or authorizing the product for final production. The objective here is to ensure that the designed device will perform its intended use as required, and that the design is correctly translated into production specifications. This stage is very important. In order to achieve this requirement you must plan your transfer activities for the production. Once you have developed the product, and have completed, reviewed, and validated all the project tasks and required tests, take some time to verify that the product will be produced as required, and ensure that the objectives of the medical device have been accomplished during production. Now is the time to develop and carry out the interface between the development and production departments. It is important that everything is clear for the production departments–that all the required controls are understood and implemented, gaps or open issues regarding the quality and production objectives of the product are resolved, and that the product is produced appropriately. Naturally, there is room for communication between the development and production departments during the later stages of the production cycle (for clarifications, inquiries, and handling certain cases).

Internal and External Interfaces

Interface between the different units or groups involved in the design and development stages are immensely important during the processes as a communicative channel. They are responsible for:

- Sharing knowledge, data, and information between the different participants
- The interrelations between various development plans on different levels of design and development
- Promoting the development throughout the different stages
- Ensuring that outputs are verified and suitable for the next phase

As a consultant to many developing companies, I personally experienced how information had failed to flow between various departments due to the lack of suitable communication channels. Healthy communication channels will obtain information transparency, and the sharing of knowledge during the developing processes. These are the top quality objectives of the development stages. Therefore, every member of the development team must be aware of the information or data that they are supposed to receive and pass on. The plan shall specify the internal and external communication channels. In order to make the interface more effective, I recommend describing the interface on a flow chart as a process explaining the relations and interrelations between the documents throughout the development stages—how documents relate to other documents, how the outputs of one document are the inputs for another, and so on. This will make it easy to identify whenever a communication is required, and to specify what information is required, between who, and how.

When defining the relations that serve the design and development process, the interface with external objects, bodies, or parties that may have an affect on the process or may take part in any of the design or development activities are to be referred. These may be customers, suppliers, authorities, or other developing teams or organizational departments. For example, when a product is developed, responsibility for the various components must be shared among the different departments. Another example is when a certain material must be purchased for the development—the purchaser must manage the purchased material and notify the relevant party when the material has arrived. Yet another example is when a component is to be delivered to another development team in order to be integrated with other components—the other team must approve the acceptance and report the integration.

Required Training for the Development Team

When appropriate, training related to the design and the development will be identified. This issue will have been already covered during your planning of human resource enhancement in accordance with requirements in subclause 6.2.2 (Competence, Awareness, and Training). You should define, in the plan, a method for the identification of training required for the design and development process. If you already defined such a method, then you refer the plan to it. The ISO 13485 Standard does not support double work.

Identification of Standards, Regulations, and Legislative Requirements

Medical devices are produced under strict regulations and external requirements. These are applicable to the design and development stages as well. The plan shall identify, indicate, and refer to requirements such as international standards, regulations, or regional directives. When defining the design and development plan, such regulations and standards are to be reviewed and particular requirements are to be incorporated into your activities. Another important aspect is the exclusion of design and development controls. The ISO 13485 Standard permits the exclusion of the design and development controls when regulations allow it. The exclusion is conditioned by the fact that these regulations dictate alternative controls to the design and development stages. I suggest reviewing the relevant regulations and examining whether you may exclude controls from your design and development plan. For further information see chapter 1.2 (Application).

Application of Risk Management during the Design and Development

Risk management activities are to be implemented and incorporated during the design and development phases. The detection and identification of hazards, hazardous situations, related to the use of the medical device should be completed as early as possible in its life cycle and that in the design and development phases. Through the introduction of risk management activities, the implementation of risk controls, and the elimination of known hazards during the design phases, the manufacturer reduces the probability of the occurrence of potential dangers. The result is the inherent safety of the product. The incorporation of risk management in the design and development stages has several goals:

- To introduce the risk management activities into the design control process and the life cycle management of the medical device
- To implement risk control measures in the final design of the medical device
- To systematically assure that required risk management elements are in the process
- To reduce the probability of a risk by improving the characteristics of them medical device
- To focus and refine the risk controls

In practice, the design and development plan shall relate to the risk management policy and method (identifying hazards, evaluating risks, and implementing risk control measures), specify the activities and responsibilities, and refer to the required documentation standards, regulations and records. The issue will be documented in the procedure.

7.3.2 Design and Development Inputs

As well as the ISO 9001 Standard, the ISO 13485 Standard requires defining inputs required to carry out the development of new products. The inputs should be determined according to the design and the development activities, and the intended use of the product. The main concept of defining your design and development inputs is simple: the inputs must relate to the medical device's intended use, functional performance, quality requirements, and safety and regulatory requirements. Within the design and development inputs requirements, the organization must refer to the following issues (Table 7.8).

The inputs for the design and development are determined according to the functionality or performance requirements, but they could also be derived from prototypes or the need to modify earlier developments:

- Request for changes
- Problem or failures with earlier versions
- Failure to comply with the acceptability criteria
- New customer requirements
- An iterative development

TABLE 7.8
Standard Requirements of Subclause 7.3.2

ISO 13485	ISO 9001
Personnel requirements	Personnel requirements
Operation, performance, and safety requirements of the medical device with reference to its intended use	Operation and performance requirements of the medical device
Outputs and results of earlier applicable designs and developments	Outputs and results of earlier applicable designs and developments
Documentation of information necessary for the development process	Documentation of information necessary for the development process
Outputs of a risk management process	
The inputs must be reviewed and approved by an authorized person before submitted for use. The approval must be documented	The inputs must be reviewed and approved by an authorized person before submitted for use
The organization must maintain records of the design and the development inputs. These records must be defined as quality records under your records control procedure, as mention in subclause 4.2.4 (Control of Records)	The organization must maintain records of the design and the development inputs. These records must be defined as quality records under your records control procedure, as mention in subclause 4.2.4 (Control of Records)

The organization will take into account the state of the art and available information such as technology and practice existing at the time of design.

Employees' Requirements

The organization is required to identify the organizational personnel responsible for the product design, development, and quality aspects during the design and development stages. The organization must refer to any role that performs any kind of activity of design and development: engineers, scientists, programmers, lab technicians, and so on. The bottom line is defining and determining which functions or roles participate in the design and development activities. The definition may be documented on a job description, a development plan, or a procedure.

In cases where the development of a certain medical device require training that was not included in the training program, such training must be identified, planned and given to the appropriate parties.

Product Characteristics and Functional and Performance Requirements

The organization must define the product requirements and functionality in order to allow identification of all necessary design and development inputs. The ISO 9001 Standard requires functionality and performance requirements, but the ISO 13485 adds another aspect to the functionality and performance—safety according to the intended use. Allow me to specify (safety shall be referred to in a specific clause):

- The intended use of the medical device refers to the purpose, operation, and utilization of the medical device and relates to the user and patient requirements (these are the intended users or patients). The intended use may include also special requirements regarding them due to the nature of the medical device. This standard requirement refers to information and outputs derived from market surveys or research, RFPs, risk management outputs, customer requirements, and a review of requirements related to the product. The definition shall include contraindications—situations where it is inadvisable to use the medical device.

- Physical characteristics of the medical device—plans, dimensions, diagrams, drawings, and samples. The definition shall refer to tolerances and limits.
- Requirements for handling and behavior with the medical device—specifying aspects such as package, storage, operation, handling, and maintenance requirements; anything that might affect the quality of the product or its intended use must be regarded during the development stages.
- Definition regarding the operating environment of the medical device—if the medical device is to operate under a controlled temperature, the customer must be aware of that. This requirement is also valid when a software must be installed and there are technical specifications for installation.
- Interface with other devices—if the medical device is to be combined or installed with another medical device or piece of equipment, and/or accessories, it shall be referred as inputs to the design and the development for functionality, performance, or safety.
- Service requirement—if you already know that the medical device will require service activities in the long term, then you must notify the design and development teams in advance. They need to plan the medical device appropriately.
- Labeling requirements—this requirement includes reference for the prevention of foreseeable misuse of the medical device.
- Toxicity, biocompatibility, or electromagnetic compatibility—this requirement refers to the compatibility of components. For example, if the medical device is constructed or assembled from various components and materials, it is required to examine the materials used in order to ensure that the different components of the medical device compete or match to one another and the risk of contamination, error, or failure is prevented. The compatibility test and proof must be documented.

Safety Requirements

The manufacturer will specify the safety requirements that are needed to serve as inputs for the development. These may affect the design of the device, and will therefore also affect the inputs of the design and development:

- Functionality and intended use: What is the functionality of the medical device? What are the operation instructions? Is there any special guidance? Where will the device be used for? Are there any risks related to the use? Who is to operate the device? Who is the target group that will use it? Is the device intended to be used with other devices?
- Performance: What are the energy requirement of the medical device? Are there any special restrictions or limitations? How long is the expected shelf life? Are there any service or maintenance necessities? What may influence the device and its performance?
- Safety: Does the device present any risk to the user, operator, or to the environment? Does the device have special requirements, such as sterilization or storage? Do any special measures need to be applied before, during, or after use? Are the materials influenced by certain conditions?

Such considerations may be expressed through data safe sheets, safety measures, training, special services, or certifications. Remember the objective the medical device should be designed to be inherently safe. For example, when the manufacturer designs a medical device for home use, several factors must accounted for:

- Special user instructions that apply to unqualified operators or users
- The electricity conditions in various geographical areas
- The home, as an operation environment, must be analyzed

Documented Requirements of Any Kind for the Design and Development

The manufacturer must identify documentation and any kind of information or specifications that are used while designing and developing the medical device. Documented requirements may include:

- Internal procedures
- Policies
- International standards or technical requirements
- Environmental standards
- Technical specifications
- Industry standards or specifications
- Legal requirements or laws (local or international)
- Packaging requirements
- Harmonized standards
- Directives

Each of the above places restrictions on medical devices regarding its performances, functionality, intended use and safety with influenced by a market or a region. These requirements are to be documented and made available. They must be first identified (such as discussed in chapter 7.2.1, where the manufacturer must define and document the requirements related to the product, In this case, however, it is specifically in relation to design and development). These requirements are to be handed to the relevant parties in the appropriate manner; through summaries, reports, charts, appropriate files, and so on.

While reviewing the documentation that may serve as inputs, you must refer to any impractical requirements (requirements that cannot be fulfilled or that the development team might have problems fulfilling). The following cases may occur:

- Requirements that cannot be validated or verified
- Incomplete information or lack of information regarding the user or the intended use
- Lack of information or details regarding the user's environment
- Any documentation related to the design and development that does not appear in the plan

The goal is to detect any future difficulties or obstacles that may arise during the development phase. It is recommended that the reviewing procedure be carried out with the customer or with the responsible party for these requirements in order to obtain their points of view.

Outputs of Applicable Earlier Developments

Where applicable, one should refer to prior similar or parallel developments that have been performed in the organization. The outputs of what the organization has already developed may be used throughout the new development. This might save time and/or resources (depending on what you are developing). The inputs may appear as:

- Documentation of applicable earlier developments
- Complaints, failures, or other events regarding previous products
- History of the organization (a knowledge center)

Development Tools of Any Kind

Here I relate to the means with which you would conduct the design and development—computer software, glass tubes, supporting tools, rulers, and so on. The purpose is to define the accessories and environment used for the design and development activities. You must define the versions of the development tools in order to eliminate the use of irrelevant or invalid tools. For example, when the organization is using software in order to develop functionalities in the medical device, it must define the current version that is used. If monitoring and measuring devices serve the development, then the validation required in chapter 7.6 of the standard will be the control over them.

Outputs of Risk Management

As mentioned in the last chapter, design development stages will include risk management activities in order to implement iterative safety. A risk analysis outputs are required in order to identify hazards, hazardous situations, and events that can cause harm while determining the characteristics of the medical device. The outputs of the risk management process are control measures, methods, and the activities needed to eliminate hazards related to the use of the medical device. These are to serve as inputs for the design and development stages. Risks management inputs may refer to the following issues:

- Control of risks that are suggested by the risk report
- Risks relevant to the use of tools and equipment during realization processes
- Risks caused by realization processes (e.g., transportation)
- Risks that derive from material components of the medical device
- Review of feedback activities, outputs complaints, surveys, advisory notices, recalls, or research regarding prior or identical devices or common areas

Depending on the particular risk management method implemented in your organization, you must identify where inputs are documented and gather the relevant information. Visualization of processes or products' characteristic (for example, a prototype or process simulations) may refine make more accurate estimations of risks of processes, a prototype of the medical device.

Purchasing

It is necessary to define what products, components, or services are to be purchased in order to achieve the development. The requirements for purchasing shall be reviewed and defined in order to serve as input for the design and development process.

Inputs Approval

The next requirement is to approve any input and to prove its competence and adequacy before introducing it to the development processes. The ISO 9001 Standard requires only the review of the inputs before introducing them into the development process. The ISO 13485 Standard, however, requires review and approval for adequacy. Naturally this approval must be documented. It is required that you appoint, for each input, the person that will control and approve the inputs. If it is an input related to the electric compatibility, for example, then let the electronics engineer review and approve it. This person will be the authority regarding debates, disagreements, or obscurities in relation to the inputs. Competence and adequacy according to the ISO 13485 Standard means:

- Inputs are complete—all the required information is where it is supposed to be
- Inputs are without any contradictions between one another
- The inputs are clear and appropriate for use
- The inputs are available

It is necessary that you review any of the input requirements mentioned above. The objective is to review their compatibility to the various design and development stages. I recommend making a list of the inputs, the relevant or responsible function appointed to the input, and a comment or remark concerning the review and the approval (a signature, for example). It would look like this (the following table is merely a suggestion and may not be suitable for all industries or types of products) (Table 7.9).

Note:

1. The Input
2. Appl.—whether it is applicable to this case
3. Which aspect of the medical device it influences: functional (Fun.), performance (Per.), safety (Saf.), interface with other devices (Int.)—mark with an X wherever applicable
4. Res.—the responsible party
5. Remark—if there is anything to remark or to add
6. Appr.—the required approval

This kind of chart may provide you with the necessary control over the approval of the inputs.

Records

The records of the inputs are to be submitted to the records control process as specified in subclause 4.2.4. The list of your quality records must include the list of the design

TABLE 7.9
Approval of Development Inputs

Input	Appl.	Fun.	Per.	Saf.	Int.	Res.	Remark	Appr.
Product Description (written and detailed)								
Intended use								
Product performance requirements								
Technology								
Regulatory requirements								
Biocompatibility								
Other								

and development inputs, and the records must be submitted to the records control process in your organization. Inputs should be: informatively defined, properly stored, under defined responsibility, retraceable and retrievable, and controlled.

7.3.3 Design and Development Outputs

The ISO 13485 Standard requires defining which outputs are expected at the end of any development stage. You are required to define, by the end of any step, what the expected outputs are. You are also required to define which information should be delivered at the end of any milestone or activity, the way in which this information will be documented, and the format in which it will be delivered. Let us review the requirements (Table 7.10).

The design and development outputs shall be defined and documented according to a method. There is no requirement to document the method. The following issues will be covered.

Verification against Input Requirements

The first requirement regarding the outputs is the need to verify them against the input requirements. The design outputs shall be realized in terms that can be verified, validated, and proved for compliance against design input requirements. Here the loop closes. A few pages back we discussed the planning of the design and development, and the sources that needed to be submitted to the processes as inputs; that is, customer

TABLE 7.10
Standard Requirements of Subclause 7.3.3

ISO 13485	ISO 9001
The outputs must be delivered in a manner that will allow verifying them against the design and development inputs	The outputs must be delivered in a manner that will allow verifying them against the design and development inputs
The outputs must be approved before release	The outputs must be approved before release
The outputs must meet the design and development requirements	The outputs must meet the design and development requirements
The outputs must specify information regarding the product realization processes, such as purchasing and production processes, and the provision of services	The outputs must specify information regarding the product realization processes, such as purchasing and production processes, and the provision of services
The outputs must introduce the product's accepting or rejecting of the criteria	The outputs must introduce the product's accepting or rejecting of the criteria
The outputs must define the product's characteristics accurately to ensure the proper and safe use of the product	The outputs must define the product's characteristics accurately to ensure the proper and safe use of the product
Records of the design and the development outputs must be maintained and submitted to the records control procedure as required in subclause 4.2.4 (Control of Records)	

requirements, regulatory requirements, documentation, employees, training, and so on. Now we are dealing with the expected results of the design and development. These results are to be attributed to the inputs. The review will be done on various levels:

- Performance—whether the performance requirements are achieved
- Functionality—whether the functionality requirements are applicable
- Regulatory—whether all regulatory requirements were referred and implemented
- Safety—whether all safety issues were covered

For example, let us assume that a company develops a medical device with material X. The government requires that development with material X will be done under regulatory specifications. These specifications require that producing a product with material X will be supported with documented training for the production teams. The training will explain how to handle such material during production processes. Thus:

- The input—the regulatory specifications
- The requirement for an output—documented training
- The expected output—documented training regarding material X

Another goal of this verification is to serve the next development stages. You are developing a product according to a defined plan (subclause 7.3.1). It is essential that you verify that any development stage will generate the required outputs necessary to move on to the next stage.

Approval of Outputs

The outputs must be reviewed and approved before their release for use or for the next design stage. The review shall be done at strategic points during the development processes, and will ensure that an output complies. The reason for this is that outputs may serve as inputs for the next design stage and therefore must first be evaluated for adequacy.

Just like the inputs, you must appoint a certain party for the review of every output. This party will be the authority regarding the review and approval of the output. One person, or a steering committee, may be responsible for several outputs.

It is required that you review and approve that:

1. All required outputs are accepted.
2. The accepted outputs are in the appropriate manner or form.
3. The accepted outputs are adequate.
4. The status of the output (the result of the verification test against input requirements)—whether the output is acceptable or usable.

Outputs as Criteria

Another objective of the outputs is to generate criteria for product acceptance or rejection. Criteria are a basis for comparison or expected results for a reference point against which the product can be evaluated (i.e., passed or failed). To put it another way, the criteria—including performance requirements—will allow you to evaluate your product quantitatively. The classic example is the determination of quality specifications for a product; you designed a product and one of the outputs shall be a basis for quality evaluation: the measurements of the product, performance or functionality, and tolerances and limits. These criteria will serve the production processes in later stages. Naturally such outputs are to be planned in advance in order to verify that they are accepted at the end of the design processes. The criteria will refer to various levels: performance, functionality, regulatory, and safety.

Outputs as Product Characteristics for Safe and Proper Use

The ISO 13485 Standard is especially concerned when it comes to the medical device's users. In order to resolve its concerns, it requires us to warn and protect the user, and to specify crucial product characteristics that may pose a threat to the user due to the use of the medical device. You are required to identify the characteristics that may threaten the user, and to supply the appropriate outputs to resolve these hazards or to instruct the user in using the medical device properly and safely (i.e., through warnings, labels, user instructions, safety instructions, health notifications, or studies). Therefore, if, during the design, it has come to knowledge that the medical device may cause injuries in certain cases where several events occur, it is required that you notify the relevant parties—the producer, controller, marketer, distributor, and end users—in an appropriate manner. The notification shall include:

1. The nature of the hazard or the relevant product characteristic
2. The parameters involved (e.g., the user, medical device, operation, and operator)
3. The event
4. The result
5. How one must avoid such a hazard
6. Additional information that may shed light on or contribute to understating the issue better

Application for Realization Processes

The outputs are to be applicable and deliver the appropriate information for later provision stages. The intention here is to ensure that the outputs will be usable for the realization processes of the product; that is, purchasing, production, and service provision. The emphasis here is on the appropriate and applicable information—information that can be used as inputs in these processes. For example, for the purchasing processes, it is required to specify the right "ingredients," or preferable suppliers, so that you may realize the product as designed. For the production it is necessary to plan the right activities in order to realize the product; and for the service it is required that you design the appropriate activities for postdelivery activities. The definition shall include the forms and tools required to deliver the information (e.g., work instructions, charts, drawings, etc).

Expected Outputs

We may encounter the following outputs: product prototype, master models, product portfolio, routing charts indicating the development stages, product specifications, process specifications, specifications for raw materials, component parts, instructions for production, quality instructions, quality procedures, control plans, engineering drawings or charts, research logs, reports, maintenance instructions, installment instructions, work environment requirements, conditions for realization, user manuals, customer training materials, code syntax, measurement and monitoring requirements, packaging and labeling specifications, identification and traceability requirements, requirements for outsourcing, and postmarket surveillance requirements.

Advice: When a prototype is an output, it is required that you document all the design and development stages of it.

Records

The ISO 13485 Standard requires that any output of the design and development stages will be documented. The standard does not specify in which format or media. The main objective of the records is to prove that each development stage was preceded according to the design requirements. You are required to define the design and development outputs as part of the quality records, and the records will be submitted to the control of record in your quality management system as required in subclause 4.2.4 (Control of Records). In practice, the list of your quality records shall include which outputs are required as design and development outputs.

7.3.4 Design and Development Review

At appropriate stages, the organization must review the design and development in a methodical way. The review objectives:

1. To evaluate the design and development results against the product requirements
2. To control the design and development processes, and to ensure that the input requirements are being answered
3. To assign all the appropriate resources required for the review
4. To carry out the control under a defined method
5. To identify difficulties or problems that occurred during the design and development processes, and to suggest solutions or necessary actions to solve these
6. To verify that actions taken were effective and reached their goals

See Table 7.11.

A Method for the Design and Development Review

The ISO 13485 Standard requires defining a systematic method for reviewing design and development. The objective is to evaluate the compliance of the design and development results (final and intermediate) to the input requirements. The evaluation is of the accepted outputs. In other words: you have defined inputs for the design and development; these inputs present requirements and goals for a product; certain outputs must be generated in order to achieve the goals; thus, it is now time to review whether the outputs are:

- Accepted as planned
- Comply with the requirements

In order to achieve this, the ISO 13485 requires that you create a process where all the design and development processes are controlled. All aspects of the review will be determined, such as:

- When the review takes place (in respect to design and development milestones)
- What are the issues to be reviewed
- The type of review (demonstrations, presentations, examinations, interviews, etc.)
- Which records and development outputs are required to be reviewed (drawings, prototypes, summaries, syntax code, results of tests, etc.)

TABLE 7.11
Standard Requirements of Subclause 7.3.4

ISO 13485	ISO 9001
The review of the design and development will be conducted according to a systematic method at appropriate stages during the design and development processes. The method for the review will be documented as a part of the design and development plan	The review of the design and development will be conducted according to a systematic method at appropriate stages during the design and development processes. The method for the review will be a part of the design and development plan
The review must evaluate the competence of the design and development processes in relation to the requirements. The evaluation would be based on the design and development outputs that are presented	The review must evaluate the competence of the design and development processes in relation to the requirements. The evaluation would be based on the design and development outputs that are presented
The review must identify problems that occurred during design and development and suggest appropriate or required ways for action	The review must identify problems that occurred during design and development and suggest appropriate or required ways for action
The review shall include appropriate and verified participants and functions relevant to the design and development processes and stages, as well as suitable and authorized by the management to participate in or to conduct the review	The review shall include appropriate participants and functions relevant to the design and development processes and stages
The participants of the review are to be the relevant parties that have (or had) affected the design and development. These functions and their duties are to be defined and documented	The participants of the review are to be the relevant parties that have (or had) affected the design and development
The organization must keep records of the design and development review. These records must be defined as quality records within your records control procedure as mention in subclause 4.2.4 (Control of Records)	The organization will keep records of the design and development review. These records must be defined as quality records within your records control procedure as mention in subclause 4.2.4 (Control of Records)

- Preceding activities for the review (setting goals, setting schedules and agendas, summons, etc.)
- The process of the review; for each reviewed milestone, the method shall indicate the exact way in which it will be reviewed
- The expected records of the review (summaries, reports, tasks, messages, procedures, updates, e-mails, etc.)

Let us assume that one of the design and development milestones is a "weekly engineer meeting" between the electronics engineer, the software engineer, and the mechanics engineer. The meeting will take place on Tuesday at 1:00 p.m. in the small meeting room. During the meeting the engineers will exchange opinions and impressions regarding the medical device, review drawings and diagrams, go through open tasks from the last meeting, such as electronic compatibility between various components in the medical device, or problems that occurred in the software's functionality. At the end of the meeting a summary will be written with conclusions, open tasks for the next meeting, and—no less important—the demand for an update of drawings and plans according to the conclusions and decisions. This meeting is a design and development activity. These details and specifications are documented on the design and development plan.

At suitable stages, which the organization will determine, there will be a review that this "weekly engineer meeting" is taking place as planned, that the appropriate outputs and documentation are generated, and that the activities promote development according to the requirements. The definition will be documented in the procedure mentioned in subclause 7.3.1 (Design and Development Planning). The milestones will already be defined in the plan. It is now necessary to define the control and review the milestones.

First of all, you are required to define when the "weekly engineer meeting" will be reviewed—once a year, once a quarter, at the end of another milestone. Next it is required that you define who will conduct the review—a head of the department, the R&D vice president, an external auditor. After the definition of the reviewer, it is required that you define how this review will be summoned, and the process of the review—a simple meeting, or maybe a quick review of documentation is sufficient (though there is no requirements that the review shall take place as a meeting).

Let us look at the review itself. It is necessary to define the data and information to be presented and studied in the review; in this case, the meeting summaries. These are the main outputs of this design and development activity. The next thing to examine is whether the meeting was held as planned. In these meeting summaries, different tasks are documented; it is required that you examine whether these tasks have been carried out—for example, examine the update of documentation development plans, and so on.

This is the process of the design and development review itself:

- When—determination of suitable stages for the review
- What—the activities required to be reviewed
- How—the information or data to be reviewed (demonstration, presentation, etc.)
- Who—the relevant parties being reviewed
- Outputs—the outputs of the review

Participants

Relevant parties that take part or have effect on the design and development processes or milestones will participate in the review (i.e., developers, scientists, researchers, quality representatives, customers' delegates, etc). The ISO 13485 Standard requires, for each reviewed milestone, a definition of the parties requested for the review. These parties will shed light on the activities and the outputs, and will:

- Explain what was done during the design and development processes
- Provide answers to any questions raised
- Offer support, when needed

The standard requires that specialist personnel will attend the review, and refers us to subclause 5.5.1 (Responsibility and Authority) and to subclause 6.2.1 (Human Resources). These references indicate two things:

1. The participants of the review must be appointed and approved by the top management.
2. The participants of the review are required to be sufficiently competent to perform the review on the basis of appropriate education, skills, and experience.

The definition can be documented in various way—job descriptions, development plans, procedures, or work instructions.

Criteria for Evaluation of Design and Development Outputs

Up to now we have discussed the process of the review. Let us now discuss the matters or issues related to the design and development that are to be reviewed. The prime objective of the review is to evaluate and determine whether the design and development are advancing according to their goals and requirements. The main question that must be asked is: will the product answer the expectations? You must examine the different components in order to answer the question.

One way to answer the question is to set criteria for evaluation. Criterion is a documented basis for comparison and reference on whether design and development outputs have achieved their objectives. The evaluation will assess all of the design and development aspects. Thus, for every aspect it is required that you determine the criteria for the success of the review. The level of formality and complexity of the review will be defined according to the nature of the medical device.

The aspects that are to be reviewed and evaluated are:

- Evaluation whether the design answers the product specifications
- Evaluation whether the product answers all requirements: performance and functionality
- Evaluation whether the product will answer other specifications (e.g., regulatory)
- Review and assessment of whether the design and development inputs deliver the appropriate information and data for the processes
- Review of the design plan's applicability for development
- Review of the design and development tasks and assignments
- Examination of whether all safety and environmental issues have been addressed
- Reference to outputs of risk management
- Examination of used raw materials and their compatibility (e.g., chemical, biological, mechanical)
- Assessment of the design and development tools
- Evaluation of the integration between the different products' components
- Inquiries on whether the different components may be replaced by others in times of need, and whether they are available and reliable
- Review of the development plan's availability for production and service processes
- Review of quality specifications

The above follows a logical design and development process; other questions and examinations could easily have been addressed. Thus, the reader should feel free to add their own.

The Use of Computer Software

When reviewing the use of software as a design for a medical device, it is required that you review whether the computer software is verified and authorized for design. The reason for this is that the software outputs (as applies to other design tools) will be used for further development stages. Verifying and validating the software will ensure that the outputs are also verified and validated for use.

Treatment of Issues and Problems

Another interesting objective of the review is the identification and treatment of issues and problems that occurred during the design and development stages. Naturally such challenges will come up when the development is discussed. In case these problems could not be resolved on their own, the standard gives you a chance to examine the problems and suggests necessary options for solving them. This is an opportunity for a resolution as participants with different skills and points of view are brought together to discuss the medical device. With such brainstorming activity, there is a strong chance that the problem would be resolved, or at least action would be proposed.

When actions or solutions to problems are proposed, it is required that you not only document them, but that you also review their effectiveness; that is, whether they achieved their objectives, and, more importantly, whether the actions or modifications met the design and development requirements. A method for the review of effectiveness must be documented on the design and development plan.

Advice: In order to make this issue of problem treatment effective and constructive, determine that all problems that occur during the design and development will be concentrated and documented in one database. The treatment and the review of effectiveness will thus be documented there as well. In the long term, this would allow you to create a knowledge center for the development, regarding problems and failures.

Handling Nonconformities

When nonconformities are detected during the review, the organization is required to submit them to the process of handling nonconformities as required in chapter 8.3 (Control of Nonconforming Products). This way, it is ensured that nonconformities that occurred during the design and development stage are submitted to a controlled process and will be resolved. Further development activities shall be approved and preceded only after all nonconformities have been eliminated or referred.

Records

As mentioned before, the review shall have outputs—summaries, reports, tasks, messages, and procedure updates. The outputs of the design and development review are to be defined on the plan, documented, and maintained.

When the outputs of the review include further actions, it is required that you follow these actions in order to verify their execution and effectiveness. This is a standard requirement. Thus, there is a need for the management of editions and revisions of the records due to the nature of the review process—the evaluation of the effectiveness.

The standard does not specify which format or media to use. This is up to you. These records will be part of the quality records and will be submitted to the control of quality records in your quality management system as required in subclause 4.2.4 (Control of Records). In practice, the list of your quality records shall include the required records of the design and development review.

7.3.5 Verification Requirements

The organization is required to perform verification activities on the design and development processes and outputs. Though design and development activities have already been performed, now is it the time to verify that the development is advancing according to plan, that is:

- All necessary inputs were delivered in the right form.
- All development tasks were performed and accomplished.

- All the required outputs were accepted.
- The design and development processes were reviewed according to plan.

See Table 7.12.

The verification activities are to be included in the design and development plan. The primary goal is to confirm that outputs meet input requirements. The verification guarantees that the design and the development activities were performed as expected, and that the outputs are appropriate and could be forwarded for later development stages or production. Bear in mind that you are not evaluating the product performances yet—you are ensuring that the required outputs are accepted. The verification shall be performed during the development processes (not after, and not before).

For example, let us assume that the organization is designing a medical device. The developer has a document of specifications with the inputs (e.g., required measurements, tolerances, and a description of the intended use). Design tasks had been assigned respectively. To each design input and developing task there is an expected output:

- Tolerances—will be backed up with descriptions of the tests and calculation charts generated from the software HAL 9000.
- Product measurements will be described with diagrams.
- Intended use will be supported by a risk management review and a list of validation tests.

The verification activities must confirm that these outputs were accepted and that they are appropriate; that is, they deliver the required information or data and can be used for later design and development activities. In such a case it is quite simple—you must review the calculation charts and the diagrams, and go over the risk management review. At this stage no one is studying the results; they are observing the method and manner. You are required to plan these verification activities—reviews of outputs, analyses, simulations, comparisons, tests (lab, chemical, mechanical, biological, clinical, etc.), reviews of prototypes, verifications of other proven products.

TABLE 7.12
Standard Requirements of Subclause 7.3.5

ISO 13485	ISO 9001
The verification of the design and development processes is to be performed according to predefined activities documented on a plan	The verification of the design and development processes is to be performed according to predefined activities documented on a plan
The verification shall evaluate the adequacy of the design and development outputs to the input requirements	The verification shall evaluate the adequacy of the design and development outputs to the input requirements
The organization will keep records of the design and development verification. These records must be defined as quality records within your records control procedure, as required in subclause 4.2.4 (Control of Records)	The organization will keep records of the design and development verification. These records must be defined as quality records within your records control procedure, as required in subclause 4.2.4 (Control of Records)

This is the exact point of time computer software will be verified according to various parameters: version, inputs, outputs.

There is no requirement to define specific verification activities for each medical device (or a part you are designing) given the fact that the same development process plans apply to all the products or components. However, the proof of outputs' compliance to input requirements is specific, and each input must therefore be verified specifically. When the medical device, its components, or its design and development processes are complex or critical, then there is a need to identify them and plan specific verification processes.

Because there is no requirement to document the verification activities on a procedure (but only to mention them), you may use a form specifying:

- Inputs
- Required outputs
- Evaluation of the accepted outputs
- Status of the verification
- Release/rejection for further use

Only outputs that were verified and approved are suitable for use and release to the next development stage.

Records

The results of the verification activities shall be documented. The results shall include the outcome of the verification activities and nonconformities (in case outputs were not appropriate). When such a case has occurred, be sure to submit this output to the process of control of nonconforming products as required in clause 8.3 (Control of Non Conforming Product)—it could be critical and mean that one of the design and development parameters has failed.

These results will be part of the quality records and will be submitted to the control of quality records in your quality management system, as required in subclause 4.2.4 (Control of Records). In practice, the list of your quality records shall include the required design and development verification outputs.

7.3.6 Design and Development Validation

The organization must validate the design and development in order to ensure that the resulting outputs and the resulting product meet the specifications of functionality, performance, safety, and intended use. The validation is a critical test intended to ensure, with objective evidence, that the medical device satisfies its users' needs. The validation is considered a prospective one; it provides evidence that the medical device and/or a realization process conform to its specifications prior to the release for realization. Another aspect of the validation is to prove that the requirements will be consistently met throughout the entire life cycle of the medical device. Naturally the results are to be documented (Table 7.13).

The main goal of the validation stage is to generate objective evidence demonstrating explicitly that the medical device is designed and developed with accordance to specific requirements, and that it will meet these requirements consistently.

TABLE 7.13
Standard Requirements of Subclause 7.3.6

ISO 13485	ISO 9001
The organization is required to define a method for the design and development validation activities. The activities will be defined in the design and development plan	The organization is required to define a method for the design and development validation activities. The activities will be defined in the design and development plan
Validation activities will ensure that the accepted product and outputs of the design and development activities meet the intended use or application requirements	Validation activities will ensure that the accepted product and outputs of the design and development activities meet the intended use or application requirements, where known
The validation process would take place prior to the release of the product	The validation process would take place prior to the release of the product, when practical or applicable
Clinical performance or safety evaluations will be integrated into the validation of the medical device, as required by regional or national regulations	
Delivering the medical device to the customer for the purposes of a clinical evaluation (for validation purposes) is not regarded as a product delivery. Validation activities must be completed before full delivery	
Where a medical device can be validated only after delivery, assembly, or installation, the validation will be completed only after these have been performed, and the medical device will be delivered to the customer only after validation activities have been completed	
The organization will keep records of the design and the development validation. These records must be defined as quality records within your records control procedure, as mention in subclause 4.2.4 (Control of Records)	The organization will keep records of the design and the development validation. These records must be defined as quality records within your records control procedure as mention in subclause 4.2.4 (Control of Records)

These requirements are predefined—intended use requirements, functionality, performance, and safety specifications. In other words, a documented guarantee that the outputs and results of the design and development process are as expected. While planning the validation activities, and examining the outputs and results of the design and development process, you need to ask some questions:

- What are we validating? What are we measuring?
- How are we to do it?
- What do we need in order to achieve it?
- What supports our activities and our decisions?
- How much is required to be examined?

- How will we decide upon the results?
- What do we need to document and record?

Answering these questions will assist you in gathering the right inputs and planning the appropriate validation activities. The validation activities will regard the following issues:

- Medical device specifications
- Medical device characteristics for validation
- Parameters for validation
- Tools and equipment used for the design and development
- Methods for validation
- Objectives for validation
- Criteria for decisions
- Definition of validation activities
- Required tools and equipment for validation activities
- Required inputs
- Required human resource qualifications

Planning the validation activities shall be done on three levels of the design and development process:

- Validation of elements used for the design and development
- Validation of the compatibility of design and development activities
- Validation of the outputs

These three levels of validation will be introduced to the process with the help of the designated tests, the gathering of data, the definition of the criteria, the method for evaluation, and the decision.

Validation of Elements Used for the Design and Development Activities

Before starting the design and development activities, you need to ensure, by establishing objective evidence, that all related technical aspects and resources that are invested in the design and development process are designed and implemented in order to achieve the specifications (intended use, functionality, performance, safety, and so on):

- They are qualified to participate in the design and development process.
- They assist in meeting the specifications.
- They deliver satisfying results.

By technical resources I mean all the technical measures that perform processes and generate products or outputs. Which technical resources are invested, and what is required to be verified?

- Development and design environment—verification that the environment is suitable for the development: safety measures are implemented, conditions are identical to the conditions where the medical device will operate, and control and preventive measures are implemented.

- Design and development tools and equipment—verification that the tools and equipment will provide the manufacturer with the appropriate services and are: calibrated, intact, used correctly, maintained as planned, and there are preventive measures implemented.
- Human resources and knowledge—verification that the human resource is able to perform the required tasks and is qualified, trained, has the required experience, and is supported.
- Documentation—verification that the required documentation is available, applicable, and brings up the correct information and data.

Parameters to be considered:

- Laboratories and laboratory equipment
- Statistical methods
- Computer equipment and software
- Training for the development team
- Documentation platforms such as forms, electronic charts, and tables
- Updated procedures
- Calibration procedures and records
- Availability of supportive data and knowledge

In some cases the accessories for development will be purchased. The manufacturer is then responsible for testing the accessories and validating their functionality. Once again the main goal is ensuring that they will deliver an output that will meet all predefined requirements.

Validation of the Compatibility of Design and Development Activities

During design and development activities, you need to ensure—by establishing objective evidence—that all design and development outputs and results comply with the predefined specifications and requirements. The validation activities shall ensure that:

- The results are accepted under the appropriate development conditions.
- The results are evaluated and compared with an approved predefined criteria.
- The evaluation presents you with the level of compliance with requirements and specifications.
- The changes on the design and the development are reviewed and implanted.

This stage would be achieved when:

- The appropriate training and qualifications are available to the design and development process.
- The inputs to the design and development process were optimal.
- The validation tests were planned according to the medical device specification and provided with a clear validation, supported with data.
- The verifications of the tests conducted as planned.
- The criteria are validated, present a suitable method for the evaluation, and refer to the medical device's requirements.
- All of the medical device's characteristics are covered.

Validation of the Design and Development Outputs

The validation of outputs is to be achieved by the provision of objective evidence that the results meet the requirements (intended use, functionality, performance, safety, and so on) consistently throughout the entire life cycle of the medical device:

- Compatibility of design and development has been achieved.
- The validation activities will be planned and carried out in the same conditions in which the medical device will operate—the intended clinical environment for the medical device.
- The criteria are to demonstrate the ability of the medical device to comply with its requirements consistently. The parameters which create the "product normality" are to be defined and simulated. The simulation will create the exact operation environment in which the medical device will function. These parameters will be the conditions of the validation tests.

The combination of the two (criteria and conditions) will create an optimal validation environment that ensures that the medical device will sustain its specifications in the long term. The necessary extent of the validation, in order to prove consistency, will also be determined.

Parameters for control will include:

- Characteristics of the parts, components, and medical device
- Contaminating environments
- Realization processes
- Software that will be used to operate the medical device
- Operation environment
- Processes that the medical device will perform
- Electrical factors
- Wear outs of the medical device
- Agronomic factors
- Training and user instructions
- Any psychological factors that may affect the operator
- The use of supplements during operation of the medical device

Data of the validation test shall be analyzed in order to identify variations. A "side effect" of the analysis will provide the parameters in which the medical device could be unstable, and thus fail to comply. This will generate a list of restrictions on the use of the product. The next phase is to plan a systematic control of the product to ensure that the medical device will meet the necessary requirements in the long term. The control system will be able to detect nonconformities and submit them for treatment.

Tests

Tests are the most common means of validation, though they need to be effective and provide objective evidence on whether the design and development has achieved its goals. The tests shall examine and validate each intended user characteristic—functionality, performance, and safety—and replicate the actual use of the medical device. The study that the test initiates shall provide a clear validation supported with data. The results shall demonstrate the success of the test and compare them to the requirements. The tests shall be performed according to clear instructions, usually referred to as validation protocols—a set of rules and events describing how validation activities will be performed. These protocols include criteria for acceptance or rejection. The tests will be assigned to various levels of the design and development, starting from a single component or part, and extending through to the entire medical device, and the integration among the components. Processes that are designed to produce the medical device must also be validated. The test protocols will be reviewed and approved by an authorized person prior to the beginning of the validation activities. The definition can be on a job description or the development plan.

When planning a test the following issues are to be considered:

- Objective and type of the test—what must be achieve by testing
- Scope of the test—products, parts, components, or processes; the areas the test is covering are to be identified
- Extent of the test—for how long or how many times must the test be done
- Supporting documentation—what documentation is required during the test (e.g., procedures, forms, diagrams, charts, drawings, material specifications, etc.)
- Responsible party to conduct the test activities and the necessary training
- Environmental conditions required to perform the test—definition of the environment, conditions, use conditions, temperature, humidity, air pressure, particles, and so on
- Sequence of the test—a complete description of the test activities and the sequence of events
- Required tools and equipment, including calibration requirements
- Supplemental parts, materials, or components that may be necessary for the test
- Required inputs for the test—what information or data is required in order to perform the test
- Tolerances and limits
- Statistical or analytical techniques and methods for results evaluation—tolerance analysis, and screening experiments
- Criteria for decision and assessment assigned to the test—a basis for evaluating the results of the test
- Expected outputs and data to be recorded during the tests, and which outputs are to be reviewed—data sheets, graphs and charts, test protocols, reports, and conclusions
- Controls to be implanted during the test
- Criteria for revalidation

Type of tests:

- Load and condition tests on components or parts throughout the realization processes: test of materials, storage, production, assembly, package, and transportation
- Integration tests among components
- Influence of environment on components throughout the realization processes: storage, production, assembly, package, and transportation
- Test of processes: performances and results
- Feasibility and applicability of processes (design rule check); ensuring that the processes are feasible and applicable for realization by analyzing the events of the process and the progress of the production—usually done by simulation software
- Tests that are necessary to qualify a medical device for use (ones which prove that the medical device answers the intended use): safety tests, functionality tests, and delivery of the medical device to users for test use
- Clinical evaluation investigations
- Assembly and examination of prototypes
- Acceptance test to decide whether the medical device is ready before release
- Retests for validation when changes where implemented

Setting Criteria for the Tests

In order conduct effective tests you need to assign and document criteria to each test. The objective of the criteria is to support decisions for judging, evaluating, and determining through facts, values, and data the compliance of the outputs to the requirements. The criteria will provide a successful validation by indicating whether the outputs of the design and development are accepted or rejected. The criteria will present a method for the evaluation. The method will be defined with relevance to the medical device's requirements. The criteria will refer not only to product, parts, or components, but also to realization processes, conditions for realization, and services.

The criteria may be objective or subjective. Objective criteria means distinctiveness, invariance, and controllability; the results are being compared to a set of determined values and a decision (accepted or rejected) is made based on the comparison. Subjective criteria are when the results are being evaluated and submitted for assimilation by an individual—a personal opinion, so to speak. It is subjected using knowledge and experience. When there is no standard or technical requirement for criteria, the manufacturer will determine and document criteria before submitting the design and development outputs for validation.

The criteria should be documented. In cases where you are implementing and using test protocols, the criteria will be documented in these. The criteria are required to be approved before submission for use. The following issues are to be considered:

- The criteria shall refer to documented product requirements; for example, material, functionality specifications, technical specifications, product characteristics, reference to drawings, and quality requirements.
- When appropriate, the criteria will use statistical methods for validation.
- Reference to the required information for evaluation against the criteria is to be defined; that is, test data, findings, and measurements.
- The criteria will be planned with relevance to the quality requirements.
- If standards, regulatory requirements, or technical specification demand the establishment of criteria, then it is required to implement these criteria into the tests.
- The criteria will be designed in order to provide alarms regarding the status of the output, and to define when the results are regarded as being nonconforming.

Clinical, Performance, and Safety Evaluations

Developing and designing a medical device according to the ISO 13485 Standard requires clinical evaluations of performances and safety. The standard requires specifically including these evaluations as product validations during the design and development stages. The organization will initiate these evaluations as required by national or regional regulations. These evaluations will analyze, estimate, and identify any necessary principles in relation to the safety of the medical device. The objective of the clinical evaluation is to validate:

- The clinical safety of the medical device—the assurance that the medical device, when used in normal conditions and under appropriate user instructions, does not pose any clinical risks to the user, patient, or environment.
- The clinical performance—the ability of the medical device to perform according to the intended use under normal conditions as specified by the manufacturer.

A clinical evaluation includes the review, assessment, and analysis of clinical data relating to the clinical safety and performance of the medical device when it is used as intended under normal conditions. The data is based upon available data, scientific works, and laboratory or clinical studies and investigations. The clinical evaluation will be conducted on those medical device characteristics that pose the greatest risk to the patient, the user, or the clinical environment where the device will be used. These evaluations will be incorporated in the risk management processes; the evaluations support risk management—when conducting risk management processes, the results of the analysis, evaluation, and assessment of risks are the controls to be implemented on the medical device. After the controls have been implemented, residual risks are left. These are to be assessed once again and to be controlled. Clinical evaluations analyze these risks, evaluate them, and validate their controls. The output is a clinical evaluation report that objectively proves the safety and performance of the medical device. The report is to be designed and planned according to national or regulatory requirements on the matter. When the medical device will be marketed in various regions, it is required that you consider the appropriate regulations for each region. In cases where the medical device was delivered for a customer for the purposes of a clinical or performance evaluation, the ISO 13485 Standards specify that it is not considered as a delivery, and the medical device is to be validated.

Historical Data from Previous Validations

Validations can be based on, or can use, historical validation activities performed on previous products, components, or processes, and the results and data that they have generated. It may also be referred as "retrospective validation," "concurrent validation," and "prospective validation." The tests could be performed by a third party that is not related to the organization, though the organization may still use the data and information. If you intend to validate the medical device using historical data, then you must verify that:

- All the required data and information is gathered.
- The historical validations are appropriate to this medical device.

Once you are using the historical data in order to validate the device, you are required to perform an analysis of the historical data and verify that the validation activities were conducted with similar or identical conditions as those required for the new validation. The method of analysis shall be defined, and the results are to be documented and regarded as a validation output.

Validation on Delivery

There are cases where the organization is unable to validate the product in the design and developing environment before releasing and delivering it to the customer. This may occur because development of the medical device includes installation processes at the customer's premises, and full validation can only be done after installation in the intended environment. In such cases, the organization shall validate the medical device after the installation has been completed. The validation will be performed under all requirements mentioned above. Only then can the organization release and deliver the product to the customer. In other words, a manufacturer may physically hand over the medical device to the customer, install it, and take the money, but as far as the ISO 13485 Standard is concerned, delivery is only considered to have been completed once all of the planned validation activities have been performed, with the results evaluated and compared to the criteria; and, where deviation has occurred, it has been analyzed, corrected, and revalidated, and the development has been approved by an authorized party. This will have to be supported with objective documented evidence.

For example, say the manufacturer designs a medical device that would be installed in a certain hospital. The requirements include specific room measurements. The thing to note is that the measurements are a design parameter, and the functionality of the medical device depends on these. In order to validate the functionality, the medical device must be installed in the specified room. Only there can the validation activities be completed.

Reference to Regulatory Requirements

Additional validation requirements may be dictated by regulatory or regional demands. When planning the validation process, the organization will refer to these requirements and include them within the design and development plan. Let us turn back to the example of the hospital, where the manufacturer supplied the medical device, validated its functionality, performances and safety, performed the required training, and everybody is satisfied. Local regulations, however, require that a certified representative will inspect the medical device and generate a certification declaring that the equipment is safe for use. This test will be regarded as a validation activity on the design and development plan, and the certificate that follows is the evidence.

Records

The results of the validation activities shall be documented and maintained. The objective of the records is to prove that the validations were completed on time, and the outputs met the medical device's requirements. The results shall include the outcome of the validation activities and nonconformities (in cases where outputs did not meet requirements and needed correction or change). It has already been said that each validation activity must have an output—these are the discussed records.

- Computer reports and printouts.
- Results of validation tests.
- Certifications.
- Results of historical data from previous validations.
- Evidence for environmental conditions.
- Clinical evaluation reports.
- Outputs of processes.
- Prototypes—registered and identified.
- Criteria—when criteria is not documented on a procedure, protocol, or any other documentation, but individually determined per test, it is considered as a record and must be maintained.
- Various reports regarding the validation activities and results.
- Charts.
- Corrective actions.

These records are to be included under the quality management system, and required for a control as specified in subclause 4.2.4. They must be registered, controlled, maintained, stored, and—not least important—retrieved in case of need. In order to manage and maintain validation records according to the ISO 13485 requirements, I advise that you prepare a list of the expected records and document:

- Range or field—to which field of the design development the records are relevant
- Responsible—who should explain the results
- Reference—for example, a procedure, a test protocol, a diagram, a set of criteria
- Type—the type of the record (according to the method of categorization used)
- Source—what source produced the record (e.g., computer software, a person)
- Location—where is the record stored

Such a list will provide the necessary control. The list will also be controlled during the verification of the design and development process. It is a record and will be referred from the design and development plan.

7.3.7 Control of Design and Development Changes

When changes occur during the design and development process, the organization is required to establish an effective control plan in order to implement the changes, but still be able to satisfy the predefined requirements. The changes should be evaluated for their influence and affect on all aspects of the medical device—the preproduction as well as postproduction. The purpose of controlling the changes is to ensure that any changes made are accepted by the relevant functions and managed appropriately (Table 7.14).

The goal of the standard is to introduce the change throughout all the development processes. The main objective is to create consistency between the medical device's requirements and the rest that follow: inputs, design, development, verification, validation and tests, and outputs.

TABLE 7.14
Standard Requirements of Subclause 7.3.7

ISO 13485	ISO 9001
Changes in the design and the development shall be identified	Changes in the design and the development shall be identified
Records resulting from control activities of changes in the design and the development shall be documented	Records resulting from control activities of changes in the design and the development shall be documented
Design and development changes shall be reviewed, verified, validated, and approved before release	Design and development changes shall be reviewed, verified, validated, and approved before release
An evaluation and control are required in order to determine whether, and how much, the changes will affect other medical device parameters	An evaluation and control are required in order to determine whether, and how much, the changes will affect other medical device parameters
The organization shall keep records of changes in the design and the development review. These records must be defined as quality records within the records control procedure, as mentioned in subclause 4.2.4	The organization shall keep records of changes in the design and the development review. These records must be defined as quality records within the records control procedure, as mentioned in subclause 4.2.4

A Defined Method

Although the ISO 13485 Standard does not demand it directly, a method shall be defined describing the control over design and development changes. The method shall cover clear topics, such as: review, verification, validation, approval, and implementation.

The ISO 13485 Standard does not require a documentation of the method. However, do not be complacent here; though you may have already written a design and development plan (7.3.1) it would not take much effort to add the control over changes on the design and development process. This will assist you. Document your "control plan."

The objective of the control plan is identifying the changes, evaluating them and their influence on the design of the medical device, approving them, and implementing them. This will be carried out under a controlled process.

Identification

In some cases changes will be demanded due to the need to modify designs, or in cases where designs have failed the verification or validation test and cannot provide the required outputs, and, as a result, the design cannot be realized. The change then occurs before the product has been released (preproduction stage). Sometimes more features and characteristics are to be added—due to a customer's request, the updating of a product, market fluctuations, or new regulatory requirements. Change is then made after the product is released (postproduction stage). Possible reasons or factors for changes:

- Results of design review; results of verification and validation activities or failures to provide satisfying results
- Failures or nonconformities detected on the medical device after release, and the need for corrective or preventive measures
- Improvements or updates
- Difficulties during the realization processes; production, installation, or service
- Regulatory or safety requirements
- Customer requests
- Postmarket reviews and experience reports

When a change is identified, it will be submitted to a control method. First, you must estimate whether it is altogether regarded as a change. Let us review the following cases:

- You reviewed your design and decided that the validation activities generated unsatisfying results. In response, the designer suggests using another type of material and then to try validating it again. This is regarded as a change—a factor in the medical device was changed.
- You decided to replace one component in the medical device with a similar component that performs the same role, but it is delivered from another supplier. This is regarded as a change—a factor in the medical device was changed.
- You performed a validation activity and realized that the results deviated from the limits. The developer checked and detected a mistake on the design plan. He suggested correcting it and performing the test again. This is not regarded as a change—you did not change anything, only followed standard requirements and validated the design. It is definitely not necessary to submit the correction to a change control.

A Review

The review will include a clear definition of what is to be reviewed regarding the requested change. The change does not occur only on the medical device itself, but on all the associated processes and documentation—design inputs, verification tests, validation activities (product and processes), work instructions, quality tests, expected records, reference to human resources, and purchase requirements and verifications. For each issue it is required that you define what is to be reviewed, verified, validated (if appropriate), approved, and then implemented. The best way is to review the product portfolio, the quality plan, or the technical file, and make sure that nothing has been left untreated, such as:

- Product requirements
- Design inputs
- Realization requirements—production, assembly, installation, service, and so on
- Intended use and user needs
- Risks from the risk analysis
- Verification and validation protocols of products and processes
- Regulatory status of the medical device
- Outputs of design and development processes
- Labeling and advisory notices
- Traceability

For example, after a request for change and the following review, it may be decided that:

- A certain validation activity is not sufficient anymore and a new one must be planned.
- The quality reports need to be changed.
- A new periodical training for the personnel must be implemented.
- Another component in the medical device needs to be changed.

These outputs are the beginning of the control plan; they are the tasks to be performed in order to evaluate and implement the change correctly; and, most important, they will be managed under a controlled plan.

There are cases where an update will have to be done on medical devices that were already delivered to the customer and are currently in use. The change, its influence, and the implementation on such medical devices is to be reviewed and considered on the control plan; first, it is required that you will define the extent of the change is, and how such medical devices will be updated.

Questions to be asked during the review include:

1. What is the effect of the change on the intended use?
2. What is the effect of the change on the medical device specifications?
3. Will the change affect the safety of the medical device?
4. Will the type of the product be changed?
5. Will the change affect other components in the medical device?
6. Will the change affect auxiliaries in the medical device?
7. Will the change affect other processes related to the functionality or performance?
8. What are the implications on the realization processes?
9. Is a new verification and validation plan required?
10. Will the new statutory or regulatory requirements be applicable?
11. Will new certifications or licenses be required?
12. Which related documents will be affected?

Responsibilities

The plan shall refer an authority for each of its stages—review, verification, validation, approval, and implementation. It is not that the ISO is accusing anyone, but the responsible party must report regarding the progress and implementation of the change.

Verification

The changes are to be verified in order to ensure that all expected outputs are appropriately accepted. During the review you must consider issues regarding the design and development; and also any suggested, decided, and determined tasks and measures needed to achieve the change. It is now time to describe the necessary steps and examinations that will ensure that the activities are performed correctly and in compliance with the control plan. The verification shall ensure that all issues are resolved: functionality, performance, safety, and regulatory. To return to the previous example:

- A certain validation activity is not sufficient anymore, and it is required that the manufacturer plan a new one—the verification will ensure that the new validation was planned, a test was designed and documented on the relevant documentation, and criteria were set.
- The quality reports need to be changed—the verification will ensure that the reports are updated and submitted to the control of documents.
- A new periodical training for the personnel must be implemented—the verification shall ensure that the training is introduced to the training program as part of the quality management system.
- There is a need to change another component in the medical device—the verification shall ensure that the new change is submitted to a new control plan of design and development change.

Validation

The changes are to be validated in order to examine the influence of each change on the medical device, other components, or parts. The validation will ensure consistency of functionality, performance, and safety.

Let us review once again the last example:

- A certain validation activity is not sufficient anymore, and it is required that the manufacturer plan a new one—the validation will check whether the results that were accepted from the test are sufficient and met the predefined criteria.
- The quality reports need to be changed—the validation will review that the new quality reports can really document the results, that no data is left unrecorded, and that the forms are submitted to the appropriate parties for review.
- A new periodical training for the personnel needs to be implemented—the validation will evaluate the topics of training and their relevance.
- There is a need to change another component in the medical device—after the new component has been designed and developed, the integration of the medical device and the component must be evaluated.

In cases where the update will have to be done on medical devices that were already delivered to the customer and are being used, it will be required that the manufacturer plan specific validations to these medical devices.

Implementation and Approval

After all issues related to the design and development change have been resolved, it is required that you implement the change in the realization of the medical device. The implementation shall include the necessary tasks and controls, and will include practices on specifications, drawings, processes, procedures, work instructions, and forms. The objective is to submit the implementation to a controlled process in order to examine whether the change is effectively implemented, the goals are achieved, the change is integrated successfully in the medical device (components, realization processes, and final product), and to provide alerts and warnings.

I suggest managing the implementation as you would a project: setting and meeting tasks and assignments, objectives, schedules, required resources, responsibilities, expected results, and recording processes.

As long as the implementation and the relevant tasks and objectives have not fully and successfully been reviewed and approved, the change is to remain under the control plan. Some organizations manage their implementations as a configuration management:

- Sole identification of the product and any of the components
- Identification of editions for any component
- Identification of the developing status
- Control of configuration—when several people work independently on the component
- Identification, tracing, and reporting for all components for all activities following the demand for a change
- Evaluation of the changes—status, verification, and validation
- Releasing the component for use

Once the implementation is complete and successful, the final approval can be achieved and the change can be fully integrated into the realization process of the medical device.

In case the change was implemented during the postproduction stage, and the medical device was updated or corrected, I suggest implementing a process of releasing the new version or edition: ensure that all issues and problems are resolved, that relevant parties approved, and the change was released and communicated to all relevant parties.

Preproduction vs. Postproduction—Implementation of Changes

The changes can occur before the product is released (preproduction stage) or after the product is released (postproduction stage). There should not be a distinction between the implementation of the two, and both should be implemented with the same controls. It is worth bearing in mind that they are a somewhat different, and this may affect the implementation process.

In case of changes in a postproduction stage, there will be probably more changes to be implemented due to the fact that they would need to be implemented on existing processes that were already released, and are already operational. In the postproduction stage the processes are not yet released.

The type and extent of documents to be reviewed and changed is different; in the postproduction stage there are documents to be reviewed and updated related to production process. In the preproduction stage there are design-related documents such as design plans, drawings, and inputs.

The review approval process by the postproduction phase is likely to be more complex and extended due to the fact that the there are more parties involved that need to be accounted for.

Records

The ISO 13485 Standard specifically requires maintaining records of control of design and development changes. The objective of the records is to prove that the change was implemented under a controlled method, and was identified, reviewed, verified, validated, implemented, and approved. When the standard requires records they must be controlled, listed, and reviewed. The records of control of design and development changes are to be specified on the quality records list, and so submitted to the control of records, as specified in subclause 4.2.4 (Control of Records).

7.4 PURCHASING

7.4.1 Purchasing Process

As a quality manager, before I start implementing quality requirements in the purchasing department, I will try to understand which process I need to control, what are the main factors that influence the purchase processes and who are the suppliers that are relevant to these processes (Table 7.15).

TABLE 7.15
Standard Requirements of Subclause 7.4.1

ISO 13485	ISO 9001
The organization shall maintain a documented procedure describing purchasing processes in order to ensure that purchased products meet the predefined requirements specifications	The organization shall ensure that purchased products meet the predefined requirements and specifications
For every type of supplier and purchased product the organization shall determine the appropriate controls	For every type of supplier and purchased product the organization shall determine the appropriate controls
The requirements and control would be suitable to the effect the purchased product has on the realization processes, the realization of subsequent products, or the realization of final products	The requirements and control would be suitable to the effect the purchased product has on the realization processes, the realization of subsequent products, or the realization of final products
The organization shall assess and select suppliers according to their performances and ability to supply suitable and appropriate products	The organization shall assess and select suppliers according to their performances and ability to supply suitable and appropriate products
The organization shall determine the criteria for suppliers' evaluations and selections	The organization shall determine the criteria for suppliers' evaluations and selections
A reevaluation shall be performed according to determined criteria	A reevaluation shall be performed according to determined criteria
Records of the suppliers' evaluations should be maintained and kept. The evaluation process would be introduced to the records control process according to subclause 4.2.4	Records of the suppliers' evaluation should be maintained and kept. The evaluation process would be introduced to the records control process according to subclause 4.2.4

A supplier is an interested party in the organization though is still independent from the organization's quality management system. This includes a supplier that may be part of the organization but maintains a separate quality management system. For example, in some corporations, one business unit may receive services and goods from another business unit; though both are paid by the same boss and have the same brand name, they manage two different quality management systems. In such a case, they maintain "organization supplier" relationships. Your suppliers include suppliers of parts or materials, consultants, contractors, and trainers—product and services that are related to the realization of the medical device. For example, if your organization purchases coffee every month, unless it is a coffee-related organization, and uses the coffee to realize the product, the coffee must not be included under the purchasing control.

Your medical device should be safe and effective; therefore, you implement a quality management system. The quality management system, however, is implemented in your organization, not within the supplier's organization. The purchasing control puts your suppliers under your quality management system.

The same extent of control applies to services too. When you purchase a service that affects the medical device and constitutes realization processes, it means that this service is a part of your medical device. Therefore it should be under control.

In some cases the supplier will be audited as part of a regulatory, quality certification process by a third party. Such a review and certification process does not affect the manufacturer's responsibility to control the supplier. Also, when processes are being reviewed and audited, if the manufacturer of the medical device determines that these processes are critical, then they are also required to audit them. The certification received may serve as an input for the manufacturer's purchasing processes; for example, if the manufacturer demands that a supplier be certified for the ISO 9001 Standard requirements.

A Documented Procedure

The extent of the control over your suppliers applies to materials or services that are related to the product.

When the organization purchases parts, components, or services that affect the medical device, a process is to be defined which describes how the organization is to ensure that the products will:

- Meet the predefined requirements and specifications.
- Determine the appropriate controls over the suppliers.
- Ensure that the manufactured medical device is safe and effective.

The purchasing process will be documented in a procedure. The main objective of the procedure is to provide the organization with a means of control in order to achieve the goals mentioned above, thus ensuring that the purchased product meets the requirements. The procedure may refer to the following issues:

- Types of products and services that are included under the process—raw materials, components, assembled parts, services, and packages
- Preliminary or introductory conditions—minimum-inventory levels, production demands, and special projects
- Preliminary or introductory requirements—regulatory or internal requirements

- The responsible parties and authorities—production managers, warehouse workers, purchase managers, account managers, and transporters
- The interrelations between the participants—what the role of each participant in the process is
- Inputs required for the process—production requirements, inventor requirements, service requirements, agreements, and contracts
- Records supporting the process—purchase orders, reports from the management system, and delivery notes
- Reference to other procedures, such as acceptance procedures and forms in the process
- A clear description of the process, such as a literal procedure or a diagram
- Risks to be accounted for during the purchase control
- A description of controls over the process—where and how will the process be controlled
- Product specifications or reference to them—they are the reference for later control
- Required outputs—documentation that the supplier must deliver regulatory certifications, delivery notes, and quality tests
- Supplier's evaluation and reevaluation

Documentation

The types of documentation related to the process must be defined. This is the documentation that the purchase process will refer to; that is, other procedures such as acceptance procedures, or forms in the process. This documentation supports the purchase processes. I divide these into three categories:

- Instructions
- Forms (which will later become records)
- Specifications

Control Your Suppliers

The extent of control applied on a supplier should be in proportion to the effect that the purchased product has on the medical device. The objective of the controls is to eliminate any potential failures that may occur with the supplier during communication with them. This topic will be discussed during the contract stage in order to ensure the supplier's engagement to the matter. One main aspect is risks associated with the purchased product, and the effect these risks have on the medical device, on its subsequent products, or on the realization processes. These risks must be identified. Here are some of issues to be regarded when identifying risks:

- Complexity of the product
- Ability to continually supply
- Ability to manage and control complex production processes
- Liability and stability of processes
- Reaction to failures and nonconformities
- Liability of products
- Qualifications of personnel
- Awareness of quality
- Availability and cooperation
- Legal status
- Capital investment and financial viability

There is no requirement for risk management when it comes to purchasing. However, the purchase has a direct implication on risk management since the purchased product are used to realize the medical device. A review of these risks will assist with applying the appropriate controls over the suppliers, and that is already a standard requirement. I highly recommend reviewing and documenting these risks.

After identifying the risks you are ready to set the controls. These controls are the quality requirements and will be applied at suitable points of the purchase process.

This is why a clear definition of the purchase process, its inputs, and the participants, is important. The controls need not only be applied when the goods are received; on the contrary, you must identify exact control points throughout the realization processes and control the supplier there.

The training of personnel is a sensitive issue. You are required to ensure that the personnel performing the realization processes are qualified, and have the appropriate skills and knowledge before they take part of the realization of the product.

Here are some examples for possible control issues where you may control your suppliers:

- Audit by the supplier's premises
- Control of further tier suppliers
- Testing of products or parts for functionality
- Measurement and monitoring of part or components
- Certificates of quality analysis
- Maintenance of management systems—quality, environmental, and safety
- Accreditation of processes—laboratory accreditation, and control over monitoring and measurement tools
- Quality specifications
- Control over equipment and machinery
- Process parameters and performances
- Quality control
- Statistical process control
- Correction processes
- Management and control of inventory
- Traceability
- Configuration of product
- Protection of customer's property
- Protection of data
- Management of documents
- Review of training performance of personnel

These controls will be defined and documented in the procedure mentioned above. Do not forget that there may be regulatory requirements to be considered when applying controls over the suppliers; it is required that you control whether the purchase of products, parts, material, or services must conform to regulatory requirements. In some cases the control shall be implemented on second or further tier suppliers. So long as these suppliers deliver parts that will end up at your premises, and be used for your medical device, you are responsible for controlling them.

Evaluation of Suppliers

A supplier shall be selected on the basis of their abilities to supply a product in accordance with predefined requirements. In order to determine what your objective opinions of the supplier are, you must evaluate important parameters regarding the purchased product. To begin with, the organization needs to determine which parameters are important for the evaluation. The assessment is conducted through:

- Evaluation of realization processes
- Evaluation of quality processes
- Evaluation of supplied products
- Review of risks related to the supplier

These parameters will constitute criteria for evaluation. The criteria will provide you with a situation report about the supplier and their performance.

The evaluation will be conducted on a periodic basis. The frequency of the evaluation must be defined. The objective is to establish an ongoing control process over the supplier in order to foresee events that might become nonconformities or quality problems. This is normally done once a year, but there are cases of purchased products that require more frequent control, depending on the risk and effect that the purchased product has on the medical device.

The objective of the criteria is to rank the supplier in a quantitative manner and to assist with deciding whether the supplier can supply a well-controlled product. The determination of the criteria is to be based on three main issues:

- The purchased product
- The intended use of the medical device
- The effect that the purchased product will have on the subsequent product realization or the final product

The evaluation criteria will derive from these and will be a combination of parameters regarding the issues mentioned above.

For example, a supplier delivers you plastic packages that must be sterilized. The sterilization is crucial for the intended use; when packages are not delivered as required, there is a threat that the medical device will fail. Let us review the issues again:

- The purchased product (the packages)
- The intended use (requirement to be sterilized)
- The effect (the intended use might fail if packages are not delivered according to the requirement)

When you are evaluating suppliers, the criteria for evaluation will derive from the issues mentioned above. These are the questions that must be asked:

- Does the supplier maintain stable sterilization processes?
- Does the supplier comply with regulatory requirements?
- Does the supplier maintain supporting documentation?
- Does the supplier maintain appropriate controls over their processes?
- Is the supplier certified for the certain processes (for example compatibility to the ISO 10993 Standard)?
- How does the supplier handle nonconformities?

Answering these questions will present a status report regarding the supplier and their performances. I recommend evaluating each supplier on their merits; each case or product has its significant characteristics, and therefore may require different parameters for evaluation. Objective evidence, information, and data regarding their performances are gathered and documented through the controls applied on them—delivery records, quality control reports, agreements, complaints, and nonconformities. You may review the results, compare them to the criteria, and draw conclusions from them.

Beside evaluation criteria regarding the purchased product, you may set general supplier criteria such as:

- Quality certifications—ISO 13485, ISO 9001, ISO 14001
- Delivering to schedules
- Credibility
- Lead time
- Delivery of sufficient information and data regarding the product—product portfolios, material safety data sheets (MSDS), and working data sheets
- Delivery of quality evidences—COC (Certificate of Conformity), certification of tests
- Appraisal of quality processes—handling nonconformities and training employees

There are many ways to rank a supplier. I will focus on a simple one in order to demonstrate the idea and objective, which is to eliminate inappropriate suppliers from the list of approved suppliers. The rank and the classification that follows represents the supplier's performance. According to this data you should decide whether you want to work with them or not.

Let us assume that your evaluation draws, at the end of the process, a simple grade ranging from one to one hundred. You may determine the next classification (Table 7.16).

You may determine that your organization is willing to order only from suppliers with a "B" classification and above. When a supplier is ranked with the classification "B–", it is required that you submit clarification and an improvement plan. After the classification, the suppliers are to be notified of their ranks. A supplier who receives a grade of 61 on the last evaluation may begin to worry, and make some enquiries regarding your last complaints. Thus, rankings can help drive the supplier to improvement.

When the evaluation failed and the supplier was found to be inadequate, you must define the necessary actions to take; for example, you may suggest an improvement plan, you may cancel the supplier and select another that has achieved an acceptable rank, or you may submit a corrective action. However, the emphasis shall be on establishing an effective action, and it is required that you assess its effectiveness over a define period of time. The ISO 13485 Standard does not specify which actions are to be taken, but it indicates that the effectiveness of such actions is to be controlled. The action will specify how the supplier intends to improve their performances, and how the organization will control the purchased product until the action is completed. The definition shall include the following factors:

1. Goals and objective of the action
2. Required inputs

TABLE 7.16
Classification of Suppliers

Final Grade (Points)	Classification
81–100	A
61–80	B
51–60	C
1–50	D

3. Correctional or preventive actions taken
4. Establishment of communication channels regarding the failure
5. Responsible parties from both sides—the organization and the supplier
6. Action and tasks
7. Target dates
8. Required outputs

The outputs of the evaluation process are to be recorded, maintained, and included under your control of records process. During later stages you will have to retain these and compare results of old evaluations with reevaluations. Plan a clear and simple form (digital or analog), and bear in mind that this is not a one-off action, but an ongoing one. This record will be updated.

Advice: If you maintain an ERP system or any other system that manages your purchasing processes, (naturally) your suppliers will be documented on the system. Some of these systems offer the option of computerized questionnaires and surveys. This is exactly what the evaluation is all about. Look for this option on your management system and try to implement it through you purchasing processes. You might want to call your system administrator now...

Although the standard does not demand a documented process specifically for the evaluation process, it does require a process to ensure that purchased products conform to specification. There is often debate between quality managers and auditors regarding the need for a documented method of evaluation. I believe it can assist you; however, when documenting the method on a procedure there are some issues that must be regarded:

- The type of suppliers that are included under the evaluation
- The parties responsible for conducting the evaluation
- Reference to the criteria
- The frequency of the evaluations
- Inputs required for the evaluation
- The type of evaluation or a description of the evaluation method—performances compared to the criteria
- Outputs of the evaluation

Documenting the process on a procedure already covers two standard definition requirements: definition of frequency and definition of responsible parties.

Reevaluation of Supplier

After you have evaluated the supplier, and have provided them with your feedback, you should, after a defined period of time, reevaluate whether or not they have improved their performance. This is an ISO 13485 Standard requirement. The frequency of reevaluations will be determined in accordance with the associated risks, and their effect on the medical device. The reevaluation shall refer directly to the last evaluation as there is a direct link between them. The results of the two should be compared. In cases where measures or actions were applied to the supplier due to the last evaluation, the reevaluation should indicate their effectiveness in the long run.

This is review of:

- Quality system records compliance to purchasing requirements
- Compliance to regulatory requirements
- Control over processes
- Meeting requirements

List of Approved Suppliers

Next, you are required to add any accepted supplier into a documented list of approved suppliers—also referred to as ASL (approved suppliers list). The supplier's rank (relating to the criteria) can be put on the list, but it is not obligatory. There is no specific requirement for a list on the ISO 13485 Standard. It is, however, a logical output of the evaluation process thus required. The requirement is that any actions arising from the evaluation should be maintained; that is, documented. After evaluation you are left with a list of approved suppliers. You shall be required to show this during the audit. This list is one of the quality records of the purchase process and needs to be controlled.

Advice: If you maintain an ERP system or any other system that manages your purchasing processes, (naturally) your suppliers will be documented on the system. You need only define, on the procedure, that approved suppliers are documented on your ERP system. Using the status of your supplier on that system (e.g., whether they are active, inactive, suspended, etc.), you may declare and document the approval. You may also produce a report from the system: a list of approved suppliers. This option may allow you to keep the list up to date.

Records

The standard clearly requires maintaining records (i.e., outputs of the processes) related to the purchasing processes under your records control method. The target of the records is to provide objective evidence that the processes were conducted, and, more importantly, that they are effective. Let us review the expected records:

- Details of suppliers: names, addresses, and contact persons
- Product specifications: agreements or contracts with the suppliers, purchase orders, and so on
- Regulatory requirements
- Inputs from the supplier; MSDS, REACH certifications, quality certifications, and internal certifications of suppliers
- Inspection of parts and products: quality tests, quality protocols, and samplings
- List of risks related to a supplier
- List of controls related to a supplier: work and test instructions, process diagrams
- Criteria for evaluation
- Records related to the purchase order
- Correspondence with suppliers: e-mails, meeting summaries
- Records of suppliers' evaluations
- List of approved suppliers

Not all of the above need be included. Naturally, the outputs and inputs of your purchase processes (the records) are to be specified on your quality records list, and submitted to a control of records as specified in subclause 4.2.4 (Control of Records).

7.4.2 Purchasing Information

Purchasing information shall indicate your product's specifications and requirements for you and for your suppliers. The ability to transfer to your supplier clear specifications regarding the product is essential. In certain cases the information will be the comparison criteria between what you have ordered and what you have

TABLE 7.17
Standard Requirements of Subclause 7.4.2

ISO 13485	ISO 9001
The information of a purchased product will define the product and its characteristics; that is, the specifications and requirements	The information of a purchased product will define the product and its characteristics; that is, the specifications and requirements
The organization shall define requirements for the control and approval of a purchased product	The organization shall define requirements for the control and approval of a purchased product
The definition shall refer to the determination of processes, procedures, and the use of tools, equipment, and procedures	The information shall refer to the determination of processes, procedures, and the use of tools, equipment, and procedures
The information shall include training and qualification requirements relevant to the purchased product	The information shall include training and qualification requirements relevant to the purchased product
The information shall regard any quality requirements	The information shall refer to quality management system requirements
Traceability requirements, as presented on chapter 7.5.3.2, are also applicable to purchasing information	
The application of the traceability shall be carried out with documents and records control as required in chapters 4.2.4 and 4.2.3	

received. The organization shall ensure that an order (or a transfer) of information contains the required details prior to delivery to the supplier. While defining the information of the purchase products, the organization would refer to the following issues (Table 7.17).

When defining the information for the purchase, the organization shall:

- Determine and document the designated supplier and add references to relevant agreements or contracts.
- Define and document all information that identifies the required product for purchase—name or description of the product or service, catalog number (internal or external), edition, edition of diagram, configuration, and model.
- Define information regarding the purchase process—required quantities, delivery dates, prices, discounts, and addresses for delivery and billing.
- Define operational requirements, technical specifications, instructions, and guidance that the supplier must follow—packaging requirements, delivery requirements, transportation conditions, development environment, operation environment, work instructions, procedures, and diagrams.
- Define quality requirements—test instructions, inspection instruction, quality records, quality protocols, tools and equipment for control, quality certifications, and statistical data.
- Identify necessary training regarding the purchased product.

- Identify any supplementary requirements—regulatory requirements, safety documentation, and so on.
- Quality management demands—ISO 13485, ISO 9001, ISO 14001, and management systems.
- Identify additional requirements needed for an effective product.
- Define necessary documentation—delivery notes, safety data sheets, working data sheets, and so on.

Requirements for Controls over the Product

As the manufacturer of the medical device, you should instruct your supplier on what the required controls are in relation to the purchased product, and provide him/her with technical requirements. This includes procedures, and work and test instructions that the supplier must follow and implement when realizing the product. The objective is to ensure the provision of appropriate products or services. The requirements will be documented and shall describe specifically:

- Production requirements
- Quality requirements
- Test and acceptance requirements
- Material handling requirements
- Handling delivered parts or components
- Product validation requirements
- Process capability and validation requirements
- Batch and lot sizes
- Handling data or patient information
- Measurement requirements
- Necessary statistical methods
- Environmental requirements (during realization)
- Storage and inventory requirements
- Packaging, delivery, and transport requirements
- Instructions in cases of nonconformities
- Documentation requirements
- Records requirements

Changes in the Purchased Product

When your supplier needs to perform changes on the product, he/she must notify you in advance, and receive your approval. The issue should be discussed and agreed upon on an agreement or contract level. Changes may occur to each parameter of the realization process:

- Material
- Production processes
- Assembly processes
- Human resources and personnel
- Equipment or machinery
- Test equipment and tools
- Documentation
- Packaging

- Storage conditions
- Transport conditions

Before accepting the change, the manufacturer needs to evaluate the requested change and its implication on the medical device. They must also validate the results of the evaluation and ensure that the change will not affect the medical device. When it will affect the device, the changes will not affect the intended use, functionality, performance, and safety.

In order to implement an effective change control, design a change control plan via a communication channel with your supplier, which they will follow when they need to implement changes. The plan will follow the following suggested sequence of events:

1. Initiating a change
2. Documenting a description for a change
3. Communicating and notifying the manufacture about the requested change and the reason for it
4. Defining a responsible party or parties from the manufacturer to review the request
5. Communicating with the supplier and announcing that the request has been reviewed and accepted
6. Establishing a review committee consisting of delegations from the supplier and the manufacturer
7. The outputs and decisions of the committee
8. Validation of the change
9. A documented approval for the change
10. Updating the required documentation
11. Implementation

Implementation includes planning the realization processes, the revised controls and validation activities, updating the relevant documentation, providing training to the appropriate personnel, and planning new storage and transport requirements.

Although it is not required by the standard, I highly recommend defining and documenting the issue on a procedure.

Requirement for a Qualification of Personnel

In some cases you will require that the supplier's personnel be specifically qualified in order to supply you with an adequate product. You may train the personnel yourself or demand that the supplier do so. Training may be applicable in the following cases:

- Special processes
- Regulatory requirement
- Changes in production processes
- New contracts
- New parts
- New suppliers
- Nonconformities
- Rework

For example, when outsourcing a process, and regulatory requirements demand that the personnel working on the process be specifically trained, it is up to you to ensure that they are. The supplier must prove that its personnel are suitably qualified to your specifications. This proof should be documented.

Requirement for a Quality Management System

The ISO 13485 Standard suggests that you demand that your suppliers maintain a quality management system. When the maintenance of a quality management system is requested from your supplier, they must provide you with the appropriate certification.

Beware of expired certifications and conduct supervision. The fact your supplier is audited by a third part body does not mean that the manufacturer is exempt from any responsibility to control its processes and products.

Transferring an Order to the Supplier

The purchasing information must to be reviewed and verified. It is necessary to determine a method for reviewing the purchasing information before submitting it to the supplier for execution. Ensure that the information is clear, correct, and complete. The check will be carried out by an authorized person. The communication channels, the information to be transferred, and interrelations with your suppliers must also be determined. Communication channels can occur as printed orders, e-mails, or by the installation of your supplier's terminal at your premises (SRM). Other interrelations can be the deliveries—air or sea deliveries. There is no requirement to document the method of transferring an order to the supplier, but there is a requirement to prove it with records.

Advice: Most management or ERP systems have a purchase module which is usually used by the purchasing manager, issuing purchase orders based on demands (or at least control them). It is possible to parameterize a purchase order so it would bear an "order category," according to the department it purchases for: production, assembly, quality, administration, and so on. It is also possible to determine that certain users may approve certain orders (e.g., purchase managers and production managers). In this way you can implement the review and control of an authorized person over the purchase orders, as well as maintain records.

Traceability

There is one crucial additional requirement regarding purchasing information. Traceability and records of traceability must be maintained. This requirement marks the difference between the ISO 9001 and 13485 Standards. The organization must introduce the purchased products to traceability control, as required in clause 7.5 and subclause 7.5.3.2. The main purpose is to provide the ability to trace back all purchased products. Traceability of the purchased products would begin from the purchasing order and continue to the medical device itself (after delivery). This is one part of the traceability chain that the ISO 13485 Standard initiates.

Where components, materials, or (purchased) processes may cause the medical device to fail to meet its specified requirements, records shall be maintained and kept; this is a general instruction. When problems arise, the organization could then trace back to where they started. All of the purchased components of the product that may cause problems or nonconformities after delivery must be included under a method of traceability.

Suppose, for example, that a medical device manufacturer releases a batch of products. After three months, an employee performs a quality test and discovers that a purchased component fails to comply and thus creates an error. As a result, the entire batch that includes this component is disqualified, and must be quickly removed. People's lives may depend on such actions. By introducing the purchasing process to the traceability control, the organization can trace back all the medical devices from this batch containing this certain nonconforming component. Traceability requirements will be discussed in more detail on chapter 7.5. In order to ensure that the organization is tracing the purchased products according to the ISO 13485 Standard requirements, the purchase information must have a reference to traceability. This requirement will be supported with documentation and records. The documentation will be under the document control process, as required in subclause 4.2.3, and the records will be under the records control process, as required in subclause 4.2.4.

7.4.3 Verification of Purchased Product

This chapter refers to the control that the manufacturer must implement over purchased products. In the last chapter we discussed information describing the product to be purchased. This information was defined and then transferred to the supplier. Once the product has arrived at the manufacturer's premises, it needs to be examined, evaluated, and compared to the desired specifications. There is a direct relation between the information delivered to the supplier and the controls that the manufacturer must now define (Table 7.18).

Types of Controls

When defining the supervision activities over purchased products, the organization shall define which product requirements will be controlled; which areas, characteristics, specifications or issues on the purchased product are to be tested, controlled, evaluated, verified and so on. The objective of this control is to verify that the purchased product meets all the requirements. The controls will be determined according to various factors:

- The nature and complexity of the product: The control over complex purchased products is to be tighter. When evaluating, the complexity or effect that the purchased product has on other components is to be considered.

TABLE 7.18
Standard Requirements of Subclause 7.4.3

ISO 13485	ISO 9001
The organization shall determine and implement controls and supervision activities to ensure that purchased products are delivered as specified	The organization shall determine and implement controls and supervision activities to ensure that purchased products are delivered as specified
In cases where the verification of the purchased product is conducted at the supplier's premises, the manufacturer will define and document the needed controls for verification, validation, and the release criteria of the product	In cases where the verification of the purchased product is conducted at the supplier's premises, the manufacturer shall define and document the needed controls for verification, validation, and the release criteria of the product
Evidence and records of the control and verification activities shall be maintained and introduced to the records control procedure as required in subclause 4.2.4 (Control of Records)	

- The risks and risk level associated with the product are to be evaluated: Where the risks and the outputs of risk analysis indicate the part may have an affect on the final product, should also considered.
- History of the purchased product: Parts or components that are known and recognized as problematic should have more control than others.

Suggested type of controls:

- Identification of the product—name of the product, the catalog number (internal or external), edition, edition of diagram, version, configuration, and model
- Controlling over delivery—packaging of the products and delivery specification
- Technical verification—the product was designed and developed in the required environment, and that it was realized in the required environment
- Implementation of requirements during the realization processes and delivery—that is, regulatory and quality requirements
- Controlling the functionality of the product
- Controlling the performance of the product
- Controlling the safety of the product
- Testing compatibility to other parts or components
- Testing integration with other parts or components
- Verifying and validating quality tests—executions and results
- Verifying certifications
- Controlling the information regarding the purchase order—delivery dates, prices, and quantities
- Verifying the required documentation—COCs and MSDS

The Methods for Control

The method for conducting the control activities are to be defined:

- Tests
- Reviews
- Samplings
- Evaluation of services

The method shall ensure that a purchased product is:

- To be isolated from other controlled products in order to avoid contamination
- Not to be released for realization processes as long as it is not controlled and validated

This definition is valid on the premises of the manufacturer as well as on those of the supplier. The method will define responsibilities regarding the performance of the controls; that is, who shall perform the control. The method will define sequences of the controls—when is the control to be carried out. There are two distinguished cases that may affect the method:

- In case components that are purchased are assembled in the medical device, the control will take place only on the final component (the purchased product). The functionality, as well as performance and safety, will be controlled and verified.
- Since it is not always possible to evaluate and verify parts, components, or services on receiving them, but only after installation or assembly, it is critical to define that these will be controlled before the delivery for use. Only then will the verification of the purchased products be considered as having been completed.

The easiest example to explain these cases is when installation is a part of the medical device and is performed as an outsourced service by a supplier. Naturally, the purchased product (the installation)—and all its implication on other components and parts of the medical device—can be verified after the installation has been completed. As far as the ISO 13485 Standard is concerned, the test control will be approved and completed only after an examination that it was done according to the requirements. Maintaining a documented procedure is not required, though it is recommend.

Setting Criteria

In order to plan the control effectively you must set criteria to support the controls. The criteria will be documented. The objective of the criteria is to support the validation processes, and to judge and evaluate (by facts) the compatibility of the purchased product to meet the requirements. The criteria will be planned with relevance to the quality requirements of the purchased product and will indicate whether the products are accepted or rejected. The criteria must be approved before submission for use.

All parameters on the product that affect the medical device are to be examined in order to plan effective criteria: the production environment, realization processes, human resources, packaging, storage, and transportation. In order to plan effective criteria you need to refer to the following issues:

- The criteria will refer to documented product requirements, such as material, functionality specifications, technical specifications, reference to drawings, and quality requirements.
- The criteria will cover not only product parts or components, but realization processes along with services.
- The manufacturer must examine whether the production standards or technical specifications require criteria for the product or processes.
- When required, the criteria will use statistical methods for validation.
- The criteria need to provide alarms regarding the status of the purchased product.

Types of criteria: drawings, tolerances and limits, material specifications, component specifications, and functionality tests.

Nonconformities

The method of the control is to relate to cases and events where a nonconformity has been detected. In such a case the purchased product will be isolated and the need for corrective action will be determined. The identification of nonconformities is achieved with the help of the predefined criteria set as a control; namely, evaluation and comparison. This relates to the issue and requirement of isolating and segregating purchased product before their review.

The Extent of the Control

How many purchased parts are to be verified? What is the sample rate or size? These are important questions that must be answered; otherwise quality control inspectors would find themselves controlling all of the parts. The extent of the control will be determined according to several elements:

- Type of the product: The type of the product definitely determines how many parts are to be controlled. Services, for example, are not the same as electronic boards. These two types of product require a different extent of control.

- Risk assessment: The extent will be determined by a consideration of the risks involved.
- Prior events related to the product such as failure or nonconformities: When such are known or experienced, naturally the extent will rise.
- History of the supplier: If it is a well-known supplier, and you know that their processes are stable and reliable, then you will determine a lower extent of control is needed than in the case of an unknown or a "trouble-making" supplier.

Controlling Outsourced Processes

When a process is outsourced, the responsibility to control these, and to verify and validate the outputs, applies to the manufacturer. Outsourced processes need to be identified. The verification and validation will include:

- The controls that the organization is to implement over the supplier
- The controls that the supplier shall implement and perform during the realization of processes

The controls will be set in accordance to the complexity, importance, and affect that the purchasing process has on the final product. Planning the controls will include reference to the risk analysis; the outputs of this analysis refer to required risk controls on certain processes. When these processes are outsourced, the controls mentioned are to be implemented by the supplier. Supplier certification is not sufficient on this case when risks are related to the processes. The organization must consistently verify and validate the performances of the supplier.

The controls will be set according to the supplier's ability to perform the processes. This ability is measured through:

- The history of the supplier
- The level of nonconformities that have occurred
- The supplier's evaluation

In order to establish effective controls over the supplier, the organization must ask itself what are the reasons for outsourcing these processes; it could be because of a lack of resources or a lack of knowledge. When it is a lack of knowledge, the organization must assess whether it can really control the outsourced processes. In some cases the organization may consider outsourcing the control over the outsourced processes. This would ensure objective control from an independent body.

The controls to be documented are:

- The controls that the manufacturer implements on its suppliers must be included in work processes or instructions, and in agreements or contracts.
- Controls that must be performed by the supplier must be delivered to them documented; that is, work instructions, specifications, test instructions, and drawings.

Records

The ISO 13485 Standard specifically requires maintaining records of the verification activities. The objective of the records is to prove that the controls over the purchased products were implemented, and that the products meet the requirements. There is also another objective: it is to close the loop of the purchasing process; that is, the purchase order (transfer of information and data), product realization (acceptance of the purchased product), and verification. The expected records are:

- Documents sent from the supplier regarding the realization of the product, such as supplier's quality tests
- Documentation related to the delivery, such as delivery notes or packaging lists
- Records of internal control and quality tests
- Required documentations, such as COC, certifications, and so on

As always, when the standard requires records, they must be controlled; that is, listed and reviewed. The records of the verifications of purchased products are to be specified on your quality records list, and so submitted to a control of records as specified in subclause 4.2.4 (Control of Records).

7.5 PRODUCTION AND SERVICE PROVISION

7.5.1 Control of Production and Service Provision

7.5.1.1 The ISO 13485 Standard: Control of Production and Service Provision—General Requirements

The organization is required to plan and perform production and service provision under controlled conditions. The control must be performed and achieved according to the planning requirements specified within clause 7.1 (Planning of Product Realization). The control would apply to all realization processes, and would include activities such as:

- Production activities
- Product release activities
- Replication activities
- Sterilization processes
- Delivery activities
- Transportation activities
- Installation activities
- Maintenance activities (support and services)
- Operation activities
- Labeling activities

For example, if the medical device is to be sold in a sterile condition, the sterilization method must be defined, documented, recorded, and validated. The planning and carrying out of controlled conditions for the production and service provision will refer to the next issues (as far as is applicable) (Table 7.19).

This chapter deals with the controls over the different elements and resources that combine the realization processes, and specifies the requirements for achieving controlled production conditions. Once again, the goal is ensuring conformance to the medical device specifications. The control shall be planned in accordance with the medical device requirements and specifications (i.e., those specified in clause 7.1). The customer, the manufacturer, and the local authority should have decided upon and documented the particular requirements and specifications required to realize the medical device. Now is the time to ensure—supported by objective evidence—that the medical device is realized and conforms

TABLE 7.19
Standard Requirements of Subclause 7.5.1.1

ISO 13485	ISO 9001
The organization shall establish and maintain the controlled conditions required to realize the product and service	The organization shall establish and maintain the controlled conditions required to realize the product and service
Information describing the product or service characteristics that is relevant or essential to the realization processes shall be made available	Information describing the product or service characteristics that is relevant or essential to the realization processes shall be made available
Documented processes, procedures, realization instructions, resources specifications, control, measurements, and test procedures necessary for product realization shall be made available throughout the realization process	Documented processes, procedures, and realization instructions shall be made available throughout the realization process
The organization shall allocate and control the appropriate equipment for the realization process	The organization shall allocate and control the appropriate equipment for the realization process
The organization shall allocate the appropriate control and measurements tools and equipment for the realization process	The organization shall allocate the appropriate control and measurements tools and equipment for the realization process
Monitoring and measurement processes shall be implemented in order to control the realization process	Monitoring and measurement processes shall be implemented in order to control the realization process
The realization process shall refer to activities of approval and release, delivery, and postproduction	The realization processes shall refer to activities of approval and release, delivery, and postproduction
The realization process shall refer to labeling, classification, and packaging activities	
Each batch shall be documented and controlled with records. The records shall provide:	
Traceability requirements as specified in subclause 7.5.3	
The amount of medical devices manufactured (in each batch)	
The amount released for distribution (in each batch)	
The records shall be verified and approved	
The records must be included under the record control procedure as specified in subclause 4.2.4	

to the specifications. A good way of doing this is via a well-controlled realization process.

Determination of Conditions

Before planning and submitting the controls, the manufacturer shall define and determine the required conditions necessary for the realization of the medical device:

- Activities
- Means and resources

The activities, means, and resources were defined as part of the quality plan while implementing the requirements from clause 7.1 (Planning of Product Realization). The planning included quality objectives, goals, product specifications, realization means, and resources. Now is the time to verify that the conditions to achieve the plan are applicable.

The conditions will be determined in accordance with the medical device specifications. The conditions are combined from the elements that influence the realization processes:

- Environment
- Machinery
- Tools and equipment
- Materials
- Human resources
- Knowledge
- Regulations

If we take a few steps back in the process and return to the development labs, we can see that the issue of controlled conditions was to be accounted for there. During the development of the medical device you will have already designed the processes and activities that will transfer the specification to a product. The realization conditions were also to be considered. The output should have included the condition requirements.

Availability of Realization Requirements and Specifications

The ISO 13485 Standard requires that the manufacturer supply all essential documentation to the realization process in an appropriate manner. At any stage during the realization documentation of production, assembly, storage, installation, service or support, and the specifications are to be available for anyone who is involved in the processes. The documentation will answer the following questions:

- What is the task or activity to be carried out?
- Who is responsible for performing it? What are the required qualifications?
- How shall the employee perform it?
- Are there any required accessories?
- What are the expected results of the activity?

The objective here is to provide the employee, supplier, contractor, or any other party that participates in the realization processes, with full access to the required product characteristics and tasks specifications. This information can be used by the relevant parties to do the job correctly; measuring performances against specifications, and verifying and validating the product. These verifications and validations will be under defined arrangements, but this issue will be discussed later. If there are questions, uncertainties, or issues regarding the realization, the enquirer will have to turn to a reference for comparison.

When would the documentation be used?

- When training a new employee
- When implementing a new device into production
- In cases of confusion or hesitation
- In discussions and exchanges of information between employees
- Where rework is required

- When there are claims, calls, or complaints from other departments
- Where there are customer complaints

In order to provide an effective set of product characteristics that will be of use when needed, and to verify that the job will be done correctly, the organization must sit down, think, and define what the necessary information will be for the verification and validation of outputs; that is, the product's characteristics, as well as activities. For example, the quality tester knows what he/she has to do to validate when testing a product; he/she has a test instruction identifying the part to be tested, the machine that realizes it, the interval of the test, the sequence of the validation (the test), and the criteria for acceptance. All the required data and information are defined, documented, and made available. When he/she performs a test and faces an issue, they may turn to the test instruction and find the answer there. To take it one step further, when the medical device is assembled, specific assembling instructions, data forms, and inspection instructions—including all the required documentation, such as diagrams and criteria—will be available at the workstation. The documents will instruct the employee in:

- How to behave in the work environment (see clause 6.4)?
- How to handle materials, parts, or components?
- Which tools and equipment to use?
- How to assemble, construct, and install?
- How to test and inspect?
- How to finish the task?
- How to label?
- How to pack?

When an acceptance or quality approval is required for parts, materials, or components in order for them to be used in the realization process, the approval will be documented and made available to the worker, and he/she will use these parts only when an approval has been given—this is control.

When training for the employee, contractor, or supplier is needed, in order to ensure that they follow the instructions, this training will documented and controlled. For example, not all employees know how to read engineering drawings and to understand what is expected. The manufacturer must verify that an employee who is using the documentation knows how to use it, so that when they required to record processes, they will know what to do. This topic is referred to in chapter 6. When outputs of risk management activities specify the need for documentation such as control requirements or safety measures, these will be made available at the workstation. Where appropriate, the training will also cover this topic.

When a regulatory requirement demands certain documentation at the workstation, it is to be made available to the employees just like any other documentation. For example, material safety data sheets (MSDS) are the internationally standardized way for documenting the hazardous properties of chemicals and other agents. In several countries, occupational safety and health regulations require the availability of such charts, when they are used during the realization.

When the documentation is exposed to environmental conditions that may harm and wear it, it is necessary to implement protective cautions, and to locate the documentation in a safe area in order to ensure its use (i.e., a pouch, in laminated files and covers, etc).

Types of documentation:

- Documented instructions
- Standard operating procedures

- Specifications
- Work instructions
- Test specifications
- Blending or mixing procedures
- Step-by-step procedures
- Flow charts
- References for measurements and monitoring
- References for measurement procedures
- Routing cards
- Operation instructions
- Packaging procedures
- Service manuals
- Process control charts
- Diagrams
- Fabrication drawings
- Assembly drawings
- Subassembly drawings
- Technical (engineering) drawings
- Exploded-view drawings
- Label drawings
- Package drawings
- Samples of finished devices/goods
- Samples of assemblies
- Models
- Reference material

Samples of products or assemblies that are given to the employee as a reference will be identified, registered, and controlled with details such as the drawing, revision, control, lot, serial and batch numbers inserted on an attached card or tag.

Tools and Equipment

Tools and equipment used during product realization must be under control. It is required that you define the controls and maintenance activities that are to be implemented. The functionality of tools and equipment is affected when they are not properly maintained and controlled. This also directly affects the medical device. The required maintenance activities of tools and equipment shall be defined, documented, and made available for the person who uses them and realizes the product with them. The goal is to ensure that the information related to the tools and equipment includes adequate information, and is available at the workstations at the realization stage. It is necessary that you identify the departments or individuals that use these tools and equipment, and that you verify that they are trained, qualified, and have the appropriate skills to operate them. When determining the control on tools and equipment, one shall estimate the affect that the tools and equipment have on the medical device. The extent of the control shall be determined in accordance with their extent of their use, and their affect on characteristics of the medical device. In cases where the issue is critical, the manufacturer will develop processes and procedures in order to increase control. This is related to risk analysis.

For example, when an employee operates equipment during the sealing process, an improper operation will result in a defective medical device. Suppose that a required maintenance activity had not been performed; the outcome will likely be a far from desirable one.

You are required to ensure that:

- The worker is trained and qualified
- The operation instructions are available to them
- The equipment is maintained and controlled

In cases where there is a risk for the safety and intactness of the tools and equipment, a measure of precaution should be implemented in order to ensure their protection.

Under tools and equipment we may encounter:

- Vessels
- Mixers
- Work tools
- Molds
- Production tools
- Computer software
- Test equipment
- Maintenance equipment
- Assembly tools
- Electronic equipment

Infrastructure and Work Environment

The infrastructures related to the product realization must be under control. The requirements for the controls are specified in clauses 6.3 and 6.4. It is defined there how one must plan and implement controls and maintenance activities into the infrastructure and work environment of the realization process. The functionality of infrastructures and work environments is affected when they are not properly maintained and controlled. This directly affects the medical device too.

The control and maintenance activities of infrastructure and work environment shall be defined, documented, and made available; once for the person who uses it to realize the product, and twice for the person responsible for maintaining and servicing it. The goal is to ensure that the documentation related to the infrastructure and the work environment used to realize the product includes the adequate information, and is available to the appropriate parties. In order to maintain it effectively, you are required to define which parameters that can affect the medical device; thus, which are essential for control.

Process parameters that are influenced by the infrastructure and work environment include:

- Cleanliness
- Sterilization
- Orderliness
- Temperature
- Humidity
- Particle count
- Electrical current
- Speeds
- Pressure
- Accuracy
- Tension
- Geometrical measures
- Machine cycles
- Technical performances

The documentation will refer to issues such as:

- Instructions for proper operation
- Machine maintenance procedures
- Schedules for activities (maintenance and service)
- Responsibilities for activities
- Setup data and procedures
- Cleanliness and sterilization between sessions
- Test instructions
- Statistical methods
- Limits, tolerances, and values for measurements
- Required controls
- Calibration requirements
- Accuracy requirements
- Tools and equipment
- Requirements for environmental conditions
- Requirements for operational conditions
- Control and verification of performance activities
- Validation activities
- Troubleshooting procedures
- Reporting methods
- Required records

It is necessary to identify the departments or individuals that use the infrastructure and work environment while realizing the product, and to verify that they are trained, qualified, and have the appropriate skills to use them. In cases where there is a risk for the safety and intactness of the infrastructure and work environment, a measure of precaution should be implemented in order to ensure their protection.

The Use of Monitoring and Measuring Devices

During the realization process, the manufacturer implements controls over the outputs. The use of monitoring and measuring devices is an effective way to validate products, processes, infrastructures, equipment, and the required environmental conditions. The selection of such devices will be done in accordance with the nature of the product, and the implementation is done in accordance with the nature of the process. The use plays an important role during the realization process. Chapter 7.6 is dedicated to this matter: how, who, and when. I guarantee you that.

For each product, process, infrastructure, piece of equipment, and work environment that need to be monitored and measured by an objective tool or piece of equipment, the organization will identify and allocate the appropriate monitoring and measuring device; for example, scales, caliper gauges, software, or particle counters. The allocation, and the link between the device and the product, process, infrastructure, equipment, or work environment will be documented as required by the appropriate standard requirements:

- Clause 6.3 (Infrastructures Requirements)
- Clause 6.4 (Work Environment Requirements)
- Subclause 7.5.2 (Validation of Processes for Production and Service Provision)
- Subclause 7.5.5 (Preservation of Product)
- Clause 8.1 (Measurement, Analysis, and Improvement)

The organization will identify the roles that are responsible for the use and operation of these devices, or are responsible for their activity; namely, quality testers, maintenance technicians, laboratory technician, and assemblers. They each use different tools to control their activities and process outputs. You must verify that:

- They are using the appropriate devices related to the processes they are realizing.
- They are qualified to use the monitoring and measuring devices.
- The appropriate operation and use instructions are available.
- Documented criteria, such as tolerances, limit, SAL, particle/m^3, weight, and the allowed deviations required to evaluate results (whether the output is validated or not) are available.
- Any required training is provided.

The use of the monitoring and measuring devices includes the activity, documentation of the results, and the reporting method of evaluations or alarms. You should define and document according to the relevant standard requirement:

- A method for documenting the results
- A method for reporting and transferring the results to the relevant parties

The control of the monitoring and measuring devices should be implemented as specified in clause 7.6 (Control of Monitoring and Measuring Devices), which will be dealt later.

Release Activities

The release activities are to be defined and controlled. The objective is to prove that the manufacturing phase has been completed successfully, and that the medical device is a finished good ready for the delivery. This will be done with the definition of final acceptance activities or tests (final release tests)—that is, activities that will ensure that the product was realized according to the requirements—and that all controls were implemented, and the product meets the acceptance criteria. The activities will be supported with records. This requirement refers to each lot production, series production, batch production, serial production, jobbing work, or piece production. It does not mean that the control is finished—only that:

- The production of the medical device is completed.
- The product went through all the required realization processes and activities.
- Each process was validated and approved according to specified criteria by an authorized person.
- The required realization records are verified, completed, and available.
- All the required validation activities (for products, parts, and processes), during and after the processes, have been completed and the results are satisfying.
- The medical device is identified and labeled as specified.
- The medical device is packed as specified, and the packaging is controlled.
- The medical device is stored in the appropriate conditions.
- All the required records are complete.
- The traceability is maintained as specified.
- The risk management activities has been appropriately implemented.
- Release of the medical device (approval that the medical device is ready for delivery).

A defined role will be designated for the reviewing of the above, and for authorizing the release of the medical device. The definition may appear in a job description, a form, or a procedure.

Advice: When the release is done digitally, it is possible to define only one user per each release phase. This way, the manufacturer can achieve injective approval through the release process.

The review, approval, and release will be documented and maintained. I suggest conducting a small audit for each batch that was manufactured. The objective of the audit is to ensure that all the required controls, which were mentioned above, were implemented during the processes at the right times, and that the results are satisfying:

- Identification of the batch and medical device.
- Verification that all the validation activities were performed and the results are satisfying.
- Verification that all processes were verified and approved by the authorized parties.
- Review of product and process controls, and verification that the results of the tests were within limits.
- Verification that the employees realizing the product were qualified (according to the work plan).
- Verification that the equipment, tools, and infrastructures that were used to realize the product are maintained and controlled, and whether there were any disturbances during the process.
- Verification that the required documentation was available.
- Verification that the package was stored in the appropriate conditions before submission.
- Verification that packaging activities were controlled.
- Verification that the product was packed in the appropriate way.
- Verification that the storage conditions are appropriate.
- Review of all the records and verification to ensure that they are complete and accurate.
- Verification that the medical devices will be delivered with FIFO (first in first out) system.

The best way to document authorization is by signature. Digital signatures are also acceptable. You may define the review on a checklist, a form, or a procedure. Another way to control the process before release is via a routing card, which is attached to the batch during the realization process, and on which every responsible party approves that the controls have been implemented and the results met. Any method that you decide upon it should be supported with evidence that the controls were implemented and the results meet the specifications; that is, test results, quality protocols, machine outputs, and so on.

Delivery Activities

The delivery activities will be defined and controlled. The scope of the definition will refer to the entire delivery process—from the point of collection to the point of final delivery to the final customer. It includes delivery of products to suppliers for processing such as sterilization. The objective is ensuring and preserving consistently the medical device's functionality and safety after it has left the manufacturer's premises. This will be achieved by creating the optimal delivery conditions. The delivery conditions were planned and defined during the determination of requirements related to the product (see subclause 7.2.1). Now is the time to implement the controls that will ensure these definitions. Transportation and delivery are critical processes, because once the medical device leaves the factory you will no longer be able to control it directly as you had in your inventory. When initiating controls over delivery processes the following issues are to be accounted for:

- The controls will ensure that the delivered medical devices are safe and secured during the deliveries, and that all transport requirements are met.
- The medical devices will be protected from influences that may affect them; for example, heat, cold, humidity, moisture, dirt, and light.
- The identification and labeling of the medical device is intact and safe.
- The medical devices are protected from damage such as spillage, shaking, hitting, or other accidents.
- There is protection against contaminations—such as contamination from other substances or medical devices, and contamination that may be caused by damage to the medical devices themselves.
- There is a protection against pests.
- There is a protection against microorganisms.
- When there are requirements for controlled temperatures, the necessary means will be provided.
- When there are requirements for special vehicles, containers, or packages for the transportation, the necessary means will be provided.

There is no requirement for a documented procedure, only a definition. You must document the method in order to achieve optimal control, and to effectively implement the delivery specifications.

There is a requirement for records and evidence that the medical device was preserved under appropriate conditions throughout the delivery process. Transportation activities, for example, are included in these conditions. The organization will define the documentation that is needed to control the medical device and its delivery conditions throughout the transportation activities. These records and evidence would be required during audits, regulatory controls, or customer complaints. The records are divided into two categories—the instructional records, and evidence of performance.

The instructional records are the definitions of controls to be implemented during the delivery process, which are needed to support the delivery activities. They include packaging instructions, delivery or transportation specifications, specifications for protection, documented precautions or warnings, and customers' delivery instructions. These records will be stored with all other documented controls of the medical device, such as quality tests or work instruction, and will be available to the relevant parties when required. One may find them in the device master record (DMR).

The evidence is a record of performances, and the objective here is to prove that the delivery specifications were met:

- Labeling and identification of the medical device
- Delivery notes, including details for delivery
- Reports of transportation or storage conditions during the delivery processes, such as data registration of temperature or moisture
- Pictures taken as evidence

These may be found in the device history record (DHR).

The organization will appoint a responsible party for the verification that the delivery activities are performed according to the specifications.

If distributors are receiving and delivering the medical devices themselves to the final customer, the manufacturer is responsible for dictating the delivery requirements to them. The distributors will have to provide the manufacturer with evidence of performance.

The manufacturer shall define what is to be done with the medical device once a deviation from the delivery specifications has occurred and there is a danger that the medical device is no longer meeting the requirements.

Postdelivery activities, such as warranties, installations, after sales, and servicing will be referred and discussed in the appropriate subclauses 7.5.1.2.2 (Installation Activities) and 7.5.1.2.3 (Servicing Activities).

Labeling Activities

The label has an important role in the use and functionality of the medical device; it provides information regarding several parameter in the medical device. The ISO 13485 Standard specifically requires defining the labeling activities, and the controls to ensure their execution. Labeling refers to issues such as:

- Identification of the medical device itself
- Identification of components in the medical device
- The status of the medical device regarding its readiness for use; that is, not released, ready for use, disqualified
- The medical device's safety, functionality, performance, and intended use

Before plunging into the labeling of the medical device as a means of identification, I would like to refer to the issue of status identification. This issue will be dealt with in depth in the subclause 7.5.3.3 (Status Identification). However, it is important to indicate that labels and labeling activities may be used to physically quarantine the medical devices according to their realization processes or conformity level, and segregate them from other products, parts, or components. This segregation is usually required in order to eliminate contamination between products with different status. Such labeling indicates the product's status regarding the use of the medical device, and prevents the shipment of unfinished devices.

With regards to labeling, the organization shall develop a policy; that is, a plan or a list of activities that will assist in meeting the labeling requirements. The policy will present a defined method and controls for the labeling activities. The controls over the labeling process, and the labels, will eliminate any confusion or mistakes that may result from labeling activities. Such mistakes may affect the medical device's safety and functionality, or wrongly identify the medical device.

There are three distinct types of labels: (1) labels that indicate the status of the medical device during the realization processes, (2) labels that are attached to the medical device which provide information regarding its components, and (3) the information that is provided on the package. All three are influenced by different needs. Labels are actually outputs of different realization processes and are part of approval processes:

- Design and development processes—model, edition, components, parts, ingredients, and intended use
- Realization processes—identification, dates, and traceability
- Risk analysis—alarms, warnings, and safety instructions

The labeling activities also refer to information and data published on the package; that is, the name, model, pictures, warnings, and user instructions (packaging activities refer to the packaging of the medical device). The label is considered to be a quality record, and will be included under your quality records procedure and submitted to the appropriate records control as required in subclause 4.2.4 (Control of Records). One important aspect, for example is the management of label revisions. Designing the controls over labeling will ensure that all the outputs will be accepted as required. A good example is the scheduling of maintenance and service activities for the medical device, which are documented with a date on the label. Uniformity and consecutiveness between the medical device and its labels are necessary to ensure that a user will be able to distinguish between different medical devices regarding the functionality and attributes; in other words, to ensure that everybody is talking about the same device.

Changes to the medical device have a direct affect on the labels. Thus, a reference and a control between the status of the medical device—its revision and edition—and the set of labels are required. This control will ensure that changes are implemented on the labels, just like any other records.

Activities of designing a label and labeling will refer to parameters such as the type, size, label structure, details, graphics, drawings, required symbols and signs, the attachment activities to the medical device, and language. All parameters will be defined and documented for each label. While defining labeling processes and labels, the following issues are to be considered:

- The label should be intact and resistible to the ravages of time, the operation environment, storage, delivery, and use.
- The label will be protected from damages during the realization processes; namely, production, assembly, packaging, storage, delivery, and service and maintenance.
- It is required that you ensure that the use of the medical device will not harm the label.
- It is required that you ensure that the label will not harm the medical device or components, and will not disturb their functionality or performances; that is, electrical currents, sterilization, or chemical reactions.
- The location of the labels on the medical device must be defined.
- Graphics, diagrams, and pictures will be controlled and maintained as quality records.
- Labels and labeling activities are to be planned in accordance with standards, technical specifications, and regional and regulatory requirements.

In some cases, when the label is a part of the package, you may need to perform a compatibility test to ensure that the materials that the label is made of do not endanger the medical device's components or processes.

The details on the label will be appropriately planned to the nature and use of the medical device, and will include information and data such as:

- Identification of the medical device and the components (i.e., name and model)
- Edition or version
- Relevant dates (i.e., production, assembly, and expiry dates)
- Identification of production and traceability (serial number and batch number)
- Process approval (e.g.,, sterilization or sealing)
- User instructions
- Performances of the medical device (e.g., electrical)
- Alarms, warnings, and safety instructions
- Storage instructions
- Delivery instructions

The symbols, structures, details, and signs on the labels will be legal according to the regulatory and regional requirements of the location in which the medical device will be marketed. The label will support traceability processes (when planning your traceability processes, you should implement and refer to the labels.

Each sector in the medical device industry has its own regulatory requirements, standards, or technical specifications for labeling. When the medical device is assembled from various components and parts, it may be that various specifications will be applicable to one medical device. Be careful that you make the right inquiries and investigations before you start labeling you products. There have been cases where medical devices were disqualified on account of labeling. These issues must be resolved before shipping.

Translating the labels must be considered under regional regulatory requirements. This is a logical demand, considering that it is a medical device with safety aspects, and that the user must be able to read the instructions and the package clearly. Translating a label refers not only to the textual content, but also to signs and symbols. The manufacturer will maintain a defined method for translating labels and packages as a part of a process control:

- Control that the content is suitably translated
- Consideration of language necessities (in some countries there is more than one spoken language)
- Review of regulatory requirements
- Review of allowed signs and symbols

Packaging Activities

The operation and activity of packaging the medical device is a critical matter and must be highly regulated. The packaging operations of the medical device—as well as the materials used in its containers and package—are to be defined, documented, and controlled. The packages and packaging operations should be planned and designed during the design and development stages. The outputs must also include the controls that are to be implemented in order to validate the processes. The objective of the control on the packaging activities is to ensure its compliance to the medical device's specifications—that is, the validation of sterilization; sealing of packages (where required); the use of appropriate materials for a package; performing the right packaging activities (which will not harm the medical device); ensuring the safety, functionality, and performance of the device; and the preservation of packages while handling or storing them. Another objective is to instill awareness of the importance of the issue among employees. Compliance with regulations could be a high production barrier for many manufacturers.

The package is considered to be one of the medical device's specifications. A package shall protect the medical device from:

- Handling, processing, and storing
- Delivery activities until the package is opened
- The environment and possible contaminations

The package must be designed in such a way that, once opened, there will be no harm done to the medical device, the patient, or the user. It should be kept in mind that defective packages are a major cause for products recalls.

Packaging processes are referred as any other realization process, and thus must be controlled; that is, there must be validation of equipment, tools, processes, as well as materials. Outsourced packaging processes, and packages that were accepted and delivered by the customer, are counted here as well.

The handling of packages and materials will be planned in order to preserve them and their characteristics during storing, processing, handling, and delivery. The activities will be documented and supported with records, which will act as objective evidence that the operations were conducted as required. You may use procedures, work instructions, drawings, pictures, or examples of packages (which are required to be controlled as any other document). The documented instructions shall relate to the packaging operations, and provide a specific description of activities to be carried out, such as:

- Identifying different types of packages
- Identifying the different materials required for the packaging process (such as adhesives and sterilizers)
- Storing and handling of packages and related materials
- Operating tools and equipment
- Handling the packages containing the medical device
- Required delivery specifications

Environmental factors are to be accounted when storing and realizing such materials. The environmental parameters that may affect the package are to be defined and controlled, including:

- The allowed level of moisture and humidity
- The allowed storage temperature range
- The allowed pressure and altitude ranges
- The lifespan of packages and materials
- Hygiene control

Such material and package specifications must be document and implemented. Controls for the verification of performance must be implemented and maintained. In other words, when the packages and materials need to be stored and handled in a specific manner, or in certain conditions, the manufacturer is required to document these and verify that the appointed persons maintain such conditions (e.g., in the storing area, it is advised that you apply a form to record parameters such as temperature and humidity). Once in a while, the manufacturer should ensure that they evaluate the data gathered on the form and verify that the conditions are as specified.

The activities of handling and working with packages will be planned and documented based on state-of-the-art methods and technologies, ensuring the specified quality of the package and of the medical device. When defining the instructions you need to refer to the:

- Identification of the medical device
- Identification of the required package and materials
- Definition of target groups that will perform the packaging activities
- Definition of required tools, equipment, or machinery, including setups and required maintenance
- The physical parameters of the package are to be defined (size and dimensions, form or shape, weight, consistency, color and graphics, and power requirements)
- A description of the packaging activities (e.g., the materials used, the packaging activities; and the operation of tools, equipment, or machinery)
- The required controls for validation

Much significance will be given to legislative and regulatory requirements, standards, and technical specifications related to the different types of medical devices. You must identify the suitable standards' requirements in relation to the packaging of the medical device; and must implement the specifications, activities, and the required controls that are detailed there.

After planning and defining the packaging activities, it is required that you validate them in order to establish with objective evidence that the activities result in a package that meets the requirements. It is important to identify the critical parameters in the process in order to apply the appropriate controls. For example, if the manufacturer is planning a sealing process, there are a lot of critical issues to attend to—physical, chemical, as well as biological. If the medical device contains wet agents such as greases, reagents or oils, it is important to plan the sealing parameters accordingly. For each parameter that may affect the package, and thus the medical device, a proper control and validation activity should be appointed. The controls will include quality assurance tests on samples of packed medical devices. The control will be carried out along with the realization processes—after packaging, in storage, and after delivery. The results will be documented as quality records. The recommended way is to perform a statistical analysis of gathered data regarding the performance of the package (i.e., sample, test, record, analyze, and evaluate). Such statistical analysis will provide validation that the package is effective. Controls will include necessary warnings regarding the packaging of the medical device and will relate to the affects that the package may have on the medical device, if any.

Communication with the distributors regarding the packages will be defined and properly transferred to them. The objective is to give instruction to your distributor concerning the safety of the package.

Documentation of Batches

The next requirement relates to the control of production batches. The organization shall document and maintain records with details of the production, review of risks, release, and distribution for each production batch. These controls will assure that the medical device was realized and released according to specified arrangements, and support the traceability processes. The records shall indicate:

- The amount of medical devices manufactured and released in each batch
- The amount of released medical devices that were distributed
- The implementation of traceability processes as specified in subclause 7.5.3

The objective of this requirement is to ensure that only approved medical devices will be released and distributed. The details to be recorded include:

- The identification and control numbers, such as serial numbers or batch numbers
- The dates related to the realization of the medical device, such as the production and packaging dates
- The acceptance records and approval of the release
- The quantities that were released after production
- The quantities that were released for delivery and distribution
- The approval of delivery

In cases where each medical device has a serial number, you will need to maintain for each batch a reference list that contains all the serial numbers related to that particular batch.

The records are to be verified and approved after each stage and before submission to the next stage; they must be reviewed, released, approved, ready for delivery, and traced. You must define the method for review, verification, and approval; that is, determine the required activities and responsible parties. The batch records are considered quality records, and will be included under your quality records procedure and submitted to the appropriate records control as required in subclause 4.2.4 (Control of Records).

The reason for this control is to verify, once more, that all the required controls suggested above have been performed, that the results meet the specifications, and that traceability is ensured. In case you are controlling the realization with a routing card, the verification and approval of a batch may appear there after each stage. The routing card will be stored and maintained as a quality record. If the processes are managed via a process management system, you may verify controls with the status of the production order. At the end of the process, define a report that indicates all the realization processes. Then review, approve, and sign this report. The report will be stored and maintained as a quality record.

7.5.1.2 Control of Production and Service Provision—Specific Requirements

7.5.1.2.1 Cleanliness of Product and Contamination Control

The ISO 13485 Standard is sometimes very straightforward in deciding whether a requirement is applicable or not. Here the standard presents us with four different scenarios in which you are required to implement control over the cleanliness of the product against contamination. The scenarios are mentioned below. Analyze these, and find the scenario that suits your realization process. Once you have one located (which is likely), you are required to implement the controls (Table 7.20).

We are still dealing here with process control requirements. On this subclause the ISO 13485 Standard relates to the control of cleanliness against contamination. Surfaces of medical devices are becoming more complex and challenging, both in terms of chemistry and in terms of geometric shapes and forms. The objective is to ensure that finished products meet the company's quality requirements, or to ensure that production processes will not contaminate the products. It is therefore necessary to develop and document actions and controls for maintaining the cleanliness

TABLE 7.20
Standard Requirements of Subclause 7.5.1.2.1

ISO 13485
The organization shall define, maintain, and document procedures for implanting cleanliness requirements
The standard specifies four different cases where the organization must maintain requirements for cleanliness and control against contaminations: a. When the medical device is cleaned by the organization before it is subjected for a sterilization process (internal or external) or delivered for use b. When the medical device supplied nonsterilized to a cleaning process before submission to a sterilization process (internal or external) or delivered for use c. When the medical device is delivered nonsterilized, but must be cleaned and cleanliness is significant to its use d. When the medical device is required to be cleaned of any process agents during the realization process
When the product is cleaned in accordance with Cases a) and b) above, the requirements appearing in clauses 6.4a and 6.4b (regarding the work environment) are not applicable prior to the cleanliness processes

of devices. The emphasis on cleanliness is important due to the relation between the cleanliness of the medical device and later complications, material failures, function failures, or harm caused to users or patients. Minimizing all contaminants is therefore crucial. The standard realizes this, and requires the submission of controls during the realization process in order to ensure that cleanliness requirements are met.

Regulatory bodies around the world are now increasing their requirements for cleanliness, and are encouraging organizations and manufacturers to implement cleaning processes and controls. The processes must be validated just as any other realization process. This will achieve:

- The implementation of effective cleaning controls over your realization processes, including sampling and testing to minimize contamination
- Identification of contaminants to be removed from the medical device
- The types of cleaning or disinfecting agents to be used
- The prevention of known contaminants or materials (such as detergent residues) from staying on the final product
- The prevention of potential contaminants or materials from staying on the final product

Let us use an example to demonstrate the importance of cleanliness control and how contamination control may affect patients (the example is taken from a real event). A company produces surgical implants. After several months, several patients reported pains where the implants were inserted. Further diagnoses of the patients indicated that they were all suffering from infections. The matter was brought to the attention of the manufacturer. An investigation by the manufacturer led to evidence showing that a change was implanted during the production process. The new process resulted in the addition of a contaminant that was not identified, and thus not treated. The implants were delivered ready for use with the contaminants on them.

Sources of Contaminants

In order to identify contaminants and maintain effective cleanliness processes and controls, it is necessary to analyze and understand the sources of contamination and their nature. The sources will be analyzed throughout the realization process—delivery of purchased products, storage of materials and components, transport between processes and organizational units, unpacking activities, human resource handling, realization processes including assembly, packaging, delivery to the distribution or final customer, and postdelivery activities including service and maintenance. Each operation and activity needs to be analyzed for the material it uses and the affect of the material on the device: microbes, detergents, rodenticides, flux on circuits, and body oils. The required controls will then be designed in order to be able to supply the product according to the cleanliness requirements. Take, for example, a clean room. The control over the clean room is restricted to the area of the room; but what happens to the product before it enters or when it leaves the room?

Which elements will be investigated?

- The material that the device is made of
- Additives or substances to processes
- Leachable substances during the realization processes

- Processing agents and any materials or substances used in, or to aid the manufacturing process
- Components or elements that may affect the device; such as packages, trolleys, cranes, or forklifts

There are a few additional instances that may require you to analyze contaminants:

- Risk analysis is an input for contamination analysis. The cleanliness may affect directly the safety of the medical device. During the risk analysis, hazards are being detected. These hazards are then evaluated and the root causes identified. From this phase you can derive contamination hazards and detect their sources during the realization process.
- Customer complaints and recalls of medical devices are an input for contamination analysis.
- Changes that have occurred in processes may be a source for new contaminations and must be analyzed.

Removal of Process Agents

When, during the realization process, a certain material is known or expected to contaminate the device, the manufacturer will plan (and document) actions in order to identify and remove this material, and will bring the medical device to a sufficient level of cleanliness. The ISO 13485 Standard refers to this as "removal of process agents." These process agents need to be identified and labeled throughout the realization process in order to eliminate processing errors. After the removal of these agents, it is required that the manufacturer validates the level of cleanliness, and ensures that the necessary quality is achieved. The removal activities, as well as the validation test, will be documented. Processing agents may include:

- Cleaning agents
- Lubricating oils
- Mold release agents
- Any substances not intended to be included in the finished device

Defining Level of Cleanliness

In order to implement effective cleanliness processes and controls, it is necessary to determine the required level of cleanliness, and to define the accepted levels of cleanliness and criteria for evaluation; that is, in terms of particulate counts, cytotoxicity levels, and total organic carbon. The objective is to provide a scale that will be used during the control for assessment. The determination will be done with the help of regulatory requirements, specifications, and standards.

Where international, national, or regional standards, regulations, or specifications for assessing levels of cleanliness are demanded by your local authorities, they will be integrated into the cleanliness process. In case the organization is not able to produce or identify specifications or standards relating to the matter, it may set them alone but will have to provide justifications for its determination.

Testing and Controls

After defining the level of cleanliness, you must determine the controls over the realization process in order to ensure that these conditions are maintained. The presence of contaminants in a product or on a product surface requires the monitoring and controlling of the production process. Bioburden testing is one example. This test is used for the estimation of the population of microorganisms on the surfaces of medical devices, or on an empty product package.

The test will be documented and will detail a sequence of events to be performed in order evaluate the cleanliness of a medical device:

- The test should be planned with regard to the characteristics and properties of the tested material, which include chemical, toxicological, physical, electrical, morphological, and mechanical properties.
- The required conditions for the test shall be defined.
- The monitoring and measuring equipment necessary for the processes are to be determined.
- The scope of the test on the medical device must be clearly defined; that is, on a certain part, component, or surface.
- The duration, frequency, and degree of the test shall be defined; that is, the quantities, sampling rates, cycles, and intervals.
- The exact stage of the realization process shall be indicated; for example, after a certain process, before packaging, or before submission for sterilization.

The results shall indicate whether the medical device complies with the cleanliness requirements according to the predefined criteria. The results shall be recorded and demonstrate the effectiveness of the processes and activities. They will demonstrate achieving objectives. This is why you must plan the output in a way that will allow you to compare them with the criteria. When necessary, improvements will be implemented. This will be discussed in chapter 8 (Measurement, Analysis, and Improvement). In case the cleanliness activities and tests affect the effectiveness of the sterilization processes to come, the controls should be planned to indicate these requirements; that is, the microbiological quality and cleanliness levels.

Documented Requirements

A cleaning process can be complex. The ISO 13485 demands specifically maintaining detailed documented procedure for cleanliness. The documentation shall indicate employees' behavior and operations with the materials, products, parts, or components. The objective is to provide the employees with proper directions and instructions on how to perform the cleaning activities and avoid contamination. The procedure will define the sequence of events and methods in order to maintain the cleanliness of the product, and avoid possible contaminations. The documented requirements will have a few properties:

- The objective and scope of the cleanliness activities regarding elements in the product to be cleaned or controlled; for example, the definition of surface
- Responsibilities, roles, and authorities to perform these activities
- Materials, cleaning solutions, and solvents to be used during the activities
- Equipment and monitoring equipment necessary for the processes
- References to documents, such as the operation instructions of equipment, documented criteria, applicable test or work instructions, standards, or specifications
- Specification of cleaning activities in order to maintain cleanliness requirements
- Tests and controls required to prove cleanliness requirements
- Policy of conducting, handling, and employees' behavior with products in the work environment—including reference to different areas where the medical device is handled

- The use of special clothing and designated accessories
- Reference to risks and necessary controls
- The frequency and interval of the activities
- Records of activities

It is important to identify any risks that may create situations that will lead to contamination. For example, processing work too rapidly may result in reduced cleaning. When performing a cleaning process, the maximum or minimum times should be specified.

Necessary accessories that support the cleaning processes should be identified and supplied; for example, cleaning solutions, racks, bins, baskets, special tissue papers, shoes, overcoat, gloves, and hangers. The shelf life of solvents and other materials used for cleaning must be controlled in order to eliminate redeposition of contaminants.

Let us review a sample cleaning process:

- Arrival of components into a realization zone.
- Registration with the barcode reader.
- Unpacking the components—wraps are to be in thrown in a bin.
- Components will be placed on trolley number YYY near the sink.
- Performing a manual wash in a designated sink—the sink must be washed first with material AAA.
- Performing ultrasonic cleaning process on device number XXX—operation instructions are available at the workstation.
- Performing cleanliness test with tool number TTT—test instructions and criteria are available at the workstation.
- If the results are not satisfying, perform the process again.
- If the results are satisfying, perform disinfection.

The requirements and the description of the process may appear on a work instruction, a procedure, or a process flow diagram. Try to create a procedure that will supply the employee with all of the necessary information and instructions. Written procedures are preferable to diagrams. The documented requirements will be available at the appropriate workstations. The relevant personnel will be trained and certified accordingly. Naturally, the procedure will be submitted to the documents control process as required by subclause 4.2.3 (Control of Documents).

Advice: In case you are already managing a set of procedures related to realization processes, and these processes are demanding cleaning activities, it is possible to incorporate the cleaning activities and the controls into these procedures. For example, if you are maintaining work instructions for assembly, and a cleaning activity is required, you may document the cleaning activity on the same work instructions.

The Relation with the Control over Work Environment

Scenarios A and B mentioned in Table 7.20 are the two first cleaning scenarios introduced to us by the ISO 13485 Standard in subclause 7.5.1.2.1 (Cleanliness of Product and Contamination Control). Clause 6.4 relates to the work environment. If you are maintaining cleaning scenario A or B, the requirements presented in 6.4a and 6.4b are applicable only from the stage of the cleaning processes.

- 6.4a. The organization is required to maintain and document health, clothing, and cleanliness requirements should contact between the human resource or work environment affect the quality of the product.
- 6.4b. The organization is required to maintain and document work environment condition requirements should they affect the quality of the product.

Two main interrelations are mentioned here—the relation between the human resource and the product; and the relation between the work environment and the product. These will be implemented from the cleaning processes only when scenarios A) and B) are applicable to your realization processes.

Records

Although the ISO 13485 Standard does not require specifically maintaining records on this subclause, the records were required throughout this chapter. That requirement is applicable here. The records to be expected include:

- List of contaminants
- Labeling of process agents to be removed
- Definition of cleanliness requirements and criteria
- Definition of cleanliness tests
- Documentation of cleaning activities
- Results of the cleanliness tests and controls
- Control records of solvents and cleaning materials

Records that support the cleaning activities are required to be available at the appropriate workstations. These may appear on forms, routing cards, charts, or other documentation accompanying the processes. The cleaning records are considered quality records, and will be included under your quality records procedure and submitted to the appropriate records control as required in subclause 4.2.4 (Control of Records).

7.5.1.2.2 Installation Activities

The ISO 13485 Standard regards the installation as a realization process but refers it to the post production phase. Therefore, the installation requirements are to be defined, documented, and controlled. There are cases where installation is performed by a third party; for example, the customer or supplier. In these cases the organization must also document the installation instructions, inspection and criteria for acceptance, the responsibilities, the relevant authorities during the installation process, and maintain skills of the installer or user that installs the medical device. The installation requirements include in Table 7.21.

TABLE 7.21
Standard Requirements of Subclause 7.5.1.2.2

ISO 13485
The organization shall define and document requirements and specifications for installation activities of the medical device, if appropriate
The requirements and specifications for installation shall include activities for inspection, criteria for acceptance, verification, and approval of the installation
When a third party is to install the medical device (an agent or representative of the organization or the customer), the organization will provide documented installation instructions, including activities for inspection, criteria for acceptance, verification, and approval of the installation
Documentation of the service activities, verification, and approval shall be recorded and included under the records control process as specified in subclause 4.2.4 (Control of Records)

The objective of this requirement is to ensure the proper installation of the medical device; the manufacturer shall determine the necessary installation activities, inspections, verifications, and approval. The purpose is to ensure that the medical device will function properly after installation in terms of functionality, performance, safety, and intended use. The organization is to define, document, and provide all the necessary data related to the installation of the medical device, such as instructions, specifications, and documentation. Emphasis will be given to the required controls, inspections, and acceptance testing; that is, the activities that will verify and validate that the medical device was adequately installed, that its requirements are met, and that the intended use is obtained.

Installation refers to the setup and adjustment activities of a medical device in its operation environment that are needed for proper function. Without these activities the medical device will fail to comply. When defining the installation activities, the organization will refer to the following issues.

Installation Activities

The stages and activities of the installation must be defined and documented as precisely as possible, in order to provide all the necessary information for installation:

- A definition of responsible roles for each activity
- Documented customer specifications
- A specific description of the installation activities and the required results
- A reference for tools and equipment, and their use
- Reference to the operation environment, customer facilities, and other devices that may affect the installation
- Supporting documentation required to perform the installation
- Tests, controls, validations, and verifications—including criteria
- Reference for schedules and time objectives
- Expected records

A list of the expected records is crucial because it provides a reference for control of the installation.

Product Preservation and Safety Measures

Activities for product preservation during the installation are critical, and will be defined and controlled. The activities will refer to risk analysis and warnings during installation activities; for example, safety measures that the installation team must fulfill in order to protect the device and the team itself (safety issues regarding the user and patient were referred during design, development, and earlier realization processes).

Documentation

The installation activities planned, as specified above, will be documented and made available. This documentation will be included in the quality plan. The documentation is divided into two categories:

In the first category is the instructional that provides specific instructions of installation activities; for example, procedures, process diagrams, instructions, user manuals, test procedures, and so on.

In the second is the documentation that supports and provides information for the activities; that is, diagrams, documented criteria, technical specifications, technical data, regulations, directives, and technical standards.

The availability of the documentation is to be defined—it may be printed, appear in a user manual, a handbook, documented trainings, or on the company website.

Regulatory Requirements

The reference to regulations or standards is critical. For each installation activity, the manufacturer must identify the pertinent international, national, and regional regulations, standards, or technical specifications; for example, electrical installation in terms of standards and safety, sterilization requirements, the setup of communication networks and software, and do on. The appropriate inquiries are to be made as there are plenty of regulations to be accounted for. When such regulations indicate or specify installation demands, they are to be implemented into the installation requirements. The availability of these specifications during the installation processes and trainings is to be maintained.

Approval and Acceptance

The installation will be evaluated and examined to ensure that it was performed according to the specifications, and is approved for use; that is, the installed medical device must be determined as being safe and ready for use. The controls and validations are to be integrated into the installation activities. Each test inspection and control will be supported with the appropriate predefined criteria. The approval provides the assurance that the medical device was delivered according to the requirements. For example, you can design a checklist that will include all the stages of the installation, including the validation and control activities. After all controls have been implemented, and all activities verified, the medical device can be approved for use. The approval of the installation will be documented.

Training

The qualifications of employees or users performing the installation activities must be defined. The first step is the identification of required qualifications and training needs related to the installation activities; the second is the development of the training methods. The necessary training activities will be incorporated into the quality management system; training program, establishing documentation, verifications, and evidence. At the end of the process you will certify the personnel as being qualified to perform the installation.

Advice: I suggest establishing a digital knowledge center regarding the installation of medical devices with the required instructions, documentations, training, and other accessories that may support the installation; for example, troubleshooting documents, known installation mistakes, and articles and resources related to installation.

Third Party Installations

When the installation is performed by a third party; under the responsibility of the customer or supplier, the organization must provide the necessary documentation to meet the requirements mentioned above. When the organization is outsourcing the installation, it is under its responsibility to control and verify it. Thus, it is required to train the supplier appropriately, certify them, and to control their installations. The supplier is obligated to perform all the installation requirements as specified for them, and to provide the manufacturer with the necessary evidence and process validations.

Records of Installation

The records of installation and verification are to be maintained. The purpose of the records is to prove that the installation had been done according to the documented definition; that it has been it was verified, controlled, accepted, and the medical device is approved for use. In order to create an effective documentation, design the records of the process according to the installation activities.

The installation records are considered quality records, and will be included under your quality records procedure and submitted to the appropriate records control as required in subclause 4.2.4 (Control of Records).

7.5.1.2.3 Servicing Activities

When an organization produces a medical device that is not perishable, it is usually required that service activities after delivery of the device be maintained. Where service is required as part of the product (e.g., support, repairs, or maintenance), the organization is to establish and maintain a documented set of processes describing the service activities. There are two main objectives:

- Assurance that after service activities, the medical device is suitable for use and still maintains its intended use.
- The information and data collected during the service activities are analyzed in order to detect quality problems (see Table 7.22).

The Scope of the Service and Maintenance Activities

The scope of the service will frame the service and define exactly the type, interval, intensity, or complexity of provided service activities, and will set up the roles and responsibilities. It is the organization's responsibility to ensure a clear and complete definition of the scope of services to be provided to the medical device, including a

TABLE 7.22
Standard Requirements of Subclause 7.5.1.2.3

ISO 13485
Where the service is defined as a requirement, the organization shall define and maintain a set of documented processes in order to provide controlled service activities
The organization will use the appropriate documentation that is needed to support the service activities such as procedures, work instructions, reference materials, and reference measurement procedures, as necessary
The definitions of processes will include the verification activities needed to ensure that the medical device maintains its intended use
Documentation of the service activities, verification, and approval shall be recorded and included under the records control process as specified in subclause 4.2.4 (Control of Records)
Service activities include repair and maintenance

division of responsibilities between the service provider and the customer. The scope of the service will be determined in correlation with the quality requirements of the medical device; that is, the functionality, performance, safety, and intended use. The characteristics of service shall refer to the following topics:

- The medical device included under the service will be identified, and the details shall indicate to the service team the exact medical device. The identification shall include details such as name, model, version, serial number, date of manufacture, batch numbers, owner, customer, and the location at the customer's premises.
- The specification of the service activities.
- Determination of the service provider (the organization or an external body).
- Reference to availability of the service; for example, in-person visits, telephone support, or periodic maintenance.
- Reference to parts and replacements of the medical device.

The service will be agreed, approved by the customer, and documented. This can be done in an agreement, a contract, or a protocol. The documentation will serve as reference for later service activities.

As far as spare parts and replacements are concerned, when determining the service scope, the organization should consider the possibility that some spare parts may not always be available. The manufacturer is responsible for providing customers with spare parts for the duration the lifetime of the medical device. In such cases, the service scope will define what other options are available.

Operation on Delivery of the Medical Device

The first operation of the medical device after delivery is regarded as a postdelivery activity. The manufacturer must ensure product preservation; the medical device's features will not be harmed during the first operation by the customer. Therefore the risks during the operation of the medical device on delivery are to be reviewed, and appropriate controls are to be implemented; for example, user manuals, training, and online and webpage support. As well as operation activities, it is necessary to define for the customer the required operation conditions—the temperature, cleanliness, and operation environment.

Maintenance and Service Activity Description

Maintenance and service activities have a defined purpose:

- Clear identification of the medical device that is under the service or maintenance
- Identification and analysis of the need, whether it is maintenance, service, malfunction, or disorder
- Execution of a defined action
- Verification of the action
- Documentation and reporting

The manufacturer will define the specific sequence of events and expected results of the service activities. The service activities shall refer to each component, and describe in detail the maintenance and service requirements; that is, an overall description of the actions to be carried out. The objective is to provide the service representative with detailed specifications regarding what has to be done in certain events and cases concerning a medical device, part, materials, or components. This will include a succinct and clear description of the objective, purpose, and components of the activity. The description will refer to:

- The definition of responsible employees that are to perform the service maintenance or support activities, including required qualifications.
- The definition of accessibility to the medical device, with locations of the medical device or the need for authorizations.
- The relation to necessary documentation, such as technical specifications, drawings, plans, or user manuals.
- The specifications of tools and equipment that are required to perform the activities.
- The treatment and handling of databases during the service activities, such as backups, data freeze, or data conversions.
- The acceptance validations and verification of service activities, including reboots.

The activities will be reviewed and approved by authorized personnel. The reason is that a repair or maintenance may affect other components in the medical deceive, and thus may also affect its functionality. In order to ensure that certain activities will not affect other components, parts, or processes in the medical device, each service activity will be reviewed by an appropriate employee in order to validate and verify it. The evaluation of the activity will be cross-referenced, and will include all relevant ranges: mechanical, biological, and electrical. This means that if a maintained component performs a chemical reaction, but with the help of another electro component, the maintenance activity will be reviewed by two responsible parties; one for the chemical reaction, and one for the electrical reaction.

Verification is to ensure that all the required service and maintenance activities were performed by the appropriate person, on the appointed time, and on the designated medical device. For example, a sticker on the medical device indicating that maintenance was performed along with the next schedule for treatment. The sticker is a classic quality record. A checklist specifying all the necessary action is also acceptable for verification. The verification will be documented.

Validation, on the other hand, is to ensure that after maintenance and service activities have been carried out, the medical device still functions according to its requirements; that is, intended use, functionality, performance, and safety. This is more complex. In order to ensure its effectivity, plan a validation test for every service activity. Measurement procedures and material references will help. The functionality of the medical device must be validated after the service activities. The validation will be documented.

Communication with the Customer

In subclause 7.2.3 (Customer Communication), you are required to define and establish communication channels between customers and the organization regarding maintenance and service, among other issues. In respect to service and maintenance, the organization needs to define communication channels, interfaces, and processes covering both information transfer and execution of activities:

- Transfer of information: definition of how a customer can contact the manufacturer or service provider in case of need—for example, by e-mail, fax, telephone call, company website—and what information must be gathered or shared in order to provide efficient service or maintenance.

- Execution of activities: definition of how the service provider can access the customers in order to perform the activities—in-person visits, service center where the device is delivered for repair, telephone support.

It may be that the organization will have to initiate contact with the customer when maintenance for the medical device is periodically required.

Responsible Parties

Since the service can be complex and have a lot of implications, each service activity must define the role that will perform it with the required qualifications. Earlier, I discussed the planning, review, and approval of the activities. I will now refer to the performance. Naturally, the suitable trainings will be define on the quality management system, as required in subclause 6.2.2 (Competence, Awareness, and Training) and incorporated into the training program. Service employees will be certified according to the personnel certification processes.

When the service or maintenance is performed by a third party (the customer or supplier), the organization must provide them with the necessary documentations answering the requirements mentioned above. When the organization is outsourcing the service activities, it is the manufacturer's responsibility to control and verify it. Thus, it is required that the manufacturer train the supplier appropriately in order to certify and control its services. The performances of the suppler during the service activities will be evaluated and included in the general evaluation of the suppliers, as required in subclause 7.4.1 (Purchasing Process). The supplier is obligated to perform all the service requirements as specified by the manufacturer, and to provide the necessary evidence and process validations.

Time Intervals for Service and Maintenance Activities

The intervals for the service activities are to be defined for each medical device, part, or component. This factor is an output of the design and development stages. The definition shall refer to the identification of the medical device, the required service or maintenance activities, documentation of the date when the service was delivered, and schedule for the next activity. Another way to define it is to maintain a service or maintenance plan.

Service Data, Information, and Report

The service activities are to be used as a means of identifying quality problems in the medical device related to postproduction phases. The issue relates indirectly to subclause 8.2.1 (Feedback), where the organization is required to implement methods and processes for collecting data and information regarding the use and performance of the medical device. Service data and records are one way to implement these. During the service activities you are required to document the problems or events, the causes or factors, and the corrective or preventive measures that were carried out. The following details for records are just a suggestion:

- The identification of the medical device
- The identifications of the service activity (e.g., service call number, service ticket number) and the date of the service
- The individual who performed the service activities
- The identification by the customer of persons who received the service

- A description of the service provided or performed
- The identification of designated tools or equipment used to perform the service, such as measuring and monitoring devices (for traceability needs)
- A list of parts or components that were repaired, maintained, or replaced, including identifiers such as model, catalog number, serial number, or batch number
- The tests and inspections which confirmed that the service reached its purposes (validation processes)
- Management of repair or maintenance history

The later appraisal of the medical device performances will include the use of statistical techniques (chapter 8.1—Measurement, Analysis, and Improvement). Therefore I suggest trying to quantify the data as much as possible in order to be able to use it effectively in later analysis; for example, categorizing the faults, problems, or treatments with codes. The records of service and maintenance will be then used for the evaluation, appraisal, and improvement of the medical device performances, and of the quality management system.

When national or local regulations require a specific data to be recorded during the service activities, this requirement will be implemented and the coverage of required data will be incorporated into the service activities. In most cases, the requirements will refer to the issue of reporting in case of malfunctions or disorders in the medical device, or on its performance if it creates hazards to users or patients. During the planning of the service activities you will need to identify which regulations (national, regional) apply to your medical device, and to implement the demands into your service processes; what information is to be gathered, how shall you report, and the subjects of the report.

The history of the medical device plays an important role when servicing or maintaining it. The history describes the functionality and performances of the medical device concerning safety and intended use. Thus, the history of servicing and maintenance is to be documented and managed, but more important is the implementation of regulatory requirements on the matter, where applicable.

In some cases monitoring and measuring devices are used to measure outputs of processes during the service and maintenance activities. These devices must be calibrated and controlled. Their use will be documented in order to prove their compatibility. Documentation may appear as an internal number, serial number, and so on.

Status Identification

During service or maintenance activities, an indication regarding the usability of the medical device will be determined; that is, whether it is usable, in repair, or defective. The status will be clearly shown on the medical device in a place or location where all users or patients may view it. It is also possible to deactivate or disable only a part, or a function, of the medical device. If you are replacing a screen or printer, it does not make sense to disqualify the entire medical device so long as the intended use, functionality, performance, and safety are not affected; but do not forget to identify the status. Of course the activity of deactivating only a part of the medical device shall be planned, reviewed, approved and documented by an authorized person before allowing a service employee to perform the deactivation.

Service and maintenance activities may create defective parts or devices. Therefore, it is required that you initiate the interface between the service and control of nonconforming products.

Changes, Updates or Upgrades of Versions

The software configuration management influences the service and maintenance activities. Software operating the medical device processes can be a crucial factor in the performance of the product, and may have safety implications on the medical device as well. The configuration management is responsible for controlling the evolution and changes made to software, which may affect components or parts, and thus processes, in the medical device. In order to ensure a smooth and safe maintenance, update, or upgrade of software, you must implement a method for configuration management and an update policy. This topic was referred to in chapter 7.3.7 (Control of Design and Development Changes) and will be covered in more detail in chapter 7.5.3 (Identification and Traceability). The policy and required activities will be incorporated into the service activities. This way the medical device that is in use by the customer, or is installed at the customer's premises, will be charted according to the configuration management, and the status of the software will be identified exclusively. The definition shall refer to all related aspects—the update activities, the required tests, the verifications, review, and approval.

I will demonstrate the importance of the issue by using a simple example. Suppose that a service activity was performed on the medical device, and, according to a customer's request, a field label on the user's application was changed. Such a change must be implemented according to a methodical process in order to plan, evaluate, verify, and document it. When the version will be updated, this change will be visible and accounted.

Documentation

The services processes and activities will be documented and available to the relevant parties in the appropriate places, and at the right times or events. The documentation is to provide the ability and means to perform the service activities according to a plan. Relevant parties may be service technicians as well as the customers themselves. Appropriate place can be the company's server, help module on the user's application, technical files, web pages, accompanying documentation for technicians, and service manuals for customers. The right time or event is the definition of the cases in which the documentation is to be used. The documentation may include (as the ISO 13485 Standard indicates):

- Procedures
- Work instructions
- Reference material
- Reference measurements procedures

If you think of anything else, you are welcome to implement it. For the record, reference material and reference measurements procedures are procedures that ensure an accurate clinical analysis and generate the statistical quality control charts that provide information. The procedures specify measurement activities, values, and criteria.

Advice: It is recommended that you add a "troubleshooting" document. This is a document that describes known, experienced, and recognized faults or problems, and suggests ways to verify and treat them. Such a document is *very* useful during use, and service and maintenance activities. It has been proven, in the long term, that when technicians and users learn it by heart they begin to solve problems by themselves. The use of such a document is highly recommended.

Records of Service

The records of service activities are to be maintained. The purpose of the records is to prove that the services have been done according to the predefined plan, were verified, controlled, accepted, and the medical device is approved for use. In order to create an effective documentation, design the records of the process according to the service activities.

The service records are considered quality records and will be included under your quality records procedure and submitted to the appropriate records control, as required in subclause 4.2.4 (Control of Records); that is, they are to be defined, maintained, controlled, and properly stored.

7.5.1.3 Particular Requirements for Sterile Medical Devices

The ISO 13485 Standard has three main objectives when a referring to controls over sterilization processes:

- The promotion of awareness of the validation of sterilization processes, and of the importance of the accuracy of these processes
- The implementation of controls related to the sterilization processes throughout all realization processes, and not only on the sterilization activities
- The identification and implementation of appropriate standards or specifications (see Table 7.23)

Sterility is an unnatural state. Thus, sterilization processes require a lot of resources due to the fact that unnatural conditions are generated; for example, preconditioning, the sterilization cycle, and aeration. Each process has a specification describing the process parameters. These parameters need to be precise and within predefined tolerances in order for the processes to be effective. The critical process parameters were determined during the design and development stages of process validations, and they assist in determining the compatibility of a product or a process.

Sterility tests are an integral part of sterility processes. The tests are to be conducted in order to determine if viable microorganisms are present, and thus the

TABLE 7.23
Standard Requirements of Subclause 7.5.1.3

ISO 13485
The organization shall maintain and document records of sterilization processes parameters for every sterilized batch
The records shall maintain the traceability specifications as required in paragraph 7.5.1.1 for production batches
The records shall be included under the records control process as specified in paragraph 4.2.4—control of records

adequacy of sterilization process parameters. The provision of sterility test data is crucial for the release of the product.

Determining the Process Parameters

Each parameter of the sterilization process, cycle, test, or activity must be examined in order to ensure that they meet the defined requirements under expected production conditions. Through these parameters, the accuracy and effectiveness of processes can be validated. As a manufacturer, you will need to identify these critical parameters as being essential to the sterilization process, and are required to do so with monitoring. Usually such parameters are defined on the validation protocols, as are the methods for monitoring them. Here are some examples for process parameters to be controlled and documented:

- Preconditioning and conditioning processes are treatments performed on devices before they are submitted to the sterilization cycle in a chamber. These processes require certain levels of temperature, humidity, and time.
- During sterilization processes the exposure time is crucial.
- After sterilization processes, sterility tests are conducted in order to evaluate the compatibility of the product. The test generates the sterility assurance level (SAL)—the probability of a viable microorganism's presence on the medical device (degree of sterility).
- Devices that are sterilized through a process of controlled exposure to ethylene oxide gases are required to be quarantined for 24 hours or longer.

Such parameters are to be documented as objective evidence. The data shall demonstrate process values and will enable you to verify that all the critical parameters during the sterilization processes were conducted according to the specifications, and within tolerances. The results will be compared to a set of determined criteria. Based on the comparison, a decision will be made regarding the process; that is, it will be accepted or rejected.

As mentioned before, sterilization control does not apply to sterilization processes alone, but is to be implemented throughout the realization processes and elements. Here are additional process parameters to be recorded:

- Work environment conditions and conditions of manufacturing locations during the processes and tests
- Equipment parameters
- Product conditions during the processes and tests are required (whether the product is packed, sealed, open, etc.)
- Employees' behaviors in the work environment during the sterilization processes are require (e.g., whether they are wearing the appropriate attire)
- Process control limits
- Software parameters
- Devices' handling requirements
- Packaging activities and systems
- Sterility testing

If certain records of earlier processes are required for the sterilization process, they will be made available and will be attached to the sterilization records. The results of such processes may determine the sterilization process, and the records may be required to commence the sterilization. For example, when cleanliness activities and tests affect the effectiveness of the sterilization process to come, the required records indicating the microbiological quality and cleanliness levels will be available. When external records provide the process parameters, they will be mentioned and included under the records list (e.g., records indicating parameters of materials or sterilants received from your supplier).

Type and Source of the Records

The records of the parameters will allow the manufacturer to adjust in situations where the processes are not satisfying. The data will be gathered in a manner that allows you to perform:

- Analysis and evaluation of process performance
- Control over trends
- Consideration for change

Thus, it is necessary to define for each process the appropriate form of documentation; for example, forms, control charts, computer software printouts, machine outputs, or test protocols. The records of the data shall be designed and planned according to the process specifications and their tolerances. It is necessary to define which process element produces the data: activities, machines, work environment controls, or human resources. The methods for obtaining and processing the data will also be determined (e.g., statistical analysis, OQ data, or mathematical modeling).

Records of the sterilization process parameters shall be included under your records control process and will be considered part of the quality management system as specified in subclause 4.2.4 (Control of Records).

Regulatory Specifications

It is required that the manufacturer identify which international, national, or local regulations or directives are applicable, and to implement their requirements. Each country and region maintains its own specifications for sterilization. These also include the requirements for records. You must identify these regulations in the region where you are active, and implement the requirements for records. When technical specifications or standards are required, the specification and guidelines will be implemented, as well as the specification for records. For example: ISO 11134, ISO 11135, ISO 11137, ISO 11138, ISO 13683, ISO 14937, ISO 14160, and ISO 13409. Each standard presents, aside from the guidelines and specifications, requirements for records. Your methods for documenting the parameters will be planned according to these requirements.

Batch Control

The standard requires that the records of sterilization process parameters will be traceable for each production batch and refers us to the requirements of control of production and service provision, subclause 7.5.1.1. These requirements will also be applied to the sterilization batches:

- Each batch will be identified with control numbers, such as serial numbers or batch numbers, in order to enable traceability.
- Each batch will bear dates related to the sterilization processes and activities.
- The acceptance activities and approval of the release of each batch will be recorded and available.

- The quantities that were released after sterilization will be documented.
- The materials, accessories, and equipment used during the sterilization processes will be documented.
- The approval of release will be documented and the person who performed the approval will be identified.

All of the above will be documented on the records of the sterilization processes. The objective is to provide the potential to track down, in case of need, each process parameter that influenced the sterilization load.

7.5.2 Validation of Processes for Production and Service Provision

7.5.2.1 General Requirements

Process validation is another control in the list of controls of realization processes that the quality management system requires us to implement. Validation means testing that expected results and objectives have been achieved. The organization is required to validate realization processes where their results and outputs cannot be monitored, measured, and verified. These are processes whose outputs cannot be controlled at the end of the process or as a finished product. It is applicable on medical devices (or services) where defects are revealed only after they have already been delivered or provided (Table 7.24).

Let us first review the fundamental definitions:

- Verification: Confirmation, through the provision of objective evidence, that specified requirements have been fulfilled. The verification will be achieved through activities such as calculations, comparing a new design specification with a similar proven design specification, and by performing tests and demonstrations.
- Validation: An approval, through the provision of objective evidence, that the requirements for a specific intended use or application have been fulfilled.
- Revalidation: A reapproval of validation in case any changes occurred within the process—a change of equipment, a change in human resources, raw material, and so on—that may affect the product.

Validation includes the process of identifying a process, planning its controls, documenting the plan and protocol, defining criteria and expected outputs, implementing measurement activities, and controlling the data. The objective is to plan controls that will ensure the delivery of processes within specified tolerances under established operating conditions. By using controls over critical process parameters, we can assure that the outputs of these processes will achieve their objectives, and provide us with conforming products. One may say that we monitor and control the stability of a process. What is a stable process? Stability can be defined by identifying the critical parameters for each process, and setting the appropriate criteria. Validation activities generate data that is used to monitor performances of processes. These performances reflect the characteristics of the medical device.

TABLE 7.24
Standard Requirements of Subclause 7.5.2.1

ISO 13485	ISO 9001
The organization shall apply validation controls on processes where results may not be validated and verified with monitoring and measurement activities	The organization shall apply validation controls on processes where results may not be validated and verified with monitoring and measurement activities
The processes include those where the deficiencies can be detected only during later stages, or when the product is being used	The processes include those where the deficiencies can be detected only during later stages, or when the product is being used
The data shall establish the ability of the processes to meet the predefined requirements	The data shall establish the ability of the processes to meet the predefined requirements
The organization shall arrange activities in order to perform validations, approval, and acceptance of these processes. The activities will ensure the planned result	The organization shall arrange activities in order to perform validations, approval, and acceptance of these processes. The activities will ensure the planned result
The activities will include definitions of parameters for evaluation of processes and the criteria for approval	The activities will include definitions of parameters for evaluation of processes and the criteria for approval
The organization shall verify that the equipment used to validate processes is qualified, approved, and intact	The organization shall verify that the equipment used to validate processes is qualified, approved, and intact
The organization shall provide evidence that employees are qualified to perform these validation processes	The organization shall provide evidence that employees are qualified to perform these validation processes
The organization shall establish and maintain methods and instructions for performing the process validations	The organization shall establish and maintain methods and instructions for performing the process validations
Records of the validation processes shall be included under the records control procedure as specified in subclause 4.2.4 (Control of Records)	Records of the validation processes shall be included under the records control procedure as specified in subclause 4.2.4 (Control of Records)
The organization shall identify processes and events where revalidation is required	The organization shall identify processes and events where revalidation is required
The use of computer software and its application for the production of product or service provision that may affect the product's quality needs to be validated. Validation shall include cases where changes to the software are performed	
The validation will be completed before implementing the software to the production process	
The organization shall establish a documented procedure for the issue	
Records of the validation of software shall be maintained and submitted to the records control process as specified in subclause 4.2.4 (Control of Records)	

Validation Circle

In order to initiate and implement effective validations of your processes, the matter must be considered by several parties related to the realization processes of the medical device. Each one will share its opinions and aspects on the matter, and together you will plan an effective validation system that will seize your processes. Who is to contribute to the circle?

- Quality management will ensure that the quality issues are addressed, and will plan the implementation of the validation throughout the quality management system; for example, through documentation such as procedures and work instructions, forms and records, training, and by implementing the verification on the internal audit plan.
- Quality assurance will be responsible for the planning and implementing of the monitoring system and processes, the analysis of the data, and the reporting and alerts system.
- Technical services will plan the implementation of the controls required on machines and equipment involved in the processes.
- Regulatory affairs will provide all the relevant inputs for the regulatory requirements that must be accounted for during the realization processes, and their effect on the process validation.
- The engineering and manufacturing team will share its opinion on how to implement the validations effectively throughout the realization process.
- Purchasing will be in charge of the controls to be implanted in relation to suppliers.
- Research and development will review that the appropriate product characteristics are being validated.

Evaluating and Identifying Processes for Validation

The first step is to examine the impact of a process on the quality of the medical device. When the influence of a process on the medical device is considerable or critical, and application of control will affect the quality of the medical device, it is needed to be controlled.

The next step in designing the validation is to make a distinction between processes that will be verified and processes that will be validated. A very famous diagram for evaluating whether a process needs to be validated or verified is included below. Sample a process and introduce it to the flow chart (Figure 7.1).

What is the different between a process that needs to be verified and a process that needs to be validated? The rule of a thumb is to ask whether a process can be verified with monitoring and measurements activities.

For each process, the specifications, inputs, resources, outputs, and criteria are defined. Controlling the process means evaluating its outputs, and establishing with evidence that the process reached its objectives. A process that can be controlled and have its outputs approved using monitoring and measurement activities is a process that can be verified; you monitor the outputs and measure them with criteria. The result is clear—the process either met or did not meet its requirements. For example, a cutting process may be measured; an employee may take the product, measure it, compare it to a diagram, and decide whether the process was done according to the specification or not. A color of a part may be compared and verified.

When is the verification not cost effective? In order to verify certain processes in an effective manner, 100% of the outputs (i.e., the medical devices) need to be tested.

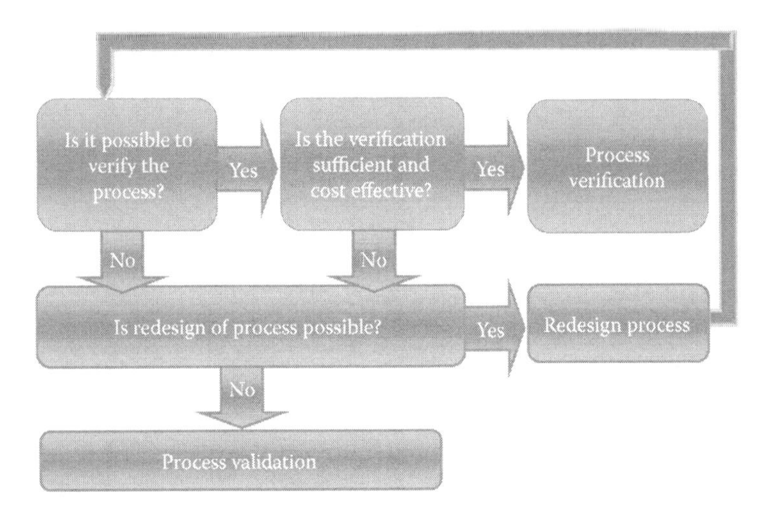

FIGURE 7.1 Distinction between processes for validation and processes for verification.

For example, the verification of sterilized sealing process is done only when the seal is opened and tested. Such verification is not cost efficient. It will not be cost effective to open each medical device and verify its sealing. The organization is left with two options—either perform 100% inspections (for every device) or validate the process. Another issue is the sequence of processes. In some cases, early processes may disqualify verifications of later processes. For example, if you are performing a CNC process that may affect the cleanliness of the medical device, you cannot verify the cleanliness by testing each of the medical devices. Once again, verification is not cost effective. Examples of processes that may be verified include:

- Manual cutting processes
- Testing for color, turbidity, total pH for solutions
- Visual inspection of printed circuit boards
- Manufacturing and testing of wiring harnesses

The level of verification must be optimal and sufficient in order to eliminate unacceptable risks. In other words, the verification must provide reliable data and a correct situation report regarding the process. If you can ensure the conditions mentioned above, you may control the process with verification activities, and submit it to the requirements of clause 8.2.3 (Monitoring and Measurement of Processes).

When the evaluation of the process has demonstrated that the process is not verifiable, there is the option of redesigning a change in a manufacturing process, and to bring it to a verifiable level. However, you will have to evaluate the process again and ensure that the conditions above are met. If redesign is not possible due to the nature of the process, or the verification is not cost effective, then a validation of the process will be designed and implemented. Verifiable manufacturing processes that were changed or redesigned are to be evaluated again in order to ensure that they are still verifiable.

The outputs of risk management and the requirements for controls may require that certain process validations be implemented; The validation is used for verifying the effectiveness of the risk control measure. These will be documented on the risk management file. The risk analysis indicates events or situations where a failure of the process could cause a failure of the device, meaning that such process need to be controlled. The level and severity of the risks will determine the required level of process confidence. One of the requirements when implementing control of risks is the proof of effectiveness. This will be achieved with the appropriate validations. Thus, when reviewing the needs for validations, the manufacturer must review the outputs of the risk management process.

All of the realization processes are to be evaluated. This is will ensure an effective process control. The evaluation is the responsibility of the validation circle. I suggest drawing a review for each process that will cover the following issues:

- The name or identification of the process
- The critical parameters that need to be controlled, and the criteria
- Relevant documentation, such as diagrams, work instructions, technical data, and specifications
- The current control, and the means with which it is being controlled
- Example of measurements such as records, evidence, relevant nonconformities, or complaints
- Resolution regarding the necessity for validation
- Approval and identity of the approver

This review is part of the validation planning and will serve as a quality record. You can design a form that will document the review. The output of this stage is a list of processes that need to be validated. Examples include:

- Sterilization processes
- Clean room ambient conditions
- Aseptic filling processes
- Sterile packaging sealing processes
- Lyophilization (freeze-drying) processes
- Heat-treating processes
- Plating processes
- Plastic injection molding processes
- Computer design processes

Process Parameters for Validation

After defining the processes to be validated, it is required that you define for each the parameters that will be controlled. Parameters affect the process performance; thus, the parameters are related directly to the quality, functionality, performance, safety, and intended use requirements. In order to implement effective validations, you must understand what the key parameters affecting the quality of the product or the performance of a process are; for example, temperature, pressure, compound of raw material, concentrations, tension, time, machine cycle, and setup conditions. Identifying key parameters will help indicate what is to be measured.

First review and analyze the effect of each process on the specifications and characteristics of the medical device; for example, a sterilization process affects the safety for the user. The sealing process affects the packaging specifications. These are critical product characteristics that must be maintained. Values and levels for these characteristics are already determined (i.e., SAL and seal strength). In order to reach these specifications of characteristics, processes must maintain certain conditions. When determining the parameters for control, it is important to correlate the inputs with the outputs. For example, by the sealing process, the temperature and the pressure are critical in order to reach the level of strength. In a plastic molding, the injection formation of the part is affected by the hold time of the part on the production tool before opening and releasing the part (a fraction of a second can be critical). The input (holding time) is directly related to the output (form of the part). These parameters will indicate the stability of a process; thus, these parameters will be controlled.

After identifying the parameters, it is necessary to relate them to process tools and elements that are influenced by these parameters; namely, machines, software, production tools, human resources, and infrastructures. These elements will supply us with the data and results regarding the process parameters.

Identification of Impact on Processes

Validation activities serve manufacturers monitoring certain characteristics of processes under controlled conditions. Failure in equipment, tools, systems, and components may affect the process and the quality of the product. The manufacturer must assess the impact of such failure on the medical device and its characteristics.

The impact may be a direct or indirect. Direct impact results in the failure of system used in realizing the product; for example, machines, production tools, raw material, and components. Indirect impact results in the failure of systems that support the realization systems, such as utilities and infrastructures, human resources, and work environments. The evaluation of the impact may assist in planning the control and validation test more effectively. Risk analysis may serve as an input for such assessment.

Desired Outputs of Processes (Acceptance Criteria)

After identifying the parameters, you need to determine, for each process, the target values and their acceptance criteria. Target values are the optimal values for the process parameter. These values will demonstrate the stability and capability of a process, and ensure that requirements are met and accepted.

The criteria evaluate the results compared to the requirements. The limits of the criteria (target values, upper and lower control limits) are based on product or process specifications. The objective of the criteria is to demonstrate effectiveness of processes and to support decisions for judging, evaluating, and determining by facts, values, and data the compliance of the processes. The criteria will support the validation by indicating the status of the parameters; that is, either accepted or rejected. The criteria will be planned according to the types of data and the statistical analysis methods. Deciding upon limits depends on the analysis method used; for example, action levels, control levels, acceptance levels, specification levels, and worst case conditions. The objective of these limits is to instruct the manufacturer in when process adjustment are required; for example, when results show that the process is deviating, then an action is to be taken in order to restore peace once again.

The criteria may be objective or subjective. Objective criteria means distinctiveness, invariance, and controllability; the results are being compared to a set of determined values and a decision is made based on the comparison—either accepted or rejected. Subjective criteria are when the results are being evaluated and submitted for assimilation by an individual. The criteria are subjected using knowledge and experience. Subjective criteria need to be supported with justifications for process conformity.

The criteria will be documented on the test protocols, and are required to be approved before submission for use. The following issues are to be considered:

- The manufacturer will develop a policy for establishing and determining the criteria: scope, relation to the processes it serves, objectives, activities, method for documentation, and methods for reporting.
- The criteria shall refer to documented product requirements or characteristics that they control—materials, functionality and technical specifications, product characteristics, reference to drawings, and quality requirements.
- Reference to the required information for evaluation against the criteria is to be defined—test data, findings, and measurements.
- The criteria will be planned in relation to the quality requirements.
- If there are standards, regulatory requirements, or technical specifications that demand the establishment and implementation of specific criteria or of technical standards for measurements for a certain type of process or product, it is required that these criteria be implemented in your tests.
- When there is no standard or technical requirement for criteria, the manufacturer will determine and document the criteria.
- The criteria will be designed in order to provide alarms regarding the status of the output, and to define when the results are regarded as nonconforming.
- Criteria that appears in the risk management plan and is required to control risks shall be incorporated in the criteria.

Worst Case Conditions

The worst case conditions must be determined. These are a set of conditions covering the upper and lower limit of process parameters. These conditions simulate possible circumstances during the realization process, which indicate a clear unwanted trend in the process (regarding its performances). The conditions will be defined according to the risks related to the process. Reaching these levels does not indicate that the process is nonconforming yet, but they warn and notify the manufacturer that the situation might pose a risk to the outputs of the process, and may impact the integrity of the product.

For example, the risk of a cleaning process is an unacceptable level of uncleanliness. You have already identified the process parameters, which influence the levels of cleanliness. You determined the values for lower and upper limits and the target results. Now you must determine the lower and upper limits in the level of cleanliness in a worst case condition.

When appropriate, worst case conditions will be the combination of several critical parameters. For example, by a sealing process there are three critical parameters: temperature, time, and pressure. A combination of the three might result in a worst case condition. You must identify the combination of these parameters and determine the levels of worst case.

These worst case conditions must be challenged, validated, and approved. At a later stage the manufacturer can decide which preventive actions and activities are necessary in order to avoid reaching these conditions.

Selecting a Method for Analyzing the Data

Methods and techniques for analysis and demonstrating parameter results for validation must be determined. The purpose of the techniques are:

- To demonstrate objectively, through data, that processes meet their specifications
- To replicate actual use conditions

The manufacturer will determine a method suitable and relevant to the type of data. Using the method will provide them with an actual accurate status report regarding its processes:

- The method will be determined in accordance with the manufacturer's analysis needs.
- The method will allow comparison to objectives and the goals of parameters.
- The method will be able to provide the manufacturer with alarms regarding the processes.
- The method will enable the manufacturer to compare new data with old data.
- When international, national, or local standards for analysis techniques are demanded by your local authorities, they will implemented.
- The use and instruction for implementing the method will be documented or referred.

There are many methods and tools that can be used for analysis in process validation. There is not sufficient space here to review them all; however, here is a short summary of the objectives that may be relevant to your processes when selecting a method for analysis (Table 7.25).

Revalidation

The need and actions required for revalidation must be determined. Revalidation is required in situations where you detected that process parameters may not provide the necessary outputs, for various reasons, and you applied an action. As a manufacturer, you must identify such events throughout your processes:

- When corrective action was implemented in a process or a product
- When changes or improvements in the product design, and thus the process, were initiated and implemented
- When the personnel operating the process were changed, and it affected the quality of the product
- When work instructions or work methods were changed
- When material was changed and affected the quality of the product
- When a new supplier is introduced to the process
- When deviations or negative trends were detected and measures such as corrective actions or changes were applied (the topic of deviation will be comprehensively discussed in this chapter)
- Changes in the packaging processes of the product
- When a certain process produces excessive defects
- Evaluation or troubleshooting of a process

While a process is validated, tools, machines, and equipment will be requalified. Requalification is needed:

- When a service, maintenance, or major repair was applied to the machines or equipment
- When production tools were amended
- When adverse trends in equipment performance occurred
- When the process was relocated to another machine or facility
- When the replacement of critical spares parts was initiated

In some cases, annual or periodic revalidation or requalification of processes, tools, equipment, or machines is required according to the: manufacturer's instructions,

TABLE 7.25
Methods for Statistical Analysis

Objective	Method and Known Statistical Technique
Determining through the product the acceptance level of the process	Sampling of a product and using this sample to decide whether to accept or reject: Acceptance sampling plan
Evaluation of the ability of a process to consistently meet its specifications by sampling its outputs	Examining the processes over a period of time by sampling outputs of the process and placing them on a control chart, comparing them to control limits and criteria: Capability study
The testing of controls implemented on process parameters in order to evaluate their performances	Creating and initiating situations where these controls would react. For example, inspecting the power backup system by shutting off the electricity, or examining the effectiveness of a visual control system by inserting a defective part in advance: Challenge tests
Identifying the cause of a differentiation between two identical process outputs (units of product)	Examining two assembled medical devices and then swapping their components, reexamining, and analyzing the cause of the differences: Component swapping study
Identifying and analyzing changes in the process and mapping their trends. The identification and examination will detect the root cause of a change	Sampling process units according to a plan and identifying and analyzing changes in the process. After the change is identified, trends are analyzed. Such a technique assists in identifying process parameters with high potential to induce a change: Control charts
Robust processes	Reducing variations of process outputs by selecting the optimal process inputs: Dual response approach to robust design Robust design methods Robust tolerance analysis
Implementation of preventive actions and control of risks	Systematic identification of possible failures in a process through the analysis of possible root causes and risks: Failure modes and effects analysis (FMEA) Fault tree analysis (FTA)
Assuring stability and reproducibility of machines, tools, and equipment	Data analysis of the precision and accuracy machines and equipment, and applying appropriate controls
Planning the optimal process output	Calculating the statistical relation between process inputs and process outputs. Using such methods can assist in identifying the optimal combination between different inputs and augment the process: Response surface study Tolerance analysis

regulatory requirements, known associated risks and changes in processes that may occur but are not detected.

The need for revalidation shall be evaluated and documented on the validation plan. For each revalidation activity a criteria will be defined according to the type of revalidation.

Validation Plan

Before we discuss the validation plan let us go through the definitions:

- Validation plan: a document that specifies the policy, strategy, and methods used for conducting the validation of products or processes in the organization. The plan will identify responsibilities, equipment, requirements for qualification (in equipment as well as human resources), and schedules.
- Validation program: an organized effort with the goal of providing the assurance that equipment and personnel are qualified, and that processes are validated with reference to regulatory as well as organizational requirements.
- Test protocol: a document reviewed and approved by authorized personnel describing the activities and their sequence of the testing of a process, system, or piece of equipment. Results of the test are documented, and serve as evidence of the performance of the process.

The objective of the validation plan is to present a documented approach, strategy, and methodology for the validation processes with reference to the relevant elements that will support the validation—in other words, identifying those processes to be validated; determining the activities, timelines, and schedules for the validation; the interrelationships between processes requiring validation; references to documentation; and timing for revalidations.

The plan will include:

- The scope of the plan; that is, which processes and products are included under its scope.
- Identification of equipment, tools, systems, and components that may affect the process.
- Description of activities and sequences of the validation processes—such as activities, timelines, schedules, and locations.
- The plan shall include reference to relevant documentation; for example, procedures, process flow diagrams, test protocols, DMR, customer requirements, instructions, technical specification, and technical details.
- Roles and functions that will be involved in the validation activities will be specifically described. In addition to defining roles, it is necessary to relate each role to its duties and specific responsibilities in the validation processes; for example, the planning and development of validation activities, executions, controls, and the approval of results. The definition shall relate the responsibility to its relevant process elements; approving documentation, development of computer software, in charge of infrastructures, operating a machine, operating a monitoring device.
- The master validation plan will provide instruction on how to detect, evaluate, and react to deviations, and will state the time interval permitted between each validation.
- The requirement for revalidation will be defined, and events where revalidations activities are needed will be identified.

The plan, as mentioned, draws the basic principles of the validation into the organization. From the plan you will derive the specific protocols that provide details regarding the validation activities; for example, control plans, or IQ, OQ, and PQ protocols—where specific procedures, equipment, personnel, and records are mentioned and related to a process. Such documents and specifications are more targeted towards a specific process, and thus will be more effective.

The plan will be reviewed and approved by the validation circle. The review will be periodic in order to ensure that any changes implemented to the realization processes were considered and referred on the validation plan. The plan will be submitted to the document control process as required in subclause 4.2.3 (Control of Documents).

Installation Qualification (IQ) Activities

IQ activities are set of actions and activities with the goal of ensuring that all key and ancillary aspects of human resources, machinery, equipment, or tools meet the required specifications, are appropriately set and installed, and are ready to operate and provide the process with the normal conditions for realization. As a manufacturer, you need to identify situations where installation conditions may affect processes, such as:

- Introducing a new product to the production
- Installation of a new machine or piece of equipment
- Relocation of a machine
- Repairing or readjusting machines or equipment
- Change on production lines
- Installing new elements on the productions line
- Production setups
- Implementing new production processes
- Changes to or new installation of infrastructures
- Changes to or repair of the work environment

Such activities require a validation of their specifications. The reason for this is that the IQ phase is based on the design specifications of the system elements. In other words, the design specifications are to be fully implemented. The tests will verify the conditions, establishing by objective evidences that all technical aspects and technical resources invested in the processes are designed and implemented in order to achieve the predefined specifications:

- They are qualified to participate in the processes
- They assist in meeting the specifications
- They will deliver satisfying results

The IQ activities have several purposes:

1. Implementation of the supplier's instructions regarding equipment, machines, and tools
2. Compliance with system requirements and specifications
3. Compliance with calibration requirements and specifications
4. Compliance with maintenance requirements and plans
5. Establishment of procedures and instructions for installation and maintenance
6. Enhancement of the human resources competence needed for the installation activities
7. Control of tools and equipment, including the systematic detection of failures and submission for correction

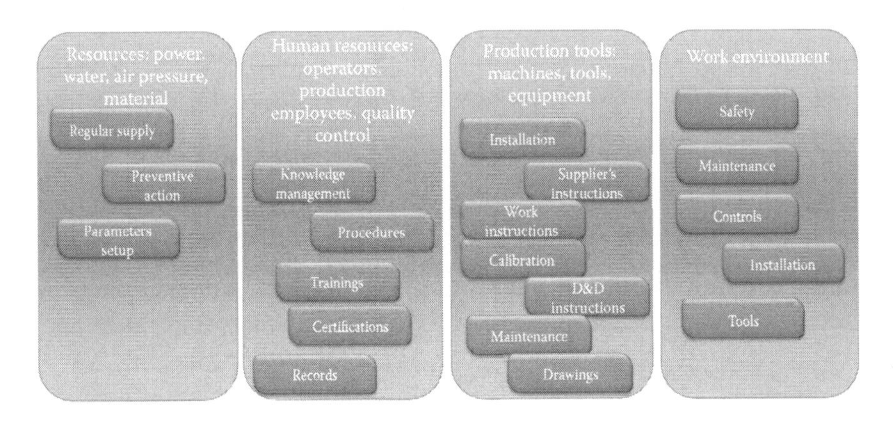

FIGURE 7.2 IQ activities.

8. Implementation of preventive measures
9. Ensuring reproducibility of processes

Take a look at the above diagram (Figure 7.2).

Each scope has its own set of activities that will ensure its optimal conditions. For each production area or issue, you must develop the controls and activities in order to verify each field's specifications and characteristics. These activities are to be verified. There are normal conditions that will ensure that tools and equipment will operate optimally. You are required to initiate such conditions through the different elements.

IQ—IQ Protocol

The IQ activities will be defined, documented, and recorded. The validation circle will establish a protocol; a set of rules and events describing how test activities will be performed. This protocol will include criteria for acceptance or rejection, identify all the elements that needed to be validated, specify for each the validation test records and the results of the test, and relate to deviations. The documentation will serve as the required evidence. The objectives of the protocol are:

- Description of the scope of the IQ activities
- Identification of the system and elements that will be tested
- Identification of the utilities that support the equipments
- Provision of specifications of the tests and test activities
- Identification of the tools and equipment, or other accessories needed for the tests
- Identification of those responsible for performing the tests
- Reference to documents relevant to the tests
- Presentation of the criteria
- Recording of results and evaluating them with criteria
- Documentation and analysis of deviations
- Signed approval of the IQ activities

Therefore, a superficial review of the installation of a new machine would be as follows:

- The installation activities will be defined; that is, the supplier's specifications and instructions.

- The installation performed by the technician will be documented; the supplier's representatives on a specific date.
- The tools and equipment used for the installation must be appropriate.
- The installation will be validated (the technician and representatives of the manufacturer will perform test runs to the machine).
- A report indicating the installation activities is expected (what was done and by whom).
- After the installation and a test report or statement of installation specifying the tests, the results and the indication that all specifications were achieved is to be produced and signed by an authorized person.

Each type of machine and equipment requires its own protocol due to the fact that each one has different characteristics, such as different elements for control, different frequencies of installation, different roles in the organization, and different tests and results. The principle, however, is the same. For a production machine, the IQ activities will have to be carried out once the machine is installed; but for a production tool that is constructed according to a need (a production order), the IQ activities would have to be done each time the production tool is requested.

IQ—Identification of Documentation

The IQ protocol will specify all the required documentation for the installation and for the maintenance activities (accepted from suppliers or internal documents)—user manuals, drawings, maintenance plans, troubleshootings, specifications, and spare parts lists. The IQ test will verify:

- That these documents are listed and accessible
- Each document for its edition, revision, approval, and location (access is an important factor)
- That each associated employee is familiar with the documentation and knows where to find it, if required

IQ—Identification and Control of Equipment

Each production tool, equipment, machine calibration device, or any other physical system component used during the process will be identified according to a defined method: manufacturer/supplier, model, serial number, internal number, location, and reference to specific product or part. The identification will be documented on the protocol. The objective defines exactly what is to be controlled. For each equipment or tool, a role or a function will be assigned for the installation, approval, and maintenance.

This document will include a report regarding the status and intactness of the equipment with relation to the different elements of the equipment. For example, in the case of a plastic mold production tool various elements must be controlled—air connections, the ejector, and the hot runner. These elements will be reviewed for their intactness according to the acceptance criteria, and then approved for use. You must identify these critical elements, define the criteria for each, and test them; they will be either accepted or rejected. The acceptance criteria are the supplier or designer specifications plus verifications that the manufacturer has decided upon. The responsible party needs to go through this list and verify that each element defined on it is as specified. For each equipment or tool, a responsible party will be assigned for the installation, approval, and maintenance.

After the review, the status regarding the usability of the equipment and tools will be documented and clearly indicated on the equipment. This will ensure that no one will use unauthorized equipment.

IQ—Human Resources

The human resource participating in the installation and maintenance activities must identified and approved. It must be ensured that:

- The personnel are competent and certified to perform the activities.
- The personnel are familiar with the processes and activities of the installation or maintenance.
- The personnel are familiar with the tests and criteria of the installation or maintenance activities.
- The personnel are familiar with the required records.

The verification and approval will be done in accordance with the training and certification methods and the appropriate customary documentation in the organization.

IQ—Installation Activities

All test activities for installation and maintenance of the equipment and tools will be defined and documented: procedures, work instructions, or process flow diagrams or on the protocol itself, with a reference to the documentation. These procedures will be controlled and submitted to the documents control process in your organization (subclause 4.2.3).

If maintenance activities are in accordance with supplier's instructions, you must maintain these instructions, document or refer to them and ensure that they are available. The performance of these activities and the results will be recorded on the protocol: who performed, when, and what has been done. If additional activities were conducted, they will be documented too. The documentation of the activities will serve as quality records.

IQ—Production Utilities

All critical utilities necessary for the operation of the equipment will be defined, reviewed, and approved: amps, voltage, water pressure, air pressure, temperature, hydraulic power, and water pressure. Such utilities are to be applied and connected in conformance with their specifications. These utilities will be reviewed for their conformance according to defined acceptance criteria, and then approved for use. You will need to:

- Identify these critical utilities
- Define for each the installation activities
- Define for each the tests, the criteria and control them (either accepted or rejected)

IQ—Work Environment

All elements of the work environment that relate to the process are to be identified and documented. The work environment is to be validated, and it is to be ensured that all necessary elements were appropriately installed and will provide an optimal work environment supporting the process:

- Verification that the installation was done according to predefined specifications is needed. This verification will ensure that the work environment conditions are according the process needs.

- Procedures and work instruction regarding the work environment will be established and implemented; for example, cleaning procedures, employees' behavior instructions, and so on.
- A maintenance plan will be established.
- Verification that all the required controls were appropriately installed, such as particle count, and temperature and humidity measurements.

IQ—Safety Measures and Alarms

All safety measures, and emergency backup systems and alarms are to be identified and documented. It is required that you verify that the installation of such systems has been done according to the specifications, and that these systems will operate as expected in time of need. One way to verify this is to perform a challenge test. The tests and examinations of such systems as well as the criteria for these controls will be defined on the IQ protocol. The results will be recorded.

IQ—Control of Monitoring and Measuring Devices

All monitoring and measuring devices participating in the installation activities are supposed to be controlled according to the requirements of clause 7.6 (Control of Monitoring and Measuring Devices); that is, they are to be identified, calibrated according to predefined standards, maintained, protected, and preserved. For each IQ activity you will need to:

- Identify the relevant monitoring and measuring devices
- Review and approve that these devices are controlled, calibrated, and ready for use

The review and approval will ensure that the devices needed for the installation are appropriate for use. The review will be defined on a form or a checklist, and will be documented on the protocol.

IQ—Deviations

Deviations are a departure from the specified requirements and may occur during the IQ activities. A deviation is, in principle, nonconformity because equipment specifications were not met. Each deviation will be evaluated for its severity and impact on the medical device. Where a deviation was applied and corrected it will be introduced to the revalidation policy as mentioned on the validation plan.

However, there are cases where the deviation is considered and accepted. Each deviation from the criteria will be recorded on the IQ protocol referring to the impact of the deviation on the installation. It is necessary to define who reviews a deviation once it has been detected. If deviation was accepted and approved, a justification for the acceptance is mandatory. The details to be recorded include: the deviation, the reason or justification for the acceptance, the identity of the approver, and a signature.

IQ—Approval of Activities

After completing all the activities a last review is required in order to approve that all specifications and requirements are met. You will need to ensure that:

- All test were conducted and supplied with satisfying results.
- All documentation is available.
- All records are accomplished and available.

- All the criteria were met, (if a system did not meet its criteria but has been approved, a justification is required).
- All deviations were either handled or accepted with justifications.
- Final approval of the IQ stage—the systems are ready for the realization processes.

The review and approval will be carried out by the validation circle in order to ensure that all aspects are resolved. The review and approval will be documented on the protocol. Once the IQ has been approved the manufacturer may proceed to the next stage. The report will be distributed to the relevant persons and functions operating the process: QA mangers, production managers, and production employees.

IQ—Expected Records

- List of all machines, equipment, tools, system and substructures that require IQ activities
- List of all documentation (internal and external) that will support the IQ activities; namely, user manuals, supplier's instructions, as well as procedures and work instructions
- Records of the certification and training of personnel performing the installation activities
- List of all activities needed to be performed, and documentation of the activities—their tests, reviews, and approval
- List of all utilities that needed to be tested and controlled; documentation of the test; and reviews and approval
- List of all the safety measures, and emergency and backup systems and alarms, that needed to be tested and controlled; documentation of the test; and reviews and approval
- List of all monitoring and measuring devices that needed to be tested and controlled; documentation of the test; and reviews and approval
- Final review and approval of the IQ stage

The records of performing the tests and the results, along with the approvals, will serve as quality records and will be submitted to the process of records control in your organization as required in subclause 4.2.4 (Control of Records).

Operation Qualification (OQ) Activities

Operation qualification activities are a set of actions and activities with the goal of ensuring by objective evidence that all process outputs and results comply with the predefined specifications and requirements; that is, that:

- The results are accepted under the appropriate production conditions.
- The results are evaluated and compared with an approved predefined criteria.
- The evaluation provides compliance with requirements and specifications.

The results of the OQ activities will allow you to identify and detect nonconformities or deviations from the specifications in real time, and react appropriately before releasing the process for production. This stage would be achieved when:

- All the process elements that may affect the process outputs are identified and controlled.
- The personnel operating the process is appropriately trained and qualified.

- The inputs to the process are optimal.
- The validation tests were planned according to the medical device specifications and provide a clear validation supported with data.
- The criteria are validated and present a suitable method for the evaluation, and refer to the medical device's requirements.
- The verifications of the tests are conducted as planned.
- Anomalies, deviations, discrepancies, and other unacceptable conditions were identified and corrected before the approval of the process.

OQ Protocol

The activities and the results criteria of the OQ will be documented. It is required that you determine and describe the tasks to be carried out, the criteria, and the expected outputs; that is, "who does what," "how it will be done," "what is expected," "what must be recorded," and "what is to be done in a particular case or event." The documentation will serve as the required evidence. The objectives of the protocol are:

- Description of the scope of the OQ activities
- Provision of specifications of the tests
- Reference to the relevant documents
- Presentation of the criteria
- Identification of roles responsible for performing the tests
- Recording of results
- Documentation and analysis of deviations
- Signed approval of the job

The protocol will include details about the process and the validation; for example, product or part, dates, participants, responsibilities, locations, and so on.

OQ—Description and Identification of All System Components

The objective of OQ activities is to qualify the important elements of the equipment, components, and system elements that affect the outputs of the process: that is, machines, equipment materials, and production tools. These were identified already during the IQ stage through:

- Processes
- Production utilities
- Components and elements of the machines and equipment
- Production tools
- Safety measures
- Human resources

These elements will need to be identified and documented on the protocol. The next stage will be to define the tests and validations for each element. The difference from the IQ activities is that the IQ verifies the installation while the OQ verifies performances.

OQ—Supporting Documents

The protocol will refer to each of the required or necessary documents relevant to the test specified on the protocol—such as, standard operating procedures, manuals, diagrams, user instructions, forms and protocols, calibration instructions, work environment specifications, work instructions, DMR, DHF, statistical techniques, or methodologies, and maintenance plans. On the protocol you must verify that all the required documentation is available, up to date, and legible.

OQ—Human Resources

The protocol will identify that personnel operating the process are trained, qualified, and certified as required. Beyond operating machines, tools, and equipment, the personnel is expected to be familiar with relevant procedures and work instructions, to know the expected process outputs, how to detect nonconformities during the process, and what is to be done when one is detected.

Before initiating the process, the assigned personnel will be validated according to the training and certification policy of the organization. Human resources that operate or are involved on the process will be trained regarding the maintenance and preservation of the IQ and OQ conditions. This validation will be documented on the OQ protocol. It is recommended that you fill out a checklist before each job in order to evaluate and verify that the personnel know all the procedures and work instructions, read the relevant part of the DMR, know all the previous nonconformities of the process, and know what to do when one is found (e.g., stopping the machine, removing the parts from the production area, identifying the parts, etc.).

OQ—Monitoring and Measurement Devices and Control Gauges

Tools for validation such as monitoring and measurement devices or control gauges that participate in the OQ phase must be recorded and validated. The validation will ensure that they are intact, registered, calibrated, and controlled as required in clause 7.6 (Control of Monitoring and Measurement Devices). Registration will include identification, such as serial numbers or other elements. Registration is necessary for traceability. Before initiating the processes, the performance of the tool will be tested and validated. The objective is to prove that the tool was intact for the OQ tests. The results will be documented on the protocol. The issue is relevant to control gauges as well as monitoring and measurement devices.

OQ—Materials

The material input to the process is to be verified and validated:

- The OQ protocol will include a list of the required material for the process. The test will verify that these materials are available for the process.
- The storage conditions of the materials will be defined and verified on the protocol (e.g., the required temperature, packaging, transportation, and safety).
- The conditioning for the material before the process will be defined and validated with appropriate documentation on the protocol (e.g., cleaning, sterilization, humidity, and temperature).
- Types of material: raw material, wrappings, containers, tubes, garments. The test, criteria for evaluations, and results will be documented on the protocol.

OQ—Machines and Equipment

The performance of machines and equipment that will participate in the process need to be validated. The validation will ensure that they are intact, maintained, and controlled. The objectives are:

- Proving that the each machine and equipment is intact for this specific job throughout the job (from beginning to end)
- Proving that the process parameters are as required through comparison to predefined criteria
- Proving process stability

Machine, tools, and equipment performances will be verified for accuracy and precision through the examination of critical parameters; for example, machine cycles, temperatures, software parameters, feeds, speeds, voltage rates, or holding time. These will be compared using analysis methods, predefined acceptance criteria, and control limits. The comparison will allow you to decide upon the capability of the machine. The activities shall cover the following issues:

- The machine's tools and equipment will be identified and registered on the protocol. The registrations will include identifications such as serial numbers, names, models and locations. Registration is necessary for traceability.
- The protocol will specify and describe which process parameters are to be controlled.
- The protocol will specify and describe the tests activities, the validations, the durations of the tests, and the quantity and frequency of the sampling.
- Acceptance criteria will be defined or referred for each test, and will assist in deciding whether the machines and equipment performances are accepted or rejected.
- The manufacturer will perform initial sample runs on the processes: machines, assemblies, function test etc. The runs are necessary to establish the baseline parameters and detect any issues related to the process and its outputs.
- The inputs of the process parameters will be determined and adjusted according to the element that operates them (e.g., machines). The test and validations needed to verify the process outputs will be then applied. The objective is to determine whether the process outputs meet the specifications. The outputs of the parameters will be reviewed, compared, and evaluated with the predefined criteria.
- The evaluation will be carried out using the techniques that were determined (i.e., statistical, qualitative, observational). The results will determine the stability of the process. If validating parts, indicate how many and when. If measuring process parameters, you need to determine how the data will be extracted, where they will be recorded, and how to compare them to the criteria.
- Normal conditions for the tests must be defined. For example, some machines need time to "warm up" until they reach their normal working conditions. Bear in mind that some systems will need to be run for hours, and be sampled for hundreds of parts until the machines reach suitable production conditions and deliver sufficient data that will allow analyzing to proceed correctly.

OQ—Challenge Tests

Challenge tests will be initiated in order to set upper and lower limits to a process. By challenging the system you are detecting where the action limits are and where the alerts are located; that is, the worst case limits and situations warning and notifying the manufacturer that process parameters might pose a risk to the outputs of the process, and may impact the integrity of the product.

Each process will be tested. The test will identify the optimal level and value targets, the upper limit and the lower limit of the process. The identification will be achieved through running the process a number of times, examining the results, and comparing them to the acceptance criteria. The starting point is establishing process parameters based on previous knowledge or experience and developing optimal parameters as the process runs advance. This is the time to apply the worst case situations, and to detect the combination of system parameters that may bring you closer to a risk. For example, the sealing process has a combination of three process parameters—heat, pressure, and time. Now is the time to calculate the combination that brings process outputs to a level of risk. The results will be a practical limitation of your process parameters. For each test you will need to determine:

- Which parameters are to be challenged
- The required extent of the test; the duration of the run, number of processes, cycles, or runs
- The sample rate; loads, parts, and units

The limits will ensure that the system operating unit is stable, and the process outputs meet the requirements.

OQ—Utilities

All utilities and their accessories will be verified. The verifications will ensure that they are functioning as specified; for example, that the air compressor and filter are constructed together, as planned. The test will be defined and will refer to acceptance criteria; that is, a diagram or documented instruction that verifies the functionality.

Critical utility parameters will be tested. For example, the air pressure will be verified for only 1 cubic feet per minute (CFM), cooling water will be verified by measuring its temperature. These will be compared, using analysis methods, to the predefined acceptance criteria and limits in order to decide upon the capability of the utilities. The tests will be specified on the OQ protocol, along with the recorded results.

OQ—Work Environment

All work environment elements that support the process or that may affect must be verified; for example, the air quality, light, humidity, and temperature. The elements that affect the process will be identified on the protocol. It is required that you set tests for each that will prove that the work environment conditions meet the criteria. The test will measure results of controls against the criteria; review results of particle counts, room temperature, and humidity. The controls will be specified on the protocol indicating which parameters are to be tested, how, with what equipment, and the results will be recorded.

Another important aspect is the consideration of agronomic and psychological factors that may affect the human resources and prevent them from operating the process as needed. For example, long-term exposure to noise may result in distractions. Such distractions may lead to inattention of the process at hand. If preventions or accessories for the human resources are defined, the test will verify their availability.

OQ—Safety Measures

Safety measures, emergency and backup systems, and alarms need to be verified. These systems will be identified on the protocol, and you are required to plan a validation test for each and provide evidence that they are functioning as planned. An effective way to examine these systems is to challenge them and initiate situations where they must be put into practice and evaluated; for example, shutting down the power and allowing the system to run on the backup power system.

In cases where the system must run under emergencies such as backup power, you are required to validate the process parameters under these conditions. This is logical as production conditions have been changed, and you must verify your process parameters under the new conditions.

OQ—Deviations

Deviations are a departure from the specified requirements and may occur during the OQ activities. Each deviation will be evaluated for its severity and impact on the medical device. There are cases when the deviation is considered and accepted. Not every deviation will prevent the medical device from meeting its requirements. Each deviation from the criteria will be recorded on the protocol referring to the impact of the deviation on the operation. It is necessary to define who reviews a deviation once it has been detected. Where a deviation has occurred and has been corrected it will be introduced to the revalidation policy, as mentioned on the validation plan. If deviation was accepted and approved, a justification for the acceptance is mandatory. The details to be recorded include: the deviation, the reason or justification for the acceptance, the identity of the approver, and a signature.

OQ—Summary Report

After completing all the activities a last documented review is required in order to approve that all specifications and requirements are met, such as:

- All tests were conducted and supplied with satisfying results.
- All the criteria were met (when a system did not meet its criteria but was approved, a justification is required).
- All documents necessary for the processes are available.
- All records are accomplished and available.
- All deviations were identified, investigated, and appropriate actions were determined with justifications.
- Final approval of the OQ stage—the process outputs are satisfying and the process is ready for the next phase.

The review and approval will be carried out by the validation circle in order to ensure that all aspects are resolved. The review approval will be documented on the protocol. Once the OQ has been approved the manufacturer may precede to the next stage—the performance qualification. The report will be distributed to the relevant persons, and functions that need to operate the process (i.e., QA mangers, production managers, production employees).

OQ—Expected Records

- List of all machines, equipment, tools, systems, and substructures that require IQ activities
- List of all documentation (internal and external) that will support the OQ activities (e.g., procedures, work instructions, test instructions, test protocols, and statistical techniques)
- List of all materials required for the process
- Records of the certification and training of personnel performing or operating the processes

- List of all monitoring and measuring devices that need to be tested and controlled; documentation of the tests, reviews, and approval
- List of all test activities that need to be performed; documentation of the activities; their tests, reviews, and approval
- List of all utilities and infrastructures that need to be tested and controlled; documentation of the tests, reviews, and approval
- Identification of related work environment elements
- List of all safety measure, and emergency backup systems and alarms that need to be tested and controlled; documentation of the tests, reviews, and approval
- Acceptance criteria and analysis technique for each test
- Final review and approval of the OQ stage

The records of performing the tests and the results along with the approvals will serve as quality records, and will be submitted to the process of records control in your organization as required in subclause 4.2.4 (Control of Records).

Performance Qualification (PQ) Activities

Performance qualification (PQ) activities are a set of test activities carried out after all the OQ activities have been reviewed and approved. The objective of the PQ is to demonstrate that a process can generate products or results that meet all specifications consistently over time and changes. Change may occur as the changing of shifts, weekend shutdowns, and the use of different operators. The process capability and stability were established and achieved during the OQ phase. It is now necessary to ensure these for the entire job. This will be achieved through the establishment and implementation of continuous tests and data analysis until a satisfying level of confidence has been obtained.

PQ—Protocol

The activities, results, and criteria of PQ will be defined and documented. It is required that you determine and describe the tasks to be carried out, the criteria for each test, and the expected outputs. The objectives of the protocol are:

- Description of the scope of the PQ activities
- Provision of specifications of the tests
- Reference to relevant documents
- Identification of the roles responsible for performing the tests
- Presentation of the criteria needed to prove the level of confidence
- Recording of results
- Documentation and analysis of deviations
- Signed approval of the job

The protocol will be designed by the validation circle in order to ensure that all aspects are counted. This is particularly important due to the fact the various parameters from various sources and fields in the realization process are involved. It is also required that you define what to do with the products during the PQ phase (e.g., quarantine).

PQ—Protocol, Scope, and Extent of the Activities

The PQ tests are to be continual until the required level of confidence is achieved. The tests will sample data and analyze it using the criteria, comparing the results with the process limits over a period of time, the number of machine runs, or the number of batches. The PQ protocol will describe the scope and extent of the PQ activities:

- The protocol will identify which processes are validated and controlled.
- The sample rate of the process will be determined in time and quantity in order to represent the process ability, and to capture the variance of the process; for example, the number of batches, number of machine runs, or units. The quantity of products to be tested will be determined.
- The tested parameters will be determined. These are the parameters that were set on the OQ phase.
- The beginning and end date will be documented. During the PQ phase each date of each test will be documented.

PQ—Identification of System Parameters

The PQ protocol will identify the critical parameters that must be captured so that the process ability may be proven. By tracing, recording, and analyzing these parameters a process may be adjusted, controlled, and corrected. The objective is to prove that process parameters are consistently reproducible for the long term. In order to capture and measure these, different controls of the various system elements are to be applied:

- The machines, tools, and equipment used in the PQ tests will be identified and registered on the protocol. The registrations will include identifications such as serial numbers, names, models, and locations. Registration is necessary for traceability.
- All utilities and their accessories that affect the process and required controls will be identified.
- All work environment elements that support the process or may affect it will be identified on the protocol.
- Different types of materials that were used in the process and which served as inputs to the process will be identified.

PQ—Human Resources

Functions and roles that participate in the PQ phase and production processes will be defined. This definition shall include the activities and tests for which the relevant parties are responsible. If certification and training are needed, they will be verified and approved or referred to.

PQ—Documentations

The protocol will refer to each of the required or necessary documents relevant to the test specified on the PQ protocol; for example, standard operating procedures, manuals, charts, diagrams, user instructions, forms and protocols, work environment specifications, work instructions, device master records. On the protocol you will verify that all the required documentation is available, up to date, and legible.

PQ—Monitoring and Measurement Devices and Control Gauges

Tools for validation such as monitoring and measurement devices or control gauges that will be used in the process must be validated and recorded. The validation will ensure that they are intact, registered, calibrated, and controlled as required in clause 7.6 (Control of Monitoring and Measurement Devices). Registration will include

TABLE 7.26
Control Table of Gauges during Jobs

Control Gauge	Job Number	Start Date	Result	End Date	Result
G2 9444	A201000334	11/08/2010	OK	20/08/2010	OK
G2 9444	A201000378	21/09/2010	OK	02/10/2010	OK

identification, such as serial numbers or other elements. The registration is necessary for traceability. Before initiating the processes, the performance of the tool will be tested and validated. The objective here is to prove that the tool was intact for this specific job throughout its life cycle (from beginning to end). In practice you will need to demonstrate that the device is intact at the beginning of the production and at the end. This will prove that the device was, throughout the entire job, appropriate for use (Table 7.26).

The results will be documented on the protocol. The issue is relevant to control gauges as well as monitoring and measurement devices.

PQ—Description of the Tests

For each of the identified elements related to the PQ, a validation test will be defined. The objectives of the test are to show that the process meets the requirements consistently throughout the entire job. Each test will be documented describing the test activities specifically. The protocol may refer to other work or test instructions.

- The scope and objective of the test will defined as mentioned above (PQ—protocol, scope, and extent of the activities).
- The tested parameters will be specified.
- The test instruction will define what the normal test conditions are; the required levels of temperature, humidity, and air quality.
- The test instruction will indicate which tools, devices, gauges, or equipment are required to measure the results.
- The test instruction will define which records are expected; which data and in what manner the data is to be recorded.
- For each test, acceptance criteria will be clear and documented on the protocol. The technique for analyzing the data and evaluating with the criteria will be defined as well.

PQ—Summary Report

After completing all the tests of the PQ, a final report is to be issued indicating that process stability and repeatability are achieved and will be maintained. The report will cover the following issues:

- The review will include a description of the tests that were conducted.
- The report will include the results and their analysis (compared with the criteria).
- The conclusion will indicate how the criteria were met, and when deviations occur, a justification will be provided.
- A reference to documentation that supports the decisions will be added.
- Where deviations were identified, documented justifications indicating the investigation and the appropriate actions that were determined will be available.

Where a deviation was applied and corrected it will be introduced to the revalidation policy, as mentioned on the validation plan.
- Non conformities that had occurred and were subjected to control measures.
- Required records are obtained and available.
- Final approval of the PQ stage—the process outputs are satisfying, the required level of confidence was achieved, and the process is ready for release.

The review and approval will be conducted by the validation circle in order to ensure that all aspects are resolved. The review approval will be documented on the protocol. Once the PQ was approved, the validation circle may release the process for production. The report will be distributed to the relevant persons and functions that need to operate the process: QA mangers, production managers, and production employees.

The records of performing the tests and the results, along with the approvals, will serve as quality records and will be submitted to the process of records control in your organization as required in subclause 4.2.4 (Control of Records).

Validation of Software Application

The ISO 13485 Standard requires maintaining a documented procedure for the validation of the application of computer software (and changes to such software and/or its application) that may affect the quality of the medical device and its ability to conform to the specifications prior to initial use. The cases in which a computer system would affect the product include:

- Record keeping
- Control of processes
- Data analysis
- Performing activities or managing processes from a process flow
- Managing service and maintenance activities

Regarding terms and definitions:

- Software verification means a review of the software or a version of software, and the verification that its functions and features answer all the requirements as specified during its characterization. A full conformance between the requirements that are documented in the specification document and the software's functions is necessary.
- Software validation means a confirmation by objective evidence, ensuring that all software functions, features, processes, and outputs answer the user needs specifications.

There is a debate regarding the scope of these requirements: to which software does it relate? Software embedded in the medical device or software used to realize the medical device? To our aid comes the ISO 14696 Standard, which provides guidance on the application of ISO 13485:2003, which specifically explains:

Software that was purchased, developed, maintained for the use of process planning, automation or control will be validated. Changes occurring on software will be managed as changes on documents, and will be submitted to the documents control process. Software released under the standard requirements is to be reviewed and approved, and a master copy of its characterization is maintained in the organization under the documents control. Any change in the software will be submitted to the document control process as required in subclause 4.2.3 (Control of Documents).

It is quite clear from the above that the ISO 13485 Standard relates to software that is used to plan, control, and carry out processes such as realization, installation, maintenance, and services. The standard specifically refers to "production and service provision" because such software may be used for other realization activities, such as service and installation. This is logical as the validation of software that is part of the medical device occurs both during and after the software development life cycle. Embedded software that was developed for the medical device itself, and that was used to manage functions of the medical device has already been validated under the standard requirements as presented in subclause 7.3.6 (Design and Development Validation). Such software serves as a function and feature of the medical device.

After clearing the debate let us discuss the documented procedure. The manufacturer is required to develop and document processes that ensure the validation of software before implementing and applying the software to the production processes. As mentioned above, the activities will be comprised of the verification of the software as well as the validation.

In order to prove verification, the manufacturer needs to develop a set of tests demonstrating conformance between characterization and specification of the software, and its actual functions and features. This may be achieved by using a checklist for reviewing the functionality, maintenance efficiency, and usability of the software according to its specifications. If you are using software to manage customer complaints, you will need to show that the software follows the process and fulfills the activities that you defined for handling these complaints.

With validation it is a bit different—validation of software requires you to identify which parameters in the software may affect realization processes and the quality of the medical device and its ability to meet its requirements. Once these have been identified you need to develop validation tests. These will be performed before the initial use. Let us take, for example, a BPM system that is used to manage production processes (a type of MRP II system). Such a system (which receives parameters such as orders, status of inventor, production durations, and human resources) relies on the database of the organization, and gives out production plans; that is, production schedules, resource assignments, production queues, and delivery schedules. One way to demonstrate validation is to compare the delivery date that was given as input to the system as a requirement with the delivery schedule that the system provided, and to check for gaps and differences. The next phase is to identify the process parameter in the BPM software that influences this calculation. Another example is software for maintenance plans—you need a validation that maintenance plans were schedules according to the technical needs of the medical device. The critical parameters include: security measures, user access, authorization approvals, change controls, backup processes, process runs, application and data recovery, protection against viruses, and maintenance.

Changes made to the software will be controlled and validated as well. Implementing the matter effectively will involve the application of a configuration control to the software:

- Injective identification of the software (e.g., name, model, date of release, and version used)
- Definition of processes that the software manages
- Injective identification of the software's accessories and other elements (e.g., directories, databases, or other external functions that assist in managing the processes)

- Applying control of changes and updates to the system; especially when the system is ran from two remote locations, and exposed to the risk that one location will be updated and the other will not be

Another effective way is to relate to the software as a document and to control its changes through its application to the document control process as required in subclause 4.2.3 (Control of Documents). The software will be registered as a document on your list of documents under the quality management system (QMS).

All of these activities will be defined in a documented procedure. This procedure will be submitted to the document control as required in subclause 4.2.3 (Control of Documents). Records of the validation activities of the application of computer software will be maintained and introduced to the records control process in the quality management system, as required in subclause 4.2.4 (Control of Records).

7.5.2.2 Particular Requirements for Sterile Medical Devices

All of the requirements mentioned in chapter 7.5.2.1 (Validation of Processes for Production and Service Provision—General Requirements) also apply to the sterilization processes. Thus, when planning the validations of sterilization processes you *must* apply all of the requirements in this chapter on the sterilization processes. In addition, the ISO 13485 Standard requires establishing a documented procedure describing the process and activities of the validations covering all the stages and phases involved (Table 7.27).

What is the difference between the documentation required by subclause 7.5.2.1 and the procedure required by subclause 7.5.2.2? First let us review the basic differences:

- A validation plan is a strategic document with the objective of stating and documenting the requirements and sequence of the validation activities (e.g., the approach and scope, schedules and sequences of activities, details regarding tasks and responsibilities).
- A validation procedure is a document describing the validation process referring to one product family or type. It identifies areas, it configures the process, sets the sequence of events (but may also refer to specific activities), refers to tools and equipment, risks, their controls and restrictions, documentations, acceptance criteria, expected results, and desired records. The standard requires that you to maintain a procedure defining the above with reference to the topics mentioned in this chapter.

TABLE 7.27
Standard Requirements of Subclause 7.5.2.2

ISO 13485
The manufacturer shall define and document a procedure describing the activities of validation of sterilization processes
The validation of the sterilization processes shall be applied before the initial use
Records for performing the validation activities and records of test results will be maintained under the records control procedure as specified in subclause 4.2.4 (Control of Records)

- The test protocol is a file documenting sterilization activities. The protocol will include criteria for acceptance or rejection, will identify all the elements that need to be validated, specify for each the validation test records and the results of the test, and will relate to deviations. The record will serve as the required evidences.

The purpose of establishing a systematic validation of sterilization processes is to initiate a routine control of these processes that will:

- Ensure that the processes are efficient, reliable, and reproducible (when process conditions and outputs are capable of being reproduced)
- Ensure compliance with the predefined specifications
- Provide confidence that there is a low level of probability of a viable microorganism present on the product after sterilization

Data and information will be gathered and recorded from each cycle. The routine control will guarantee for each cycle that process specifications are met through the demonstration of process parameters and the presentation of validations tests results. These will cover all the relevant issues, activities, and elements that are related to the medical devices submitted to the sterilization processes; for example, the relevant equipment is maintained, conditions for sterilization processes are validated before use, and the performances of the sterilization process are monitored. The procedure will define which data and information, as well as the intervals, will supply the following evidence:

- Microbiological status of incoming raw materials and/or components submitted to the process
- Loads brought to the process conform to the predefined conditions
- Work environment related to the processes
- Tools and equipment used in the process
- Human resources performing activities related to the process
- Packages and raw material used for the packaging
- Planned process activity to be performed (actions and sequences)
- Condition and activities of storage
- Key process variables
- Information regarding the condition parameters during the different stages and activities of the process (e.g., times and durations, temperatures, and pressures)
- Information regarding sterilizers

Sterilization processes require the systematic validation of their efficacy and reproducibility. This will be accomplished through the provision of documented and accurate evidence of process conditions, parameters, and SAL. Thus, thorough documentation is extremely important to the success of validation efforts. The recorded results would be measured with predefined acceptance criteria, and tolerances will prove that accepted results are satisfying. An effective procedure will describe the process, activities, and intervals, provide as much details as possible, relate the user to the appropriate topics, issues and documentations, specify methods for auditing the effectiveness of the sterilization activities, and verify that the accepted results are as required. As mentioned above, designing the validation processes will be done according to the requirements mentioned in chapter 7.5.2.1.

Below is a review of a few distinctive quality management issues that should be referred when planning your process for validation of sterilization processes.

Conditions

The procedure shall identify and relate to the appropriate condition needed for the processes:

- The definition shall refer to the product type or family, its container and the size of the sterilization load, and the location on the surface of the medical device on which sterility is most difficult to achieve. Process parameters related to these definitions shall be determined. These factors are to be defined on the procedure or the procedure will refer to other controlled documents indicating these factors.
- Cleaning processes, microbiological quality, and the cleanliness of the devices before submission to the sterilization process shall be determined. The procedure will demand verification with acceptance criteria, including the inspection of records. For example, the level of contaminants on the medical device before submission to the process will be determined and documented. Before submitting the devices to the sterilization process, the concentration of contaminants will be validated and recorded. Such a test will be defined on the procedure or shall be referred by it.
- When software is used to operate equipment or control a sterilization process, parameters that may affect the process and the sterilization of the medical device will be validated prior to the initial use as specified in chapter 7.5.2.1.
- The IQ, OQ, and PQ activities, tests, and verifications will be defined, performed, documented, recorded, and validated as specified in chapter 7.5.2.1.
- Restrictions related to sterilizers, sterilizer agents, or the use of related equipment will be specified including their controls.
- Communication, training, and the certification necessary to implement the procedure are fully accomplished and recorded. The procedure will refer to the appropriate documentations for the verification.

Human Resources

Roles and functions participating in the sterilization processes and performing activities will be identified and appointed for each of the following activities:

- Design, development, implementation, and approval of the process including the definitions of the documentation and records (activities and tests)
- IQ, OQ and PQ activities and tests
- Performing the sterilization processes
- Monitoring, measuring, and analyzing the processes
- Approving the results and releasing the medical devices

The procedure shall relate to the authorization and qualifications of the personnel, and will define where these are documented (e.g., on a job certification). The objective is to limit the number of employees participating in the process to the qualified ones.

Resources needed for the qualification and trainings of employee will be defined on the procedure, and the verification that they are available to the process will be planned. For example, one can plan the documentation of the sterilization with identities and signatures indicating who performed each particular activity during the sterilization processes.

Regulations, Standardization, and Documentation

The process shall identify and refer to the relevant standards, regulations, guidelines, and documentation appropriate for the sterilization processes and type or family of the medical device. These are the documents necessary to perform the process. The procedure will detail:

- Standard operating procedures or test instructions needed for the operation of activities
- Manuals, user instructions, or diagrams necessary for the operation of tools and equipment
- Standardization related to process; for example, ISO 11137, ISO 11138, ISO 14161, and ISO 11737
- Studies and associated researches, such as studies regarding the biological compatibility of the package to the medical device
- Applicable local, national, or international regulatory requirements related to the sterilization processes

The procedure will define the verification for the availability of these documents during the processes. For example, you may plan a check that a certain standard or relevant document is available at the workstation, and another check indicating that the employee has studied it and will act upon it. These documents will be submitted to the control of documents as required in subclause 4.2.3. The control is particularly necessary for the update.

Reference to Tolerances and Acceptance Criteria

For each validation test during the sterilization process, acceptance criteria is to be defined with the objective of confirming that the results recorded during the process met the sterilization process specifications, and of demonstrating the process reproducibility:

- The criteria will be adjusted to the type and product family or nature of the process, and will suit the type of the parameters it is evaluating; such as SAL, temperature, system functionality, performance of maintenance activities, availability of resources, humidity, and pressure.
- All criteria will be documented on designated documentations and will be referred on the appropriate procedure as well as on the test protocols; that is, process limits, charts, tables, checklists, and tolerances.
- The technique used for the evaluation will be defined and documented. When required, the procedure will refer to the appropriate documents for support.
- Wherever possible, the criteria will be planned as a numerical assessment of process rather than a qualitative one. For example, criteria that provide results within action limits are preferable to criteria that indicate whether a process has passed or failed. The criteria will set scales for acceptance and rejection of cycles such as catastrophic, critical serious, minor or negligible. The classification shall be derived from the results of the risk analysis.

- Processes, where the variation of the process affects the sterilization process, will be submitted to appropriate criteria demonstrating that all products sterilized achieve the required SAL.

Work Environment

The requirements regarding the work environment mentioned in subclause 7.5.2.1 are applicable to the sterilization processes. The extent of the affect of the work environment on the process and its effectiveness will be identified. The procedure will specify the required controls and measures. Where regulations require the control of the work environment, they will be identified, documented on the procedure, and implemented throughout the processes (e.g., the prevention of infection through the establishment of work instructions or protocols).

Control of Materials

The procedure shall relate to the conditions and requirements of materials and accessories used in the process:

- Parameters such as shelf life, identification, storage conditions, and transportation will be identified or referred on the appropriate documentation; manufacturer instructions, regulations, guidelines, MSDS, safety data sheets. An example of guidelines is the instructions that are specified on labels of agents for a process. Before submitting the material to the process, the conditions will be verified and approved using acceptance criteria. Such a test will verify that they met the conditions when introduced to the process (e.g., a checklist that reviews storage activities, storage conditions, and validation dates).
- The procedure will refer to maintenance or specific storage controls (including the inspection). Once again, such activities will be verified and approved before submission to the sterilization processes.
- Outputs of risk review and analysis regarding the material and the process will be implemented on the process; for example, difficult surfaces for sterilization. These risks controls, including their verification, will be defined on the procedures.

The next stage is the implementation throughout the process. The procedure will define how the materials will be properly introduced to the process, referring to issues such as the safety of employees, the medical device, and the work environment.

Packaging

The purpose of the package is to ensure that the medical device remains sterile and protected during and after the process until the package is opened. The procedure will relate to the following issues:

- Packaging materials and their storage activities and conditions brought to the processes will be verified, and the controls will be validated (before submission to the process).
- The safety, integrity, and attributes of the package will be ensured throughout the sterilization process. Parameters that may harm the package (e.g., temperature, humidity or mechanical disturbances such as vibrations). A good example is the handling of the packaging throughout the realization processes.

- The package shall ensure the safety, integrity, and attributes of the medical device and the procedure will refer to studies regarding the biological compatibility of the package to the medical device.
- The procedure shall refer to standardization and regulatory requirements applicable to the packaging.
- In some cases, for maximal validation, a challenge test for the package is to be defined.
- Elements and control required by risk management necessary to ensure the integrity, functionality and safety of the package and thus the device shall be related.

In order to ensure all of the above, the procedure is to refer to the relevant process validation tests, the acceptance criteria, or tolerances, and shall indicate which records are required in order to verify the performances and validate the results.

Tools and Equipment

The requirements concerning the work environment mentioned in subclause 7.5.2.1 are applicable to the sterilization processes. However:

- The procedure will identify each of the tools and pieces of equipment participating in the process as required in subclause 7.5.2.1.
- The procedure will describe the operation of systems, tools, and equipment supporting the process in order to eliminate damage to the medical devices.
- The required controls over risks related to tools and equipment are to be fully addressed on the procedure; for example, a chamber is exposed to the risk of corrosion as a result of materials and pressurizing activities. Such risks are to be identified, the criteria is to be defined, the accepted levels are to be determined, and the appropriate controls are to be applied.
- The effect that materials have on tools and equipment will be referred on the procedure, and the required control tests will be defined and documented. The test results will be recorded.
- While defining the tools and equipment used on the process, the procedure will relate to any necessary ancillary items including materials of construction.
- The composition of different material in the process will also be referred; such as sterilizing agents, gases, and the microbiological status of incoming raw materials.

Review and Approval of Validation

Data and information from each sterilization activity and cycle will be recorded and collected. The review and approval is required in order to confirm the acceptability of the results against the acceptance criteria (for each of the sterilization activities), and to approve that all process specifications are met. Each activity will be evaluated and approved. The result of the review will be recorded on a validation report. The objective of this report is to demonstrate the different variables and process parameters during the different sterilization stages, conditions, and activities, and to compare them with the acceptance criteria and tolerances (e.g., time, temperature, humidity, vacuum, and pressure). At the end of the report a confirmation that all process specifications were met will be documented with a name and a signature. The procedure will determine the responsible party for the review and approval.

This report will serve as a quality record and will be submitted to the control of records.

Process Release

The release of each load will be reviewed and approved. The procedure will define which verifications are required before the release. Each check or test will be compared to predefined criteria. This verification will be supported with records and evidence. The procedure will describe exactly which records are expected. The test will include:

- Verification that the equipment used in the process was identified for traceability purposes, and that the equipment is maintained, calibrated as planned, and that it performed throughout the processes as specified (IQ).
- The qualification of personnel that participated in the process will be reviewed and approved.
- Evidence that all OQ and PQ activities were accomplished and verified.
- Evidence that all safety specifications were applied during the process.
- Evidence that all the necessary documentation was available during the process.
- A verification that all the required data is obtained and records are maintained as required.
- Evidence that the results of the validation test are within the tolerances and conform to the acceptance criteria.
- Evidence that the conditions of the product after the process are as specified (e.g., no growth of test organism from any biological indicator, if used).

When products are detected that do not meet the specifications they will be referred to as nonconforming, and will be submitted to the control of nonconforming products as specified in clause 8.3. It is required that you define special requirements for the release of products that were used for the validation of the process, and are intended to be delivered to the customers.

Requalification

The procedure will define the need for requalification of a sterilization process:

- Intervals for the requalification will be determined. The interval will be justified.
- The procedure will define the activities for requalification.
- Each requalification activity will be validated (i.e., tested) and the results will be compared to acceptance criteria.
- The activities and test results will be recorded.

Changes

The procedure will define how changes will be identified or assessed and implemented in the process. Changes may occur to the process, activities in the process, personnel performing the activities, regulatory requirements, process parameters, packages, products, equipment or tools, and materials used in the process (such as sterilizers):

- The procedure will describe a method for introducing a change to a process.
- The assessment will verify that the process delivers the specifications after the change has been applied.
- The related process elements and documents that need to be updated will be identified.

Records

Records and evidence of the sterilization processes, tests, and validation will serve as quality records and will be submitted to the process of records control in your quality management system as required in subclause 4.2.4 (Control of Records).

7.5.3 Identification and Traceability

7.5.3.1 Identification

The ISO 13485 Standard separates the issue and implementation of activities and means of distinction, management, and control of the medical device into three main topics: identification, traceability, and status, describing specific requirements for each. In the spirit of the standard we will discuss each in specific detail.

Identification is a serious issue that does not receive enough attention throughout our daily productive lives. I have often encountered items and products in production and storage halls where it was difficult to tell what their status was, when were they were produced, and to whom they belonged. This meant that I needed to conduct investigations and interrogations, and to trouble many people in order to receive the desired answers. Fortunately the ISO 13485 Standard demands the exact definition and documentation of the all activities and elements related to identification (Table 7.28).

According to the ISO 13485 Standard, the manufacturer is expected to establish the systematic identification of its business activities and process outputs throughout the material flow into categories and characters that are in accordance with predefined needs. The objective of the identification is to ensure that products at all levels and stages of the realization process will be identified regarding their production, change, and quality status. The identification shall also eliminate the risk of mixing products, parts, or materials from different origins or with different status. Products

TABLE 7.28
Standard Requirements of Subclause 7.5.3.1

ISO 13485	ISO 9001
The product will be identified by appropriate means and techniques throughout the realization process	The product will be identified by appropriate means and techniques throughout the realization process
A documented procedure shall be planned and maintained describing the activities and conditions of the identification	
The organization shall plan, implement, and maintain a documented procedure describing activities to ensure that medical devices returned to the organization will be identified and distinguished from other products. The purpose is to prevent any product contamination as specified in subclause 6.4d	

with incorrect identification could be incorrectly submitted to a process, delivered to the customer, or may initiate contamination of other products. Through the assignment of activities, means, measures, and identifiers throughout the material flow—such as codes, tags, or product serial numbers—they will be uniquely identified. The production elements that are to be identified include:

- Raw materials, components, and parts
- Materials used for the production
- Lots or batches
- Finished goods
- Defective or returned goods

A correct definition and implementation of identification will provide full transparency regarding the medical device:

- It will allow the identification and tracking of all of the elements mentioned above throughout the realization processes until the delivery or disposal of the medical device; that is, storage of raw materials, components and other materials used for production, tracking inventory in process, storage of finished goods, distribution installation and service.
- In case quality problems occur, the identification shall support the traceability of the medical device, facilitate fault diagnosis, and assist the organization in detecting defective products.
- The identification shall provide information regarding the product's usability status and (where applicable) shall relate to the expiry date or shelf life of materials.
- Identification will ensure that those realizing the product use the appropriate materials, components, or items.
- The identification shall eliminate the risk of mixing products with different status.
- The identification shall indicate to the user when the product was manufactured or assembled, how it was done, and by whom.
- The identification will answer risk management requirements. For example the ability to identify product characteristics related to the risk analysis or the ability to relate risks, typical hazardous situations, the associated harm and controls to a medical device through identification.

Planning the Identification

The identification of the product is regarded as the collection of related information throughout the supply chain management. Thus, it is necessary to identify which information and data are needed, which activities generate the data, by what means can the data be collected, and the final stage is linking the product or element to this data. When planning identification methods and activities, bear in mind that some questions need to be answered when a person samples a product from a process or a location:

- What is the origin of the item?
- When was it manufactured?

- From what is it constructed, and are the materials or components that construct it approved?
- Where should it be stored?
- Where is this item heading? What is its next stop? To whom does it belong?

The identification details and references shall be planned according to the properties, attributes, and characters of the identified element or item. Each element has its own identification needs and possibilities. For example, the identification of a raw material must refer to its expiry date, MSDS (material safety data sheet), date of manufacture and of arrival, storage conditions, and COC. A plastic injected part shall be identified with the catalog number, marking date of production, editions, models, lot or batch numbers, and relevant quality protocols. The identification shall allow access to appropriate references. The identification will be integrated into the work processes and activities, and may be used by several means or techniques; for example, a tag with a number could be fixed on a pallet. This number will serve as the identifier in designated software. In addition, each device that is packed on the palette will have a barcode sticker attached with a serial number providing specific information about the device, and which will refer it to a specific batch. A quality report will also be attached to the pallet. In this example, four techniques were used to identify the product—a tag, computer system, quality approval, and a barcode. Each relates to another set of information, and will serve a certain cause. However, the identification will always have physical contact with the product; on the product, on its package, and on the product's location.

Another aspect to be considered is the effect and type of relation that the identified element has on the medical device. A well-planned identification is a prerequisite for effective traceability, and will allow tracking back products, components, parts, or raw materials when required (e.g., customer complaints, or a recall). For example, it is necessary to identify cleaning material used on cleaning activities. Such material has a significant effect on the medical device, its safety, and its intended use. In order to explain the importance of relation, I will use the bill of materials; a medical device may be constructed or assembled of several components and parts which relate to its safety and functionality. When these have an affect on the medical device and are related to identified risks—or bear residual risks themselves—they will need to be traced, controlled, and thus identified.

Integration of Risk Management

When planning the identification means and activities, the outputs of risk management shall be referred; and when the controls of risks are to be implemented through certain identifiers, they shall be applied; for example, serial number, model, version, production date, and expiry date. On some parts or areas of the medical device residual risks may remain and require a routine control. In order to implement the control effectively, specific identifiers are to be attached to the medical device. Such requirements may appear on the risk management plan.

Customer and Regulatory Requirements

When required, the method of identification shall integrate customer requirements for identification with its identification and traceability methods—requested labels, barcodes, qualities, protocols, or markings. In some cases, the identification will be part of the packaging instructions. When the customer delivers materials, parts, or components for assembly or use in the realization process, they will be identified. International standards, directives, or regulations related to the realization of medical devices such as the ISO 11137, ISO 11140, ISO TR 17665, or the ISO 10993, specifically require the implementation of identification methods of the materials, products, process entities, or agents that are under their scope. Requested documentation such as specific forms, and test or work instructions shall be planned and implemented. Records that are needed to prove the performance of the requirements will be maintained.

A Documented Method

The ISO 13485 Standard requires a documented procedure describing identification activities and techniques. The documented method shall be implemented at manufacturing sections, sites, locations, or areas. The prime objective is to eliminate the mixing together of products, parts, or materials with different status at all stages of the material flow (sterilization is a classic example). Here are issues that the procedure may relate to:

- The procedure will define what the inputs for the identification requirements are: customer requirements, regulatory requirements, risks management plan, supplier instructions, design and development requirements.
- The method shall determine the areas, scopes, materials, products, parts, components, or finished goods that are under its scope.
- The method shall determine in which processes or activities the products are to be identified. The identification shall provide the required information regarding the status of a product on a process, and the meaning and significance of this status to the product: controlled material before processing, sterilized products, products or packages provided by the customer, batch before release, devices for delivery, defective parts, and so on. Where applicable, the identification shall instruct the user on how to handle the product, parts, or materials. If a product has completed a process and must be submitted to another process, the manufacturer may use the identification as an indication. For example, the identification of products shows that they have already been released from a sterilization process. The significance of this identification is the indication that these products are to be submitted to special further treatment according to specific planning. So there are cases where the procedure of identification may refer the user to other process flow diagrams, work, or packaging instructions.
- The procedure must specify the information and details that the identification shall include: type of product or material, quantities, units of measure, reference to documentation or process certifications, batch numbers, serial numbers, details of production, manufacturer details (including addresses), and communication details.
- Suggested methods for identification: serials numbers, article codes, part numbers, lot and batch numbers, dates of production, barcodes, number of diagrams or technical drawings, catalogue numbers, revisions, or versions.
- The procedure shall indicate to the user the exact means and activities necessary to fulfill and maintain the identification as well as the records. This may appear on the medical device or on the batch, on the transporter, a designated area, or at a stage in a process. When needed, instructions of identification will be available at the workstations. When the identification is located on the medical device, it should be clear, visible, and accessible by all. Means of identification include: stickers, tags, segregation areas, specific locations, routing cards, bracelets, test protocols, certain containers, markings, indications or signs, packages, use of

different colors, shipping documents, labels, etiquettes, quality indications, and physical barriers.

- The means of identification shall be planned in a way that will not harm the medical devices, its properties, or its packaging. The procedure shall indicate the exact manner with which the identification is to be applied. For example, some stickers that need to be attached may harm the packaging of medical devices at a specific location, and thus affect its functionality. The procedure will relate to such issues, or will refer to appropriate documentation which offers instruction on them.
- The procedure shall indicate the responsibilities and authorities required to perform the identification activities. The issue of product identification shall be integrated into the training and certification process of the relevant personnel in order to ensure that they are aware of it.

The procedure is an obligation of the ISO 13485 Standard, and will be submitted to the document control process in the quality management system, as required in subclause 4.2.3 (Control of Documents). Records such as stickers, barcodes, and tags will serve as quality records and will be submitted to the process of records control in your organization, as required in subclause 4.2.4 (Control of Records).

Work Environment

The next requirement refers to the identification of returned medical devices. The ISO 13485 Standard requires establishing and maintaining documented procedures for the identification and segregation of returned medical devices, and refers us to clause 6.4d (Work Environment, Elimination of Contamination). Allow me to briefly review this requirement—the organization shall plan and implement special arrangements, activities, and measures for the control and management of returned, contaminated, or potentially contaminated products in order to eliminate the contamination of the work environment or personnel. The relation to the identification is clear. Returned medical devices may contaminate, pollute, infect, or trigger any other illness that may affect the work environment or personnel. When such products are detected, the organization is required to plan and implement identification activities. The procedure shall indicate activities such as accepting returned medical devices, as well as identifying, separating, segregating, distinguishing, storing, registering, and investigating them. However, we must try to avoid drifting toward the control of nonconforming products and remember that the traceability is to support the processes requested in clause 8.3. The description can appear in the "control of nonconforming products" procedure. According to subclause 4.2.1, a single document may include requirements of one or more procedures. In the event that you are including the requirements in an independent document, be sure to include them under the control of documents, as required in subclause 4.2.3 (Control of Documents). Records of identification, or distinction of returned medical devices, shall serve as quality records, and will be submitted to the process of record control in your organization, as required in subclause 4.2.4 (Control of Records).

7.5.3.2 Traceability

7.5.3.2.1 Traceability—General

Conducting an effective traceability allows the manufacturer to trace back the medical devices from both sides of the supply chain (backwards and forwards), and enables the identification of all elements that participated in the realization of a

TABLE 7.29
Standard Requirements of Subclause 7.5.3.2.1

ISO 13485	ISO 9001
The product will be traceable throughout the realization processes until its disposal	The product will be traceable throughout the realization processes until its disposal
A documented procedure shall be planned and maintained describing the extent of traceability required to be maintained, the means with which the product will be traced.	
Traceability methods shall support quality activities required from clauses 8.3 (Control of Nonconforming Products) and 8.5 (Improvement)	
Where traceability is a requirement, the manufacturer shall implement and control it, and document the distinct identity of the medical device	Where traceability is a requirement, the manufacturer shall implement and control it, and document the distinct identity of the product
The procedure shall specify the records and evidence needed to maintain the traceability. The records will be submitted to control of records as specified in subclause 4.2.4	The records of traceability will be submitted to control of records as specified in subclause 4.2.4
Note: Traceability could be maintained with a configuration management.	Note: Traceability could be maintained with a configuration management.

unique product. Auditors expect the manufacturer to be able to reach the last grain of raw material when it comes to the traceability of the medical device (Table 7.29).

Traceability is the means used to trace the history, location, or status (of a product or activity) by recorded identification, usually indicated on the product (physically or logically) or a linkage to the product. Traceability must be performed from both sides of the supply chain. One end is traceability of devices delivered to customers—delivered medical devices (to distributors and to end users), and installation of the device or service provision. Such traceability is also known as device tracking. The other end is the traceability of delivered raw materials, components, parts, work and activities, installations, and services—anything that was purchased or used during the realization processes. Traceability:

- Enables you to follow up on the status of the medical device from various critical process levels; such as processing history, identification of components and materials that construct it, verification that all the required activities were applied, the necessary validations, usability and development status of a single product element, and its quality condition.
- Increases the product liability through the ability of the manufacturer to identify distinctively the products, parts, and components.
- Reduces the extent of nonconformity and potential damage through the identification and provision of access to suspected products, parts,

components, or materials from various locations on the material flow and supply chain management.
- Supports risk management activities and establishes completeness of the risk management process.

Traceability as Requirements

The input requirements for traceability may be:

- Risk management control measures
- Customer requirements
- Internal or organizational requirements
- International, national, or regional regulatory requirements

For each requirement you must define the information that needs to be provided by the traceability, the method that may be implemented, the extent of the traceability throughout the realization, and the required records.

Planning the Traceability

Traceability shall be planned and implemented throughout the realization process. It is required that you define, for each phase of the process, the information that needs to be traced. In principle, the ISO 13485 Standard requires maintaining traceability from the moment that the most basic raw material was ordered (traceability of purchasing information) through to its arrival, the transfer for production processes, the packaging, delivery, transportation, distribution, and so on, up to the point of use or disposal. The process elements, data and information, and resources that participate in the realization of the processes on each phase need to be identified and related to a unique medical device. Traceability:

- Serves as the link between the different product characteristics and parameters (e.g., materials, processes, activities, and human resources).
- Follows and collects data concerning the status of the elements and resources while the medical device evolves through its life cycle.
- Refers the manufacturer to the appropriate evidence and records (e.g., certifications of materials, batch numbers, validations of processes, quality tests, delivery notes, guarantees, and distribution details).

The above are maintained through critical product parameters. As a manufacturer you must identify what the critical parameters are:

- The supplier of raw material or components
- The manufacturing date (of raw materials, etc.)
- The identifiers of the medical device, such as control number, batch number, or serial number
- Reference to quality tests
- Reference to evidence of processes, such as process validation or batch release
- The identification of parts, materials, or components
- Reference to risks

Where applicable, certain processes and management techniques shall be integrated with the traceability. For example, the implementation of the FIFO (first in first out) system for inventory management supports traceability. Such a system reduces the risk that devices from different batches and with different manufacturing dates will be mixed and delivered at the same time. The FIFO system will be implemented on all levels and stages of the material flow, and will be accompanied with the appropriate records. Another example is the segregation or separation of batches. This generates transparency concerning the materials used for the production, and eliminates the mixing of products with different status. More process elements that the traceability must refer to include:

- Traceability shall be integrated in the logistics and transportation processes and activities.
- Traceability will allow the control of monitoring and measurement devices that are used to verify and validate processes and products.
- Products or packages that were supplied by the customer shall be submitted to traceability requirements.

Reference to Risk Management

When planning traceability, the outputs of risk management will serve as inputs for the requirements. Traceability is necessary in order to demonstrate that the risk management processes have been applied to each identified hazard. These requirements are available in the risk management report:

- Traceability of elements is a main issue in risk management and is used to verify that medical devices were submitted to the appropriate control measures.
- Traceability allows the control that the device was realized by trained and certified personnel.
- It may be that parts, areas, scopes, components, or materials used in the medical device require periodical inspection or control of any residual risks.

Regulatory Requirements

Planning the traceability will be done with reference to appropriate regulations. Make sure that you identify, for each type of part, the components and materials that constitute the medical device or are used during the realization of the appropriate regulation. The regulations usually refer to the techniques and means of traceability, such as packaging, barcodes, and labels.

Configuration Management

Configuration management is a means through which the manufacturers may trace their products and maintain information regarding them. Here is a short review of the configuration management principles:

1. Documented definition of the configuration method is necessary.
2. A unique identification of the elements that construct the unique device is to be planned (e.g., material, components, and parts).
3. For each element on a unique device, the version or edition is to be identified.
4. For each element on a unique device, the status of the realization is be identified.
5. For each element on a unique device, the required verifications and validations must be documented, recorded, and approved.
6. For each element on a unique device, the changes, repairs, or updates that were applied are to be identified and recorded.

Implementing the configuration management shall provide full transparency of status and the components of which a device is comprised. Anyone who inspects the medical device could extract the information that was documented and trace its history. Another objective is to eliminate the possibility that wrong components could be applied to the product.

Reference to Measurement, Analysis, and Improvement

The standard refers us to certain subclauses, and requests that the traceability will support these requirements:

- 8.3 (control of nonconforming products): the requirement for managing traceability of nonconforming products
- 8.5.1 (improvement—general): the requirement for implementing the traceability of products that advisory notice was issued for, that were involved in a customer complaint, or that a recall was initiated and listed upon
- 8.5.2 (improvement—corrective action): the requirement for implementing the traceability of products that are included in a corrective action
- 8.5.3 (improvement—preventive action): the requirement for implementing the traceability of products that are included in a preventive action

All of the above are examples of quality processes that handle products with a special status. These kinds of products are to be traced both within the organization and outside it. When planning traceability definitions and activities, beside the determination and traceability actions for "normal" products, you will also refer to these products. For example, when an emergency plan is designed in order to retrieve products on a product recall, the traceability is a main issue to be considered and integrated. For each of these cases you are required to manage a documented procedure. Thus, you have two options—documenting the matter on a designated procedure for traceability, or including the traceability activities and details on a designated procedure according to the standard requirement (8.3 or 8.5).

Documented Procedure

The establishment of a documented procedure describing the methods, activities, and records of the traceability is requisite. The documented procedure shall define:

- The areas and scopes on the medical device that are that need to be traced; that is, the components, parts, packages, areas, and zones
- The information that needs to be gathered and recorded at each stage
- The processes, activities, means, and techniques used to implement the traceability or with which the traceability is executed; such as computers systems, identifiers, serial numbers, catalog numbers, article codes, part numbers, lot and batches numbers, dates of production, barcodes, number of diagrams or technical drawings, revisions, or versions
- Reference to the appropriate documentation
- Those responsible for performing the activities; for example, production workers, logistic workers, distributors, and so on
- The required records

The procedure may be planned as a process flow diagram, with reference to documented requirements such as forms, checklists, documentations of batches, and so on.

The procedure shall be submitted to the documents control process in the organization as required in subclause 4.2.3 (Control of Documents).

Advice: After defining, documenting, reviewing, approving, and releasing the procedure, it is recommended that you validate and ensure that the definition on the procedure covers all the realization stages, so that with it one could trace back all the product and process elements; such as purchase orders, human resources, materials, activities and processes, tests—everything. During external audits, the issue is considered to be very sensitive and the most likely to be tested. In 50% of cases, a rejection is given because the auditor did not find the definition sufficient, the definition did not correlate with the reality, or that the definition was not fully implemented.

Records of Traceability

The objective of the records it to allow the manufacturer the ability to relate a unique medical device to its historical information; one may sample a medical device and, through the identification on the device, track its records and data effectively.

- The information that is to be recorded will be defined on the documented procedure.
- The type of records of the traceability activities shall be defined; for example, tags, tickets, stickers, packages, signs, forms, and the device history record (DHR).
- The records of the traceability will be planned with reference to the retention time as specified in subclause 4.2.4 (Control of Records).
- The records shall be submitted to the records control process in the organization as required in subclause 4.2.4 (Control of Records).

The DHR has a role in the planning of the traceability, and of the records. The DHR is a file containing all the records related to the realization processes of one specific model or version of a medical device—that is, the certification of materials, quality test reports, and delivery notices—and it refers to a batch production lot or a specific medical device. So, by reviewing a single medical device, one can trace back (through a logical link with identifiers and numbers) all the records related to the realization of the medical device. These records contain information regarding the procession of the medical device, and the resources used for processes: manufacturing dates, registration and tracing the serial numbers of medical devices, the quantities that were delivered from each batch, and evidence of packaging and storage activities.

7.5.3.2.2 Particular Requirements for Active Implantable Medical Devices and Implementable Medical Devices

When the organization produces and markets active implantable medical devices and implementable medical devices, the traceability requirements are a bit clearer. The requirement takes the traceability one step deeper. Meeting this requirement would help trace the medical device back even further (Table 7.30).

Identification of the Device's Constituents of Active Implantable Medical Devices and Implementable Medical Devices

The organization is required to include, under the traceability definitions and activities, all the medical device elements that may affect the quality of the product, generate

TABLE 7.30
Standard Requirements of Subclause 7.5.3.2.2

ISO 13485
When components, parts, or materials that construct the medical device may cause it to not meet its requirements, the organization shall define special traceability activities
The organization shall define records needed to trace parts or materials that construct the active implantable medical devices and implementable medical devices
The organization shall define records to trace conditions of the work environment during the realization of such devices
Distributors of the medical device are to maintain records of the distributions to enable a traceability of such devices. The records shall be available to the organization
The organization shall maintain records of deliveries, including the names and addresses of entities that received such devices
All of the records required above will be submitted to control of records as specified in subclause 4.2.4

malfunctions, and cause it not to meet its requirements; functionality, safety, performance, or intended use. Among the elements we may encounter are:

- Components, assemblies, subassemblies, and parts which assemble or were incorporated into the medical device
- Materials comprising the medical device or used during the realization processes
- Work environment conditions in which the medical device was realized
- Human resources that participated in the realization processes

The requirement is necessary in order to eliminate unnecessary explantations of implanted medical devices from a user when a quality problem arises. A problem that was identified in the medical device, or in one of its components or parts, may require removal and an explanation of the medical devices to users. By uniquely identifying all the components and elements in a single device, the manufacturer may reduce the extent of the explantation of the exact faulty products. Thus, the manufacturer will evaluate which of the above may cause the medical device to fail to meet its requirements. Inputs and criteria for the evaluation include:

- Results of risk analysis and evaluations
- Residual risks
- Regulatory requirements
- Results of clinical evaluations

For each element constructing the medical device and identified as having the potential to cause the medical device to fail, all the traceability requirements of subclause 7.5.3.2.1 and the requirements of subclause 7.5.3.2.2 are to be applied.

Work Environment Conditions

When conditions of the work environment may affect materials, parts, or components in the device, and cause it to fail to meet the requirements, the organization shall include these under the traceability. This requires another review and assessment on your behalf regarding the extent of the effect that the work environment has on the components of the medical device. The review will relate to the conditions in the work surrounding and the parameters that create these conditions. When the results show that the effect may impair the medical device, the traceability shall relate to them. The traceability shall refer to records and evidence indicating the status of the environmental conditions during a specific realization activity, batch, or manufacturing lot. The reference will be carried out with an identifier (batch number, serial number or date of manufacturing). The status will be demonstrated with data of appropriate parameters; such as temperature, humidity, particle counts, and SAL. Thus, in a case where there is a quality problem, the manufacturer may review a device and, according to the identifier, may trace back records indicating the conditions in which it was manufactured.

Reference to Human Resource

Activities and actions of human resources during the realization processes may affect certain materials, parts, and components in the device, and cause it not to meet the requirements. The matter is ensured through training and certifying personnel to perform specific activities. Once again, you must review all the activities during the realization of the medical device and identify which human resource activities may impair parts or components. For actions that were indicated as crucial to the integrity of the medical device, the identification of personnel that performed these activities will be included under the traceability. The issue could be easily resolved by a simple registration of the identity of personnel on designated forms; for example, production orders, quality protocols, or backing notes of inventory for storage. An ERP system may store records of personnel (if it has a human resource module). Another means is the periodical working plan or shift schedule. However, make sure to relate such records to a specific identifier of the medical device (e.g., manufacturing date, serial number, lot or batch number, etc.).

Reference to Purchased Product or Services

Purchased products and services may also affect the medical device and cause it not to meet its requirements. When the realization of the medical device involves purchased elements or products, they must also be reviewed and included under the traceability; for example, sterilization materials, packages, installations, machines, tools, and equipment. The matter is less complicated than it seems. It requires definitions of details that are to be recorded, collecting the data and information, and reference to the appropriate records.

Distributors

The organization must demand from its agents and distributors, local or international, that they maintain records that will enable them and the organization to trace delivered products to the end user. The records are to be available for the organization upon request. The requirement will enable the organization:

- To inspect these records
- To communicate advisory notices to the end users
- In worst case scenarios, to recall products that were identified as having malfunctions

The data and information regarding the products that your distributors may maintain shall suit your processes and needs: batch numbers, models, versions, manufacturing dates and delivery dates. You must determine which information is needed for the traceability. One example is to have your distributors keep track of which lot numbers were delivered to certain customers. It may be that you will need to define your distributors and agent distribution procedures in order to maintain your requirements. I suggest anchoring the matter on the agreement or contract. Another suggestion is to prepare a template of a form that your distributors will implement, and use it to capture the data. A good way to maintain this requirement is to develop a supplier relationship management system and to provide your distributors with a web system in which they can input delivery information.

Maintaining Addresses and Names

Shipments and shipping packages of active implantable and implementable medical devices must be recorded and traced. A link or reference between the shipment and the content (the medical devices) shall be maintained. The information shall include:

- Names of persons or organizations that received the package
- Addresses of persons or organizations that received the package
- Details regarding the shipment—such as date, identifier number, and the person that prepared it
- Internal identification of the shipment

A simple delivery notice may serve the purpose as long as its content was planned according to the nature of your processes and the requirements of this subclause. Bear in mind, however, that this delivery notice has a role in the traceability, and you need to be able to access it when in need. The records of the shipments shall be submitted to the control of records.

Records

The records expected by this subclause are divided into two types: records required by the traceability requirements, and records required by other subclauses of this standard but that will include a reference to the traceability:

- Traceability records of the medical device's materials, parts, or components
- Records of environmental conditions (shall include reference of traceability)
- Records of active human resources during the processes (shall include reference of traceability)
- Registrations of shipments
- Records of distributions

The records shall be submitted to the records control process in the organization as required in subclause 4.2.4 (Control of Records).

7.5.3.3 Status Identification

The objective of status identification is to distinguish different materials, parts, components, or products with different characteristics from the different stages of the realization process. The management of a product's status shall be implemented throughout the realization process (Table 7.31).

Product status is the position of an element in a particular point of a process and the certain characteristics it bears at this point. A good example is to describe a product that has gone through its basic production processes, the cleanliness processes have been applied, and it is waiting in the line for the sterilization processes.

TABLE 7.31
Standard Requirements of Subclause 7.5.3.3

ISO 13485	ISO 9001
The organization shall define an identification and recognition method for the product's status	The organization shall define an identification and recognition method for the product's status
Status of products will be determined with regard to monitoring and measurements requirements	Status of products will be determined with regard to monitoring and measurements requirements
The status management shall ensure that the product passed all the required tests and inspections, and is released or supplied under the appropriate concession	
The status of the product shall determine its usability	
The identification of the product's status must be maintained throughout the realization processes; that is, purchasing, production processes, storage activities, delivery, installation activities, maintenance, and service and repair activities	

- Process status in the realization processes: after cleanliness, before sterilization
- Production status: finished good—production characteristics are approved
- Marketing status: forbidden

As you may notice, there are few process elements that may influence or determine the status of a product:

- The situation of a product regarding its realization
- Activities that were applied on the product
- Results of inspections and tests that the product has undergone

Applying status management ensures that medical devices, their components, parts, and materials are being controlled and introduced to the necessary activities, tests, inspections, or concessions before they are released to the next stage (i.e., introduced to a process, packed, delivered, or installed). More objectives of the status management include:

- The status management shall eliminate the possibility of mixing materials, parts, components, or products with different status.
- The status shall situate the product in its life cycle.
- The status shall provide information regarding the fulfillment of the product's requirements.

Reference to the Quality Plan

The determination of the status shall be integrated with the quality plan, and shall cover the entire life cycle of the product: material, development, production, storage, installation, and servicing. The status shall indicate where the product is situated regarding the plan. Another way to put it is that the progress of a product in the life cycle determines and indicates its status. As a result of this logic, a status of the product indicates its history. To explain further: when I pick a product with a certain status, it means that the product went through different realization stages through which it earned its status.

The status management shall be integrated with the identification and traceability methods and techniques used in the organization. The status shall be identified using auxiliary tools such as routing cards, labels, usability tags, signposting, and serial numbers. The important thing is that the status must be clear to all users and personnel participating in the realization processes. When the status cannot be indicated physically on the product (due to the product's nature and characteristics), it is necessary to define other methods to identify its status; for example, the location or segregation of products or logical management.

Types of Status

The different product status shall be determined in order to clarify the significance and consequences of each status. The definition will determine how products receive their status classification (e.g., their microbiological level, undergoing a certain process, being comprised of certain materials, being defective, being given quality status after assembly, or before packaging, etc.). In case it is applicable, criteria shall be assigned to the transition from one status to the next.

Reference to Monitoring, Measurement, and Validation Activities

Releasing a product or a component to the next stage, or changing its status and updating its usability is done through a set of predefined verifications and validations. Monitoring and measurement activities, as well as process validations, determine the status of process outputs. These tests, inspections, and controls carried out during the sequence of the realization provide the comparison between the product's specifications and the actual results of processes, and their influence on the product—its status. Analyzing and comparing the results of these tests and controls helps set the status of the product; either accepted or rejected. This is true of all stages of the realization process. If you view it from the other side of the material flow, the status of a product indicates which inspections the part underwent—whether they were successful or not, and whether the part meets its requirements or not. For example, the approval of IQ and OQ protocols determines the status of the process outputs; that is, products or parts. In order to put it into practice: establish and integrate a relation between your verifications of products and parts and validations of processes, and the status of the product; each time a product, a batch, or a lot passes a quality test, the status is updated. This will ensure that only products with the appropriate status reach the next stage.

Usability of the Product

The status of the product will indicate its usability and will determine the allowed activities for a component: can it be used in certain conditions; is it allowed to be assembled; does it need to be reworked or rejected; does it need to be disposed. The standard suggests a few types of usability:

- The product is approved for use and realization.
- The product is approved for use but with restrictions.

- The product is suspended or put on hold.
- The product is rejected.

The approval of a product with restrictions is a state where the product does not fully meet its requirements; but, under the appropriate concessions, the use of the product is still approved. These concessions are to be documented and approved.

- It will be defined under whose responsibility it is to review and approve a concession. The definition may be on the job description.
- A reference to the suitable records shall be available; for example, the justification of concessions.
- The approval will be accompanied with the identification of the approver.

A good example for the concession of a product is when a process was performed, but with deviations. These were reviewed and it was decided that they were not crucial, and therefore the product was approved. Such concession may create a special status for the product.

Status Identification of Serviced Products

During the service or maintenance activities, an indication regarding the usability of the medical device will be determined; that is—usable, in repair, or defective. The status will be clearly shown on the medical device in a location where all users or patients may view it. It is possible to deactivate or disable only a part or function of the medical device. As already mentioned, service and maintenance activities may create defective parts or devices. Therefore, it is required that you initiate and define the status of nonconforming products.

7.5.4 Customer Property

You must be careful, cautious, straight, and responsible with regard to customer property. These are the main objective of subclause 7.5.4. The customer's property may play a main role in the realization of the product, and may gravely influence the later production stages and quality of the medical device. As a manufacturer, you must take the necessary precautions in order to preserve the device's quality (Table 7.32).

Customers' properties are goods of a different kind, which were delivered cost free to the manufacturer by the customer for further processing; for use during the realization processes; for incorporating into the medical device; or for the support of realization processes. The owner of these goods is the customer. The requirement applies for anything that the customer provides:

- Raw materials or components supplied for inclusion in the product
- Packaging materials
- Products supplied for service, repair, maintenance, or upgrading
- Products supplied for further processing (e.g., sterilization or testing)
- Design and development tools and software that the customer lent for a defined period of time
- Production tools, molds, and equipment delivered for work
- Monitoring and measuring tools and equipment for the measurements of particular products

TABLE 7.32
Standard Requirements of Subclause 7.5.4

ISO 13485	ISO 9001
The organization shall handle any customer property under its responsibility with care, caution, and consideration of customer requirements	The organization shall handle customer property under its responsibility with care, caution, and consideration of customer requirements
The organization shall define a method for the identification and verification of customer property designated for realization or for use during the realization	The organization shall define a method for the identification and verification of customer's property designated for realization or for use during the realization
The organization shall define activities and controls for the protection and safety of customer property	The organization shall define activities and controls for the protection and safety of customer property
The organization must define communication channels with the customer to notify them when property has been damaged, lost, or found unsuitable for use. The organization shall record the notification, and the records shall be included under the records control procedure as specified in subclause 4.2.4 (Control of Records)	The organization must define communication channels with the customer to notify them when property has been damaged, lost, or found unsuitable for use. The organization shall record the notification and the records shall be included under the records control procedure as specified in subclause 4.2.4 (Control of Records)
Intellectual property or confidential health information may count as customer property	Intellectual property may count as customer property

- Knowledge in any form or kind, and on any media or carrier
- Diagrams, product plans, and technical specifications
- Customer's intellectual property
- Customer's premises when a service or installation are provided on the premises of the customer, including the use of customer's facilities and information
- Customer's property that has been delivered to the organization for service activities
- Personal data
- Confidential health information
- Trade secret information
- Intellectual property such as texts, patents, or professional contents

Confidential Health Information

The ISO 13485 Standard additionally states confidential health information as customer property. The difficulty arises when personnel of the organization have access to intimate patient information. Maintaining such records increases the risk of unauthorized use, access, and disclosure of this information. The organization must protect the privacy of patients and treat the information confidentially. There are several principles that may be implemented:

- Confining access to patient health information to authorized individuals only
- Developing and communicating policy and guidelines regarding confidentiality, security, and release of health information
- Review of regulations or international standards and their implementation
- Developing and documenting methods and procedures of handling and releasing such information
- Nominating authorities for the approval of use of such information
- Introducing the personnel to the importance of the matter through training
- Preparing a disaster recovery

Agreement

The most effective way to define the scope, conditions, restrictions, and requirement regarding customer property is to limit the issue within a contract or an agreement signed by you and your customer. This will ensure that both sides have reviewed the matter and the requirements; have defined the needs, controls, and activities; and have reached an understanding regarding the care and exercise of customer property.

Verification of Property

The manufacturer shall define acceptance and verification activities of customer property. Once the customer's property enters the organization, these activities will be carried out, and a documented approval will be produced. The objective is to create control of ingoing customer property before it is submitted to the realization processes. If problems will arise, they could be detected earlier. For each type of property, the manufacturer shall define a specific ingoing test. The definition shall relate to issues such as:

- Responsibility: For each type of customer property, a responsible party shall be assigned for the control and verification. Naturally, the responsibilities shall be assigned according to the type and nature of the property.
- Compatibility of the delivery: The first test would be to examine that the expected or agreed goods are really what was delivered (do not be afraid to get into details).
- Quantity: An examination of quantity will be defined.
- Intactness after transportation: An inspection is required for the verification that nothing was damaged during transportation.

These requirements shall be documented on designated forms or checklists. Fulfilling this requirement would save you a lot of debate later on.

Identifying the Property

All customer properties must be identified throughout the organization premises, and for each type of property it is required to define the type of identification. The method for identification shall be determined according to the nature and characters of the goods. If you are managing a customer's mold for plastic injection, a tag or a sign that will be visible on the mold can be applied. However, if you are saving a technical diagram on the company's server, it is required that you identify the folder where it is filed and ensure that when this diagram is printed out, it carries identification details enough to assign it to a specific customer. If the customer delivered the diagram without details you may add a staple or write it by hand. A product number on the diagram may serve as an identifier. However, you will then have to define (e.g., on the records control procedure) that customer property of type diagrams is identified with a product number. I am not reviewing records control here, but pure identification and relation to a customer.

The issue may be incorporated into the identification and traceability methods of the organization as required in subclause 7.5.3. It will, however, be indicated and identified that materials, product, or any other identified element, belong to the customer.

Protection and Preservation of the Property

The organization shall plan and implement protection measures for customer property in order to safeguard it from any harm, danger, or potential danger. Dangers for customer property may come in various manners and cases. In order to fulfill these requirements, a few measures will be initiated:

- Identification of risks that property may be exposed to while being stored, realized or used
- Capturing specific customer requirements for handling the property, such as instructions for use, treatment, storage, or maintenance
- Defining specific requirements for internal or external transportation

These requirements could be crucial—for example, when service is provided at the customer's premises. The requirements are to be documented and available to the relevant personnel in order to implement and control them effectively. When it is required by the customer or regulations, the organization shall maintain the proper records as evidence.

Storing of Customer Property

For each type of customer property, you shall define the storage activities, conditions, and controls. In particular, the manufacturer shall consider the environmental conditions in which the property is stored. It may be that you will need to evaluate the type of goods and conduct a small scale risk analysis in order to examine which environmental conditions may affect the quality and integrity of the products or equipment. It may be the case that the customer will deliver goods of a new type and nature to you that require special conditions.

Where maintenance activities are required, they will be identified and documented. This requirement is most applicable when the customer delivers equipment or tools for realizing the medical device and they need periodical maintenance. In such cases, you need to clear the matter with the customer and identify all the maintenance needs. The appropriate personnel shall be identified, and the requirements will be available. Such requirements may be integrated into the control of infrastructure as required in clause 6.3.

Service Operations

Handling customer property refers also to service and maintenance activities that are performed, whether in the manufacturer's facilities or at the customer's premises. If medical devices are delivered for service and repair, the requirements apply to them too. The property of your customers must be properly identified, safeguarded, and preserved. The organization must define how it shall maintain the requirements:

- If you are operating a service team that visits the customer's premises, it shall exercise care and caution when handling the medical device, and the surroundings where operations are being conducted.

- If you are operating a service center that receives medical devices for service or maintenance, the personnel that operate the center will be introduced to the controls of the customer's property.

Service is a complex issue with a lot of consequences. It is advised that you conduct a review of your service activities in order to examine how you may deal with customer property and to define the appropriate controls. It would be a shame to receive a rejection or nonconformity in the audit simply because the service team did not know how to behave during service calls. The matter can be integrated with the service procedure or work instructions as required in subclause 7.5.1.2.3 (Control of Production and Service Provision—Servicing Activities), although these are two different requirements that deal with two different areas.

Notification to the Customer

The standards demand that you to notify the customer in cases where their property has been damaged, lost, or found unsuitable for use. The matter requires that you develop a communication channel with your customer concerning the issue:

- The organization shall maintain the customer details needed for the establishment of the communication.
- The organization shall appoint an authorized person for the notification.
- Records of this notification and approval must be kept and included under the records control procedure as specified in subclause 4.2.4 (Control of Records).

Notification may be performed with any of the traditional documented communication tools: fax, mail, e-mail. Telephone notification alone is not sufficient since you are required to maintain records. In which cases are you required to notify the customer? The general principle is very clear: where property is damaged, lost, or found unsuitable for use. However, the question is which actions or activities may create such situation? These include:

- Damages occurred as a result of transportation activities
- Delivery from the customer of wrong goods or wrong quantity
- Delivery from the customer of defective goods
- Quality problems occurred on the goods, or goods do not meet the requirements
- Goods with expired validity date
- Goods that require rework
- Damages occurred during the realization processes or storage
- Safety issues (goods were harmed or stolen)

Documentation

This chapter covers a lot of suggestions for documentation that might support and assist you in protecting your customer's property:

- A list of verifications for ingoing goods from the customer
- Instructions for handling and protecting confidential health information
- Instructions for storing and maintaining customer property
- Traceability and identification of customer property
- Instructions for handling and protecting customer property during service activities

The ISO 13485 does not demand documented requirements; but the issue is directly related to the requirements in chapter 7.5.1 since the customer's property is used during the realization processes. This is why it is recommended that you document all these requirements and submit them to the control of documents as required in subclause 4.2.3 (Control of Documents).

Records

The objective of maintaining records is the provision of evidence that you exercised the property with care and caution, as requested. Such evidence includes:

- Agreement and contracts with the customer
- Delivery or consignment notes
- Records of goods verifications
- Records of storage and maintenance activities
- Records of customer notifications

7.5.5 Preservation of Products

The requirements for preservation of products apply to all realization processes. The organization is required to preserve the product, its conformity, characteristics, and integrity so long as it bears the responsibility for the medical device. It begins right away when materials or parts are received in the organization, and ends when the medical device is delivered to the customer. In some cases the control may be extended to service and maintenance activities. That means that distributors, agents, and service suppliers might be included under the requirements (Table 7.33).

Controlling and maintaining preservation of the product signifies the identification and management of all factors that may adversely affect the medical device or its constituents: personnel, infrastructures, or work environment. Damages may occur due to realization processes, transportations, storage, time deterioration, service activities, or other harmful factors, such as:

- Sterility factors: temperature in the aeration area
- Mechanical factors: movement, vibration, shock, or abrasion
- Cleanliness factors: segregation from other products, dust, and particles
- Environmental factors: corrosion, temperature variation, electrostatic discharge, or radiation

Note: Since the responsibility for the preservation extends until the moment of delivery, the manufacturer must define when exactly that delivery occurs.

Documentation

The organization is to establish and maintain procedures and work instructions for the control of product preservation. The objective of the documentation is to provide structural requirements of product preservation. The standard specifies exactly in which cases or situations procedure and work instructions shall be implemented. The reason is that the issue of product preservation is related to other standard paragraphs that already require the establishment and maintenance of these. For example:

TABLE 7.33
Standard Requirements of Subclause 7.5.5

ISO 13485	ISO 9001
The organization shall act in order to preserve the product conformity during the realization, storage, and transportation processes. Preservation of the product shall be maintained until the delivery of the product at the intended destination	The organization shall act in order to preserve the product conformity during the realization, storage, and transportation processes. Preservation of the product shall be maintained until the delivery of the product at the intended destination
The organization shall maintain documented requirements on procedures or work instructions, describing the activities required to maintain preservation of the product	
Preservation activities include identification, handling, packaging storage, transportation, and protection	Preservation activities include identification, handling, packaging storage, transportation, and protection
Preservation of the product refers to the materials and components that constitute the product, as well as materials or components used to realize the product	Preservation of the product refers to the materials and components that constitute the product, as well as materials or components used to realize the product
The organization shall plan and maintain documented procedures or work instructions describing the activities for control of products with limited shelf life. The organization shall maintain records proving the performance of such conditions. These records shall be submitted to the records control process as required in subclause 4.2.4	
The organization shall plan and maintain documented procedures or work instructions describing the activities for the control of products with special storage conditions. The organization shall maintain records proving the storage of the products in the appropriate conditions. The records shall be submitted to the records control process as required in Subclause 4.2.4	

- When the preservation of the product is related to the behavior of personnel around the work environment, the controls and activities are to be defined in procedures or work instructions (6.4a).
- When the product preservation is related to the work environment conditions, the controls and activities are to be defined in procedures or work instructions (6.4b).
- Procedures or work instructions shall be implemented for the control of segregation between conforming and nonconforming products (6.4d).
- When the control of a purchased product is relevant to the preservation of the product, procedures or work instructions shall be implemented (7.4.1).

- When the control of production and service provision contributes to the preservation of the product, procedures or work instructions shall be implemented (7.5.1).
- When identification of the medical devices is needed to support the preservation of the product, special procedures or work instructions shall be implemented (7.5.3).

The documentation shall be planned in accordance with the nature of the medical device, or the work processes, and will:

- Identify products that are required to be preserved, or areas that are required to be controlled.
- Identify responsibilities and authorities.
- Describe activities for preservation.
- Define the requirements for records and evidence.

All the requirements and activities of product preservation, and the relevant documentation, shall be implanted in the training and certification processes of personnel.

Risk Management

When planning the activities for product preservation, the manufacturer must review the outputs of risk management activities and implement the suggested controls and protective measures in order to reduce risks related to product preservation. The risk control measures are recorded in the risk management file.

External Parties or Delegates

All of the requirements mentioned in this chapter are applicable to external parties that may take part in the product realization:

- Suppliers of services, processes, storage, or transportation
- Distributors that store, provide services, or transport and deliver the medical device

These parties are obligated to implement the required activities, use the documentation, and provide the appropriate records.

Service Activities

All of the requirements mentioned in this chapter are applicable and relevant to service and maintenance activities performed by the manufacturer or its delegates, when such may affect the preservation of the product.

Storage Activities

The storage of the medical device will prevent it from mix-ups, contamination, or any other adverse effects that may harm the product or its characteristics. Storage requirements shall relate to all materials, parts, components, packages, and accessories related to the realization of the product, and that may affect its quality. The storage conditions must be defined and the following issues shall be referred:

- Work environment and storage parameters—such as temperature, humidity, cleanliness, and dust (particles count)—shall be defined, documented, and maintained.

- The storage facilities will not harm the medical device, and will provide it with sufficient protection to maintain its characteristics (i.e., intended use, functionality, performance, and safety).
- Special tools or equipment required for the storage of different types of parts, components, or materials shall be defined and allocated.

Storage may be implemented using segregation areas, special areas, and the identification of products and products' usability status. Where it is required, environmental control systems shall be installed. When storage is outsourced and the organization uses suppliers, they must be included under this control and the measure shall be implemented at their premises too. The supplier must provide evidence that they have followed all the requirements.

Packaging

Packaging activities, operations, and conditions must be verified in order to ensure that they do not harm the medical device or influence its quality. For example, when you are packaging the medical device in a container, you are required to prove compatibility between the container and the medical device; that is, perform a test that the container does not harm the medical device or alter its characteristics. In some cases the matter must be validated and supported with scientific research. However, there the manufacturer is required to implement controls and verify that the product is packed according to the specifications. In chapter 7.5.5 the manufacturer is required to control the packaging operations and verify that they do not harm the product.

Security, Safety, and Protection

Security and protection of the medical device must be defined. Activities such as handling of medical devices, components, materials (and all other items related to the product that may affect its quality); controlled access to products; and safety measures shall be implemented:

- Identification of devices, components, parts, or materials is needed in order to indicate their usability status, and allow the implementation of suitable preservation measures.
- Authorization and access to the medical devices, components, parts, or materials shall be defined and implemented according to organizational functions.
- Safety measures shall be taken regarding the storage facilities.
- Protection measures to preserve the medical device during realization processes are required.

Appropriate measures and definitions shall ensure the safety of the medical device and the use of tools and equipment, and the installation of an alarm system shall be considered. You may define and document for each activity the appropriate tool or equipment that can be used.

Transportation

Transportation conditions must be defined and documented. Preservation of the product during transportation means undertaking all necessary measures in order to protect the medical device and its package, and preserve their characteristics:

- The medical device, its characteristics, quality, and package shall be protected from external factors during transportation.

- Special tools, equipment, or accessories required for the transportation activities shall be defined and controlled.
- Only certified employees may perform certain transportation activities (cranes, forklift, etc.).

Transportation refers to external transportation, such as by air, sea, land, or internal—that is, performed within the premises of the organization (as by forklift, or between processes). Each transportation type shall be analyzed and suitable actions and activities shall be planned. Requirements for certification may appear in a job description or in work instructions. The definitions shall be appropriate to the nature of the medical device.

Product with a Limited Shelf Life

Special reference is given to products that bear a limited shelf life. The objective is to eliminate the use and distribution of products whose characteristics have been damaged or altered. The characteristics and quality of products with an expiry date deteriorates over time. Such products have a defined period of life with an exact date indicating when the status of the product changes and the product can no longer be used—in other words, the exact date on which the product is declared as nonconforming. From this date on the product shall be treated, handled, and disposed of according to your specifications of control of nonconforming products, as required in clause 8.3. This requirement refers to products that the organization produces and realizes, as well as purchased goods stored in the organization facilities (that have a limited lifetime). These products will be identified, indicated, and treated with different (documented) measures. The documentation shall ensure that the organization:

- Identifies these products.
- Plans and implements effective control activities over these products.
- Evaluates their usability according to defined time limits.
- When the date expires, the status of the product changes and the product is disqualified for use or distribution (nonconforming product).

The documentation may appear on a procedure or a work instruction—filling out forms is not sufficient in this case. The documentation is to include and describe specific control activities. These shall be submitted to the control of documents as required in subclause 4.2.3. Records and evidence of maintaining the requirements shall be kept and submitted to the control of records as required in subclause 4.2.4. All records or copies related to the expiration date of the product, parts, components, or materials may be saved in the DHR. Types of possible records include:

- Labeling on the products
- A designated log
- An inventory management system with alarms and warnings
- Signing and posting

If you are maintaining processes via an ERP system with a product data and management module, you may define, trace and control the validity dates of product through the system. When the medical devices are distributed or delivered by an agent of the organization or the distributors, they must follow these requirements:

- The appropriate documentation shall be available to them, or they will maintain similar documented requirements.

- They shall provide the manufacturer with evidence that these requirements have been applied.

To remain on the safe side, the organization may verify the disposal of products by distributors and agents with the assistance of traceability, maintaining the records of end customers, and through developing a designated communication channel for the issue.

Advice: In order to ensure the delivery of products in a sufficient time interval before their expiry date, the organization can manage inventory turns or stock rotations according to the expiration dates. Implementing the FIFO inventory system (first in first out) may also reduce the risks of using products with expired dates.

Products with Special Storage Conditions

Special reference is given to products with special storage conditions. These are products whose characteristics or qualities have deteriorated due to a failure to provide them with specific and defined storage conditions; thus, the status of these products changes, and their use is forbidden. In other words, failing to comply with these specifications may result in a situation where the product will be nonconforming; and since a manufacturer cannot allow such situation, they must ensure the implementation of all necessary measures in order to create the optimal conditions and, of course, provide suitable evidence. Special conditions may be required during the storage, realization processes, or transportation activities. The requirements refer to products that the organization produces and realizes, as well as purchased goods stored in the organization facilities. The requirements refer to materials, parts, components, or packages. These products will be identified, indicated, and treated with different (documented) measures. The documentation shall ensure that the organization:

- Identified these products.
- Identified the special storage conditions.
- Planned and implemented measures in order provide with these conditions.
- Defined and allocated tools, equipment, or facilities necessary for maintaining these conditions.
- Planned and implemented effective control activities that maintain these conditions.

The documentation may appear on a procedure or a work instruction. The documentation is to include and describe specific control activities and shall be submitted to the control of documents as required in subclause 4.2.3. Records and evidence of maintaining the requirements shall be kept and submitted to the control of records as required in subclause 4.2.4. All records or copies related to special storage conditions may be saved in the DHR, such as:

- Environmental conditions
- Performance of activities
- Signings and posting examples

When deviations or departures from these conditions are identified, the product shall be reevaluated, and the usability status reexamined. The examination may be performed according to a specified criteria or designated quality tests. The reevaluation shall be documented and records shall be maintained.

When the medical devices are distributed or delivered by agents of the organization or distributors, they must also follow these requirements:

- The appropriate documentation shall be available to them or they will maintain similar documented requirements.
- They shall provide the manufacturer with evidence that these requirements were applied.

7.6 CONTROL OF MONITORING AND MEASURING DEVICE

The ISO 13485 Standard treats monitoring and measuring devices very seriously. They are considered by the ISO 13485 Standard as an important element of the realization process. Therefore, the requirements are quite specific and logical (Table 7.34).

TABLE 7.34
Standard Requirements of Clause 7.6

ISO 13485	ISO 9001
The organization shall determine the necessary monitoring and measuring activities required to provide evidence that products and processes meet their requirements and specifications. According to these activities the organization shall determine the necessary monitoring and measuring devices to provide the evidence	The organization shall determine the necessary monitoring and measuring activities required to provide evidence that products and processes meet their requirements and specifications. According to these activities the organization shall determine the necessary monitoring and measuring devices to provide the evidence
The organization shall establish and maintain a documented procedure describing methods and activities to ensure that the monitoring and measuring activities are performed according to the requirements	The organization shall define processes, methods, and activities to ensure that the monitoring and measuring activities are performed according to the requirements
Monitoring and measuring devices shall be calibrated or verified prior to their use. Calibration shall take place at specific predefined intervals	Monitoring and measuring devices shall be calibrated or verified prior to their use. Calibration shall take place at specific predefined intervals
The calibration will be traceable to international or national standard measurements. In cases where such standards do not exist or are not applicable, the calibration and the basis for the calibration process (physical or calculating) shall be defined, justified, and recorded by the organization	The calibration will be traceable to international or national standard measurements. In cases where such standards do not exist or are not applicable, the calibration and the basis for the calibration process (physical or calculating) shall be defined, justified, and recorded by the organization
Each of the monitoring and measuring devices shall be identified in order to determine the calibration status, validity, and intactness	Each of the monitoring and measuring devices shall be identified in order to determine the calibration status, validity, and intactness
The monitoring and measuring devices shall be safeguarded and protected in order to eliminate any situations or conditions that would invalidate the measurement results	The monitoring and measuring devices shall be safeguarded and protected in order to eliminate any situations or conditions that would invalidate the measurement results

TABLE 7.34 (Continued)
Standard Requirements of Clause 7.6

ISO 13485	ISO 9001
The monitoring and measuring devices shall be protected from damage, environmental conditions, and deterioration that might affect the calibration during storage, handling, and measuring. In cases of need, maintenance activities shall be defined	The monitoring and measuring devices shall be protected from damage, environmental conditions, and deterioration that might affect the calibration during storage, handling, and measuring. In cases of need, maintenance activities shall be defined
When a monitoring and measuring device is found inappropriate for use, or its calibration proves to be inaccurate, the organization shall evaluate the validity of the accepted results, along with the ability of any products that were released with this device to meet their requirements.	When a monitoring and measuring device is found inappropriate for use, or its calibration proves to be inaccurate, the organization shall evaluate the validity of the accepted results, along with the ability of any products that were released with this device to meet their requirements.
In cases of need, the organization shall trace back and recall products for remeasurement where the issue is critical. Appropriate measures shall be applied to products and outputs of processes that were influenced by nonconformity	In cases of need, the organization shall trace back and recall products for remeasurement where the issue is critical. Appropriate measures shall be applied to products and outputs of processes that were influenced by nonconformity
Records of calibration and maintenance activities and of device identifications are to be kept and included under the records control process, as required in subclause 4.2.4 (Control of Records)	Records of calibration and maintenance activities and of device identifications are to be kept and included under the records control process, as required in subclause 4.2.4 (Control of Records)
When computer software is used to perform or support monitoring or measuring activities, its ability to provide appropriate results shall be validated prior to initial use	When computer software is used to perform or support monitoring or measuring activities, its ability to provide appropriate results shall be validated prior to initial use
Note: Control and management may be planned with reference to the ISO 10012-1 and ISO 10012-2 Standards for guidance	Note: Control and management may be planned with reference to the ISO 10012-1 and ISO 10012-2 Standards for guidance

Calibration Procedures

The ISO 13485 requires establishing and maintaining a documented procedure in order:

- To control the monitoring and measuring devices
- To ensure that measurement and monitoring activities are planned according to requirements, and are performed respectively

As much as a lot of people think a general description in a procedure of the devices, departments, or the calibration intervals of the tools is not sufficient. That is achieved through the documented requirements. The ISO 13485 takes the issue one step further and expects there to be guiding principles regarding the implementation and control of measurement and monitoring devices. The procedure will describe the policy of the organization in planning the measurement and monitoring activities:

- Measurement and monitoring needs—the procedure will describe how a process or a product is being reviewed, and measurable characteristics will be identified. The procedure shall describe the inputs to be considered when reviewing a process or a product; that is, customer requirements, regulatory requirements, intended use, risk management, safety, and performance specifications.
- Definition of monitoring and measurement activities—the procedure will define how the measurement activities are being determined and refer to issues such as instructions, frequencies, areas, measured materials, products, and processes. It is possible (and recommended) to use statistical methods for the demonstration of compatibility through a statistical relation of tools and equipment to certain characteristics of material parts or processes. Design and development outputs may serve as inputs to the determination.
- Determination of the appropriate criteria—the procedure will define how the manufacturer set the criteria for measurement results; for example, tolerances, limits, expected test results, customer requirements, regulatory requirements.
- Standards—the procedure is to define the parameters for the identification of the appropriate standard for comparison or assessment of the results. The issue shall refer to the planning and maintenance of internal standards.
- Allocation of tools and equipment—the procedure is to define the allocation of devices and accessories (where applicable) needed for the measurements. Importance will be given to the appointment of a device to the predefined criteria; the device shall be able to provide the expected results. The procedure shall refer to the purchase of such devices; when the matter is of importance; the types of devices; the identification of suppliers; the parameters for decision making; and a review of price quotes.
- Identification of devices—the procedure shall specify the method for identification of the devices in the organization; for example, names, types, serial numbers, catalogue numbers, and locations.
- Human resources—the procedure shall relate to the identification and allocation of suitable human resources and responsibilities of monitoring and measurement activities. When applicable, the procedure shall define the required qualifications or certifications for the operation of tools and equipment.
- Controls—the procedure shall define how the required controls and validations of such tools and equipment are determined; for example, through calibration activities (external and internal), maintenance, storage, and handling.
- Nonconforming equipment—the procedure shall define clearly the handling and measurement of tools and equipment that were identified as nonconforming. The issue shall cover the disposal of such devices.
- Documentation—the procedure shall describe the types of documentation that support the monitoring and measurement activities; that is, work instructions, user manuals, test instructions, and forms. It is important that the definitions and references shall relate to the availability of the documents at the work stations or other applicable locations.
- Records—the procedure shall specify how the measurement records will provide the necessary evidence.

The procedure shall be submitted to the documents control process as required in subclause 4.2.3 (Control of Documents).

The standard refers us to chapter 7.2.1 (determination of requirements related to the product), knowing that the requirements of this chapter include critical information concerning the monitoring and measuring processes and activities that might serve as inputs, such as:

- Customer requirements
- Requirements that were not stated by the customer
- Regulatory requirements
- Additional requirements set by the organization

When determining the monitoring and measuring processes, it is necessary that you review the issues mentioned above and identify where monitoring and measuring activities may support the manufacturer verifying and confirming that the materials, products, or processes meet these requirements.

Reference to Risk Management

The issue of monitoring and measuring processes and products is one of the tools for the implementation of controls of risks and the measurement of their effectiveness. The monitoring and measuring devices may serve the manufacturer in controlling and validating results of processes and in verifying that risks were reduced to a desired level (by providing objective evidence). During the design and development of the product, areas and scopes—where control of risk is needed—are determined. The reference is to be found on the risk management plan. The outputs of risk analysis and control are inputs for the identification and allocation of appropriate devices.

Identification of the Device

Each device shall be identified, and the identification shall appear on the device itself—a number, color, serial number, name—according to the nature and type of device. The identification is important for the traceability of products that were tested and approved with the device. If, during the later stages, it is discovered that the device is defective and the measurements conducted were incorrect—you will have the ability to trace back the "infected" products through a link to the monitor and measuring device. Managing the identification will also assist in managing the status of the monitoring and measuring devices. The monitoring and measuring devices may be identified with reference to variables such as internal number, manufacturer's serial number, location, or the responsible party. For example, tools for validation (such as monitoring and measuring devices or control gauges) that participate in and validate processes must themselves be validated and recorded. The issue is widely discussed in subclause 7.5.2 (Validation of Processes for Production and Service Provision).

Controlling

The objective of the control of monitoring and measuring devices is to provide information regarding their status. The control will manage the tools according to various parameters (the focus here is on characterization rather than manners or methods):

- Category—try to sort the monitoring and measuring devices according to a family type; that is, according to use, range, department, process, or product. The more detailed the division is, the more control you will have.
- External or internal calibration—define for each monitoring and measuring device its external and internal calibration requirements.

- Location—document where monitoring and measuring devices are stored, and under whose responsibility. When the monitoring and measuring devices are used by more than one party in the organization (for example, production halls, labs, different departments), it is recommended that you manage their locations in order to maintain sufficient traceability.
- Calibration interval—define for each monitoring and measuring device its calibration interval. This may be determined according to time periods or the amount of uses; for example, for every 100 batches, the device must be calibrated.
- Calibration status—indicate whether the monitoring and measuring device is: calibrated and permitted for use; not calibrated and not permitted for use; or permitted for use, but under restrictions.
- Owner—you may receive monitoring and measuring devices or gauges from your customers in order to perform measurements on special products. In this case you are required to document them under the customer property requirements.

The main idea is to manage a list of your monitoring and measuring devices. Choose the way that is most suitable to you (e.g., electronic chart, form, or ERP system).

Advice: Where organizations lay down a lot of control and measurement devices that no one uses, these devices are either: old; were purchased by previous employers; or are not relevant for the production anymore. There are plenty of other reasons too. However, they should always be calibrated before the external audit because it is a standard requirements that all monitoring and measurement devices in the organization must be calibrated. This results in high expenses. Here is my suggestion:

- Separate the used tools from the unused.
- For the unused, define a status as unusable (not necessarily not calibrated).
- Wrap or pack them in a way that any tampering or use of them is immediately noticeable.
- In time you should be able to reduce the number of control and measurements devices without failing to meet the requirements.

Documented Requirements

The documented requirements refer to documentation that supports the control of monitoring and measuring devices as suggested on the procedure:

- The list of the monitoring and measuring devices in the organization
- Internal calibration instructions
- Work instructions of how to use and handle the devices
- Forms for control of the devices
- List of approved calibration laboratories (can be included under the list of approved suppliers)
- Documentation for the disqualification of devices

Table 7.35 in an example control list for the follow up of the calibration of devices:

Assumed date: 01/06/2010. These documents shall be submitted to the control of documents as specified in chapter 4.2.3 (Control of Documents).

Calibration

Calibration is comparing an instrument's accuracy to a known standard—for example, the length of a ruler A can be calibrated by comparing it to a standard ruler B, which

TABLE 7. 35
Calibration Follow Up Table

Internal Number	Description	Size/Type	Calibration Internal/ External	Calibration Interval (Months)	Status	Last Test	Next Test	Location
C04A	Digital Caliper	0–150 mm—digital	External	12	Calibrated	10/10/2009	10/10/2010	Quality Dep. Cabinet1
C05A	Caliper	0–600—mechanical	External	12	Not calibrated	23/05/2009	23/05/2010	Quality Dep. Cabinet1
C06A	Depth Gauge	300 mm	External	12	Calibrated	10/10/2009	10/10/2010	Production
C07A	Control Gauge	Part No. 90012343	Internal	6	Calibrated	01/01/2010	01/07/2010	Quality Dep. Cabinet3

has a known length and was tested and approved according to a predefined standard. Once the reference of ruler A to the standard is known and determined, ruler A is calibrated and can be used to measure the length of other things. Calibrated tools and equipment are necessary to achieve product quality objectives, and to ensure that processes will meet their requirements. The medical device (or processes that realize it) has measurable characteristics that must be controlled, verified, or validated. Through a set of operations the calibration ensures that measuring devices conform to the requirements of their intended use.

The calibration of tools and monitoring and measuring devices shall be traceable to predefined criteria. The criteria may be either international or national measurements standards, internal standards, or a predefined and documented basis established by the manufacturer, customer, or a regulatory requirement. Where required, the results of the calibration shall be traceable to international standards. This is normally (and effectively) achieved by sending the devices to certified calibration laboratories that have the knowledge and the tools to perform, correct, standardize, and calibrate devices according to international standards. The most common example is labs that are certified to the ISO/IEC 17025. When calibration is performed externally, the manufacturer will receive a document indicating the standard to which the tools were calibrated. This is the evidence for traceability to such a standard.

When such international or national standards are not applicable, and the organization is calibrating according to an independent or internal requirement for calibration, you are required to document these calibration requirements as reference. If you are using a gauge delivered by the customer in order to verify a part's characteristics, you need to establish a master or a reference part for the calibration of the gauge before each batch. In this case it could be a product that the customer approved as a master product. By testing the gauge you can ensure that it meets its intended use. This issue shall be documented (for example, on the test instructions of the part). Supplier's or manufacturer's instructions may serve as calibration requirements. Bear in mind, however, that these instructions must be controlled.

The records of the calibration are to be defined and maintained. The records shall cover the following details:

- A unique identification of the device tested
- A description of all the measurements and calibration activities that were performed for a single device
- Details regarding the measurements; that is, the date, location, conditions (if required), the person that performed the tests, and the tools and equipment used during the measurements
- A specifications of the standards or criteria
- Reference to documentation (if applicable)
- The results of the measurements
- The status of the device
- Corrections, modifications, maintenance, or adjustments (if made)

You must define where you document the results, and are required to maintain the records. These records shall be submitted to the records control process in the organization, as required in subclause 4.2.4 (Control of Records).

Protection and Prevention

The ISO 13485 Standard specifically demands that you protect the devices from adjustments that would invalidate the measurement results. The intention here is not for the usual gauges (which can be stored in a plastic box); it relates to the sensitive and more complicated gauges that require greater attention and care. Bear in mind that the main objective of the protection is not to prevent scratches on the surface, but rather to protect:

- Its intactness and functionality, including deterioration over time.
- Its status of calibration—the device shall be protected from any cause that may alter or damage its calibration status.

When defining the protection, you shall refer to parameters that may affect the device and its calibration status; for example, temperature, humidity, transportation, operation, or storage. In some cases you could conduct a small-scale risk analysis and identify the risks regarding monitoring and measuring devices. The extent of the protection depends on the device itself. Usually the manufacturer of the tool provides instructions regarding the protection of the device. You may transfer these into a procedure or refer to them. If such instructions are not provided, you should contact the manufacturer. In any event, you are required to prove the ability to protect the monitoring and measuring devices, their intactness, and their calibration status. Naturally, this issue will be referred to in the procedure.

Software

When computer software performs the monitoring and measuring activities, the organization must validate the ability of the software to perform the measurements. Software configuration may serve as calibration activity. The validation is to be carried out before the initial use of the software. Calibration is usually perceived as a nonrelevant activity for software, but this is not the case. When the organization makes use of software for measurements for product validation, it shall:

- Assess the effect of the software's activities on the product and its quality
- Manage the configuration of the software in order to control any changes that may affect the accuracy and fitness of the measurement
- Manage the configuration of the software in order to identify the software as a monitoring and measuring device

Which of the software components shall be controlled?

- The data evaluated by the software—ensuring that the data is valid
- Safety and reliability of data—ensuring that data is protected
- Integrity of software's processes and features—ensuring that the software's processes and algorithms assist in achieving the objective of the measurements
- The hardware—ensuring that the hardware is intact
- Any equipment connected to the hardware—ensuring the this equipment is intact

Traceability and Recall

Monitoring and measuring devices plays an important role in their approval—according to the measurement results it is decided whether the product met its requirements or not. However, you must prepare yourself for the possibility that monitoring and measuring devices will be found to be defective, inaccurate, with malfunctions, or not calibrated. This means that there is a possibility that products that were released, based on measurements made with the defective devices, do not meet their requirements and specifications. When such situations occur, the manufacturer must evaluate the affect of the inaccurate measurement on the quality of the product.

That is the reason why the ISO 13485 Standard requires that you maintain full traceability after every medical device that is released; and after any of its components, materials, or process elements, as they may also affect the quality of the product. This relates to control and measuring devices as those that were used in order to realize the product are considered process elements. The use of inappropriate of defective monitoring devices may suggest that a quality problem, a fault, or a nonconformity, have not been detected in time. How can you tell which tool is defective? This is where the traceability is vital. Each device that was used to monitor and measure products or processes should be recorded. A detailed example for documenting the devices during the processes is given in subclause 7.5.2.1 (in paragraph "PQ—Monitoring and Measurement Devices and Control Gauges"). When such cases occur:

- It is necessary to trace back all the products that were tested with the defective device, or all the products that are related to a process controlled with the defective device.
- It is required that you assess the affect of the measurements on the quality of the product and whether a potential nonconformity could occur as a result of the improper measurements.
- It is required that you specify which measures were applied; for example, the recall of the product for remeasurement, the issuing of an advisory notice, a sample remeasurement, maintenance or service actions, and so on.
- The matter shall be recorded as a nonconformity with information such as the devices, materials, products or processes, and the actions that were taken.

Reference to the ISO 10012-1 and ISO 10012-2

The ISO 13485 Standard refers us to the ISO 10012-1 and ISO 10012-2. These are standards for guidance on developing, planning, and implementing effective measuring equipment and measurement processes. The basic purpose of the ISO 10012-1 and ISO 10012-2 Standards is to:

- Establish a measurement management system for planning, implementing, and managing the monitoring and measuring processes and activities.
- Determine the level of control needed for the effective execution of implementation.

It is not required that you implement the ISO 10012-1 and ISO 10012-2 Standards, but it is suggested that you consult them when planning your monitoring and measuring activities.

Records

Naturally, a detailed control and management activity produces a set of records and evidence, such as:

- Lists of approved, disqualified, external, or internal monitoring and measuring devices used by the manufacturer
- Records of internal or external calibration activities, including results of measurements
- Certifications of monitoring and measuring devices according to specific standards
- Lists of approved laboratories for calibration of monitoring and measuring devices

- Records of service and maintenance activities applied to the monitoring and measuring devices, including repairs or adjustments
- Records required to maintain traceability of monitoring and measuring devices

The records of calibration and evidence that the monitoring and measuring devices meet their requirements shall be submitted to the records control process as required in subclause 4.2.4 (Control of Records).

8 Measurement, Analysis, and Improvement

8.1 MEASUREMENT, ANALYSIS, AND IMPROVEMENT—GENERAL

The objective of the measuring processes is to collect, analyze, and report data that are relevant to the medical devices and realization processes. The analysis shall strive to support the processes and maintain the effectiveness of your quality management system, as well as the quality of the medical devices. The measurement and the analysis shall promote the organization on an effective course toward improvement. Note the common use the word of the word "effective" throughout this book. If this was a book regarding the ISO 9001 Standard, the word "continually" would have substituted the word "effectively." The ISO 13485 Standard, however, demands an effective quality management system. This is unique to the ISO 13485 Standard. In order to optimize effectively the quality management system, the organization must prepare an improvement plan with objectives, execution controls, and a systematic review of results against the objectives (Table 8.1).

The objective of clause 8.1 is to establish measures for improvement throughout the organization. These measures will collect data through defined intervals (a period of time, a number of batches, or a number of products) and extent (what and how many) regarding the realization processes and products. The collected data will be analyzed according to a defined method and parameters related to the effectiveness of the medical device—product as well as realization processes. The analysis, data resolution, and conclusions will support the effective management of processes and quality management systems.

Performing the above will generate improvement. Chapter 8 introduces us to the ISO perception of quality improvement, where the organization must assess the effectiveness of its processes; that is, in terms of realization and quality. The assessment will provide a status report regarding your quality objectives. These objectives were defined in the quality plan—the processes, procedures, and controls applied for the product realization (now all the loose ends are starting to be tied up). According to the status report you will decide whether an improvement is necessary. Remember that the ISO 13485 Standard requires maintaining effectiveness rather than just implementing and measuring it. Maintaining means the implementation of measures that will systemize effectiveness. The reason for this is that maintaining effectiveness would surely help achieve the desired improvement. Allow me to add that effectiveness is the extent to which planned activities are realized, and planned results achieved; you planned something, and you test the extent of the results against the expected objectives. This is performed in order to achieve a systematic improvement.

TABLE 8.1
Standard Requirements of Subclause 8.1

ISO 13485	ISO 9001
The organization is required to plan and implement controls, to measure and monitor its realization and quality processes	The organization is required to plan and implement controls, to measure and monitor its realization and quality processes
The measurements and controls will demonstrate product conformity	The measurements and controls will demonstrate product conformity
The measurements and controls will demonstrate quality management system conformity	The measurements and controls will demonstrate quality management system conformity
The measurement, analysis, and improvement shall maintain the effectiveness of the quality management system	The measurement, analysis, and improvement shall continually improve the effectiveness of the quality management system
The organization will determine methods for implementing and applicable methods for measurement, analysis, and improvement. Where appropriate, the methods will include statistical techniques	The organization will determine methods for implementing and applicable methods for measurement, analysis, and improvement. Where appropriate, the methods will include statistical techniques
Where regulatory requirements demand the establishment and maintenance of documented procedures or methods for identifying and implementing necessary statistic techniques, such procedures shall be maintained	

By submitting a process or a product to a control, and gathering data and comparing it to predefined objectives, you will evaluate their effectiveness. When the objectives have not been achieved, you will implement improvements and continue to measure them until the objectives are achieved. Thus, we have:

- Measurement—we collected data.
- Analysis—we analyzed the data and compared it to objectives.
- Improvement—we identified and implemented opportunities for improvement.
- Maintenance—by performing it over and again, maintenance is achieved.

When defining the controls over the processes that will serve the measurement analysis and improvement it is necessary to:

- Determine an appropriate method for control, such as statistical tools or techniques for each process or product.
- Determine the scope or extent of the control—what, when, and how many will be measured.
- Determine the means with which the control will be implemented and utilized throughout the organization.
- Assigning the responsible for gathering the data and authorities to be reported.

The above are also valid for service processes. Now let us discuss the practice. The control measures are to prove two things:

- The conformity of the processes and the product to the requirements
- The conformity of the quality management system to its quality objectives

The Conformity of the Processes and the Product to the Requirements

Finished products, product characteristics, parts or components, and realization processes will be evaluated and proved for their conformity using acceptance activities and validations. Examination activities may be samplings, inspections, tests, observations, or applied controls over processes. Each will generate data that will be validated against the product requirements with the help of criteria. The validation will prove whether the requirements were met and whether the product conforms to them. The data will be gathered and analyzed according to defined methods; that is, statistical or qualitative evaluations. Bear in mind, however, that you will have to justify the method that you chose and relate it to the nature of the medical devices and the realization processes. In other words, there is to be a correlation between the realization processes, the data collected, and the statistical methods you used to analyze them. Employees and personnel that perform these activities will be appropriately trained and qualified.

The best example is the quality tests where the products or processes are sampled and evaluated with criteria. The evaluation (statistical or subjective) determines whether the process has achieved its objective and produced a suitable product, or whether the process has to be held and an investigation is required regarding its results.

Let us assume that the results of a quality test showed that the assembly of a component is not carried out according to the specification, and thus the medical device fails to comply. Let us assume further that this happens just too often. The process is stopped, corrections are applied, and defective medical devices are removed. The matter was documented as a nonconformity. As far as the ISO 13485 Standard is concerned, the product does not conform—the process is not stable and a defective medical device can evade control. This is where the measurement steps in; assuming that the related data is recorded, it will be possible to analyze the reason for the machine disturbances. This is where the analysis can help; after an extensive investigation, the reason was detected. Eventually the improvement takes over; a production parameter was reviewed, changed, verified and validated, and measured again.

If we analyze the case we see that:

1. A quality problem was detected—the assembly process was not stable.
2. The process was measured—production data was recorded.
3. The data was analyzed—the problem had been analyzed and the reason was detected.
4. The improvement was implemented—a production parameter was optimized and the change was implemented.
5. The effectiveness was reviewed—the process is to be reviewed for a period of time in order to prove stability.

This was a very simple example of how measurement analysis and improvement control the processes—it is more complicated in practice.

The Conformity of the Processes and the Quality Management System

To quote subclause 5.4.1 (Quality Objectives):

> The top management shall determine appropriate quality objectives that would ensure competence to the product's requirements and shall ensure that the objectives are determined and transferred to the appropriate and relevant functions throughout the organization.

You are asked to verify that the objectives are achieved and that they are effectively improving the quality management system. I will give another example in order to demonstrate this requirement.

The top management decided after a very intense year on an improvement plan—training all production personnel to perform sterilization processes. This objective is the result of a higher quality objective that could not be achieved: supplying the medical devices according to schedules. The investigation showed that there is always a bottleneck by the sterilization processes. This is because there are not enough employees trained and qualified to perform the process.

The decision was made in the management review, and the right documentation was established. The assignment was placed in the hands of the production manager, budgets were allocated, and training was scheduled. After half a year as part of an internal audit, the quality manager will examine the progress made. He will do this on two levels: the first will be to verify that the training has been completed; he will review qualification records, documentation of training, and review whether each production employee is certified to work on the sterilization machine. Let us assume that all production employees were trained as required. The second level of investigation will be to review whether the higher objective was influenced; that is, whether the delays in supplying the orders are reduced. The investigation shows that the delays were only 50% reduced. The result indicates that the plan was not effective and that the quality management system had not improved.

If we analyze the case, we see that:

1. Quality objectives were set—the reduction of delays and the training of production employees.
2. The process was measured—through the internal audit.
3. The performance and data were analyzed—the verification of the training, and the analysis of the delays.
4. The effectiveness was reviewed—the review whether there was a connection between the sterilization processes and the delays.

Identification of Required Statistical Techniques

The ISO 13485 prepares us for the possibility that national or regional regulations might require us to plan and determine a procedure for the identification of necessary statistical methods or techniques to be implemented throughout our measurement and analysis processes. When such requirements exist, you will need to:

- Determine and document the method for the identification of necessary statistical methods or techniques.
- Implement and utilize the method throughout your realization processes, as required.

8.2 MONITORING AND MEASUREMENT

8.2.1 Feedback

The organization is to continually and systematically evaluate whether the medical device meets the requirements throughout its life cycle, and that residual risks are controlled constantly. While the ISO 9001 Standard demands the evaluation of customer satisfaction, the ISO 13485 Standard does not, but requires the evaluation of feedback regarding the use of the medical device:

- Does the medical device meet the intended use requirements?
- Does the medical device meet the regulatory requirements?
- Are residual risks still controlled and have new risks been identified?

The objective is to plan systematical methods that will provide early identification of quality problems and warnings related to the medical device. When such are detected, they will be analyzed, evaluated, and submitted to improvement processes. The idea is to detect the problem before the medical device may harm a patient or a user (Table 8.2).

The objective of the feedback, simply put, is: to define, document, and implement methods for monitoring and controlling the product using data that were collected in the postproduction phase, or by means of postmarket surveillance, in order to detect quality problems. Once quality problems are detected they are handled and submitted to improvement processes.

TABLE 8.2
Standard Requirements of Subclause 8.2.1

ISO 13485	ISO 9001
Feedback	*Customer Satisfaction*
The organization shall determine and implement methods for the obtaining and assessment of information indicating whether the organization has met customer requirements	The organization shall determine methods for the obtaining and assessment of information related to the customer's perception, indicating whether the organization has met customer requirements
The method shall evaluate the quality management system performances	The method shall evaluate the quality management system performances
The organization shall develop and document in a procedure a system for receiving customer feedback applications about the medical device relevant to issues and warnings of quality problems. The system will integrate processes of improvement, and preventive and corrective actions	
When regulatory regulations require the organization to maintain reporting procedures regarding events that occurred on the postproduction phase, the system for obtaining the feedback will be used	

By measuring feedback, importance is given to the fulfillment of the medical device's requirements rather than the perception of the customer as to whether the organization has met their requirements. Customer satisfaction is a subjective matter, whereas achieving medical device or regulatory requirements are objective issues that can be assessed and measured. A customer satisfaction survey may turn out to be diverted, and therefore may provide inaccurate results. However, the feedback will indicate the status of the medical device compared to its requirements. Feedback could be positive or suggestive—it need not be only negative regarding the medical device.

Another objective of the feedback is to assist the manufacturer in implementing improvements in the medical device or in the realization processes that, in the end, will allow the product to meet its requirements optimally (and customers' as regulatory). This will be achieved through four sub-objectives:

- Early identification of problems concerning quality, performance, functionality, and safety
- Creating communication channels allowing data to flow
- Defining and collecting appropriate data that will support the analysis of the root causes
- Initiating an interface between the problems and related data and the improvement processes for analysis, treatment, and correction
- Improving quality management system performances

Using defined systematical methods to collect data regarding the use of the medical device, the manufacturer will identify—in advance—quality problems related to its functionality, performance, intended use, and safety, and will submit them to a controlled process for handling. The purpose is to detect these problems before they can cause harm to anyone. The source of these problems may originate in the design of the medical device or the realization processes.

In some circles feedback may be referred or compared to postmarketing surveillance (PMS); that is, the search and detection of problems in the medical device that were not identified or recognized before submission for marketing.

The methods for conducting and collecting feedback data and information will be defined and documented in a procedure. This will be discussed further later.

How one can measure customer feedback? Feedback consists of a systematical gathering of information related to the use of the medical device and its affect on users or patients in the postproduction phase; for example, transportation activities, storage, installation, service, and use. The information shall be collected in various ways (which will be detailed later). You are not obligated to implement all methods, but you will be required to justify the exclusion of methods that were not implemented. Bear in mind that the data collected via feedback methods are to be used at later stages as inputs for processes of analysis of data (as required in clause 8.4 (Analysis of Data)). Thus, it is recommended that when you plan the gathering activities and characterizing the types of data to be collected, you should consider future analyses. The objective of the analyses is to demonstrate the suitability and effectiveness of the quality management system, and to evaluate whether improvements of the effectiveness of the quality management system are needed.

Distributors

Before reviewing feedback in detail the following remark regarding distributors should be noted: when a distributor is delivering the medical device to the final customer, the organization will integrate the distributor in any feedback method it has decided upon. You are required to define (and document) to the distributor the communication channel and means of reporting between the dealer and you (e.g., a dealer report).

Customer Surveys

Customer surveys are a good tool to collect data from customers regarding the use, performance, quality, delivery, service, or other issues concerning the medical device. The customer supplies you with information or data according to predefined questions. It is very important to identify the perceptive subjects and issues related to the quality, functionality, and performance of the medical device. The target group of the questionnaire is to be defined; that is, patients, users, and other authorities on the matter. Their opinion will shed light on the quality, functionality, and performance of the medical device. The questionnaire can be printed and filled out manually, or it can be digital. The latter is recommended because data from the survey may serve later on for analysis purposes. Today, most management systems provide the possibility of electronic questionnaires.

The interval of the survey must be defined. There are organizations that send the questionnaire once or twice a year. However, you must identify and define the interval that suits your medical device. It may be that you are positioning a new development in the market or evaluating a significant change in your medical device. In such a case you would ideally follow the change or development closely, meaning that the interval must be more frequent than once a year. Each case must be evaluated on its own merits.

The survey may be performed as a meeting or an interview with the customer. This is a more proactive approach, where you are sending your representatives out to the field to sense the customers' reactions. In this case you need to plan the interview and questions in advance in order to obtain the required information. Once again, the target must be defined—sending out representatives costs money and resources; thus you should ensure that you do it correctly.

Suggestions for topics and issue to be assessed in a survey:

- Product labeling
- Product packaging
- User manual
- Compliance with regulatory requirements
- Safety of the medical device
- Functionality of the medical device

Service Calls

The organization may use service calls, maintenance activities, and field visits to customers as means to collect data regarding the use of the medical device. The data collected will be analyzed from various aspects: functionality, performance, intended use, and safety. The manufacturer shall evaluate the device's competence in relation to its requirements through the data. In addition, you may plan that the service technician may perform a technical review of the medical device during the service or maintenance call for an assessment of whether it still meets its requirements.

Products Reviews and Audits

The manufacture may order or initiate reviews or audits regarding the medical device. The purpose is to objectively examine the functionality, characteristics, and performances of the medical device. Another kind of review (regarding the medical device) is one that the customer carries out independently in order to identify quality problems.

Published Literature, Journals, and Article Reviews

It may not be the most reliable source of information, but in some cases it may shed light about certain tendencies. The information gathered in such documentation will be brought to the appropriate personnel or employees for verification. For example, say that an article was brought to your attention indicating that a new risk was identified on another medical device, active in the same field as your product. The ISO 13485 Standard expects you to evaluate whether this risk is relevant to your product and its scope. The conveying and review of such information is to be systematic or methodic. This means that if you are relying on such reviews from published literature (books, journals, or articles), you must define which ones, what the intervals of review are, and the responsibilities to gather the information.

Researches, Postmarket Clinical Evaluation

Clinical evaluations are the review, assessment, and analysis of clinical data relating to a medical device required to verify the clinical safety and performance of the device when used as intended under normal conditions. The clinical evaluations are conducted on those medical device characteristics that put at risk the patient, the user, or the clinical environment where the medical device will be used. The output is information that objectively proves the safety and performance of the medical device, and may serve the manufacturer in identifying quality or safety problems. The information gathered in such evaluations will be brought to the appropriate personnel or employees for evaluation and verification.

Postmarket Clinical Follow Up

Postmarket clinical follow up is another way to gather information about the medical device. After a clinical evaluation had been done, a postmarket follow up must be performed on a regular basis and confirm that the results obtained in the initial clinical evaluation are still valid. The data gathered by the manufacturer in the premarket clinical evaluation (during design and development validations) does not allow identification of occasional complications or events that may occur in routine and widespread use of the medical device. The postmarket clinical follow up is a plan for:

- Identifying new risks to the user or patient.
- Evaluating residual risks.
- Verification that the functionality and performance of the medical device are maintained for the duration the medical device's shelf life.

It is a strategy that allows the organization to verify whether the results of the clinical evaluations are still valid and whether new risks were detected during the use. The evaluation calculates various parameters that affect the product. The results are compared to predefined criteria and provide the manufacturer with quantitative information about the compatibility of the medical device.

The postmarket clinical follow up is to be done in various cases—such as:

- A change in the design of the device
- The principles of operation and use or the material composing the medical device are new or novel
- New claims made by the manufacturer
- Significant changes are made to the design of the medical device
- Residual risks are at a high level; the use of the product poses a high risk to the user
- Open issues and questions have been left unanswered
- Evaluations of life expectancy of the device and events resulting from the use of the medical device

The data and conclusions resulted from the follow ups are inputs of the postmarket surveillance and give a status report on whether the medical device is continually meeting its requirements. More relevant to our case of feedback, however, is that it will provide information regarding the medical device during use. It is important to mention that the information derived from these studies will serve (in cases of need) as inputs for corrective or preventive actions. Therefore, you should create the appropriate link between the two activities; that is, conclusions of the postmarket clinical follow up, and corrective or preventive actions. This means that the ISO 13485 Standard expects a method for:

- The acceptance of data from the postmarket clinical follow ups
- The evaluation of the data
- Submission to the CAPA process in cases of need

Customer Complaints

A complaint is an effective way of receiving feedback. A complaint is an application communicated to the organization from a customer regarding events or the disturbances of performance, functionality, intended use, or safety of the medical device during use. It serves as an indication that the medical device has not reached its purpose or met its requirements. Thus a complaint is one of the most reliable sources of feedback regarding the medical device, its design and development, and its realization processes. Each complaint must be handled under a controlled process. The issue is dealt with in more detail in chapters 7.2.3 and 8.5.1. The complaint will be received, documented, evaluated, and investigated. The process will be defined and documented in a procedure. The organization shall focus on complaints that relate to the functionality, characteristics, and performances of the medical device. In other words, the organization is not required to refer to complaints such as "The medical device's color does not match our operating room. Is there any chance you can color it blue?"

The concentration of complaints under one database will provide the necessary information for feedback. In order to introduce the handling of complaints as a means of attaining feedback regarding the product, it is necessary to verify that effective communication channels and processes are initiated between the complaining party and the organization (e.g., the requirements of clause 7.2.3), and that there is an effective interface between the process of handling complaints and improvement quality processes (e.g., corrective and preventive actions).

Recalls of Medical Devices

A recall is an action taken to address a problem that occurred in the medical device that exceeded the norm and accepted tolerances. Such problems can put the patient or user at risk, and thus must be removed from shelves and be forbidden from use. The manufacturer is to study recalls of medical devices and investigate their occurrence. Usually the manufacturer recalls the devices with the help of distributors or other responsible parties. However, there are cases where a local authority requires the organization to recall its devices.

There are three levels of risk where the manufacturer must recall its medical devices:

- Where there is a reasonable chance that a risk detected in the device is significant and is a threat to the health and safety of the user or patient
- Where there is a possibility that a risk may pose a significant threat to the user or patient
- Where the medical device may pose a risk with low severity to the user or patient

The mandate for the recall depends on local regulations. Usually the first two require a mandatory recall of the medical device; the third requires a voluntary recall.

The recall is done according to a defined and documented plan or a procedure with objectives, implementation measures, simulations, analysis, and, of course, the submission for correctional measures. This will be addressed in subclause 8.5.1 (Improvement—General). The recall process generates data and information regarding the use of the medical device, and that is what matters here—the systematic collection of data and the analysis and submission for improvement. In order to implement the process effectively in your feedback processes, there are a few issues that must be referred to:

- The identification of relevant regulations in accordance with the region where you are active (i.e., producing and distributing).
- The implementation of the requirements in your recall plan and processes.
- The creation of effective communication processes and channels between the organization and the subjects of the recall plan and processes; for example, customers, users, distributors, and other responsible parties (such as authorities). The requirements for an effective communication channels are discussed in subclause 7.2.3 (Customer Communication).
- The initiation of an effective interface between the recall processes and plan, and the quality improvement processes (corrective and preventive actions).

Relation between the Feedback and the Corrective and Preventive Actions

One of the main goals of gathering feedback data is the transfer of quality problems to quality improvement processes; that is, corrective or preventive actions. The ISO Standard demands this. As far as it concerns the CAPA processes, this means that information and data from feedback activities are to act as CAPA inputs. For the feedback activities, this means that one of the data evaluations will be the need for a corrective or preventive action.

In practice, this means that after analyzing data and information received from the feedback activities, you must examine the need for further actions. For example, if, after the postmarket clinical follow up, you discovered that the level of a residual risk had increased and that as a result you were required to improve the control over this risk; the action to take then would be to plan a measure and issue an advisory notice to your customers (so long as the risk did threaten the user and the patient significantly)—this may account as a classic preventive action. Therefore, the conclusion of the postmarket clinical follow up is the need for a corrective action—a permanent change or amendment to the medical device. This is to be defined and documented for each feedback method or technique.

A Documented Procedure

The ISO 13485 Standard specifically requires a documented procedure describing your methods for collecting and analyzing information regarding feedback and the transfer for improvement (the CAPA processes). The objective of the procedure is to document and control the methods for collecting feedback data—in other words, introducing the feedback methods into practice. The procedure shall cover:

- The scope of the methods—which organizational elements the process covers: the quality management system, realization processes, safety of the medical device, performances, and so on
- The description of the methods systems and its activities for collecting the data and sources of the information—which methods are implemented in order to collect feedback data: customer surveys, customer complaints, postmarket clinical follow ups, and so on
- The authorities and roles responsible for collecting the data
- The authorities and roles responsible for analyzing and evaluating the data
- The interface and relation to CAPA processes
- The controls and verifications that the methods are being performed on a regular basis; for example, an internal audit
- References to relevant documents, such as procedures and work instructions (e.g., procedures for handling customer complaints, recall plans, customer survey templates, etc.)
- References to records that indicate that the activities were performed

On the matter of records I suggest a table that will specify what the expected records are for each method (Table 8.3).

Each of the records shall bear a decision referring to the analyzed data, and a reaction plan in case it is needed. On this subclause, records are not required to be submitted to the records control process; but, if analyzed, each of the records of the feedback methods is yet required to be controlled. The requirement appears elsewhere in the standard. I recommend controlling all the records and including them under the records control process. When a record is under the records

TABLE 8.3
Expected Records of Feedback Activities

Method	Expected Records
Customer complaints	Records of customer complaints and records of the investigations
Customers surveys	Records of questionnaires
Service calls	Service reports for analysis
Published literature, journal, and article reviews	List of relevant literature, journal, and article reviews
Product audits	Records and findings of audits (external and internal)

control, it is certain that it will receive the appropriate attention (control, updating, distribution, etc.).

8.2.2 Internal Audit

One of the most effective activities that organizations may implement in order to monitor, analyze, control, and improve its quality management system (QMS) is the internal audit.

The audit's main goal is to give a status report regarding your quality management system. The tactic of an audit (external or internal) is to evaluate the organization's performances with reference to any kind of requirements. Your organization is required to maintain several activities. The audit evaluates whether the activities are performed and how well they are performed (Table 8.4).

The Auditor

The auditor must be objectively related to the organizational unit or function that they are auditing. Beside their personal approach, the auditor must have a minimum acquaintance with the field of the organization in order to evaluate the processes and their results beyond the working procedures, work instructions, and documentation (the documented criteria). That kind of knowledge can give them the ability and the consideration to evaluate situations while they identify any nonconformities or faults. The ISO 13485 Standard refers us to the ISO 19011 (guidelines for quality and/or environmental management systems auditing). The ISO 19011 specifies the required auditor qualities:

- Ethics: Auditors will possess personal characteristics like credibility, integrity, and honesty, and provide reliable information and results regarding the unit they are auditing.
- Open minded: Auditors will be willing to listen, learn, and accept new ideas, and to reflect them on the situations or requirements. Sometimes they may encounter new approaches or opinions. Auditors must have the ability to assess and to accept different ideas as long as they achieve the requirements.
- Diplomatic: Auditors will be polite and good mannered; they are representative of the top management.
- Observer: Auditors will have the ability to recognize and evaluate what they see, and to understand and interpret events without deep interrogation.
- Perspective: Auditors will have the ability to evaluate situations beyond their appearance, and with a systematic view of things. They will have the ability to understand the organizational consequences of the evidence they find.
- Versatile: Auditors will have the ability to mobilize from one situation to another without losing direction. One moment they may audit one field; the next moment it may be another. They must be able to stay focused.
- Structured: Auditors will advance and progress the audit according to a defined method or a plan.
- Persistence: Auditors must be persistent with their objectives, so that when they ask a question, they must receive an answer to it and not to be diverted by interferences or disturbances.
- Independent: Auditors shall have their own opinions on things and will not be influenced by the environment.
- Decisive: Auditors must be ready to make decisions even when they are hard or will not satisfy the auditee.

TABLE 8.4
Standard Requirements of Subclause 8.2.2

ISO 13485	ISO 9001
The organization will conduct internal audits at defined periodic intervals in order to assess the performances of the quality management system	The organization will conduct internal audits at defined periodic intervals in order to assess the performances of the quality management system
The audit shall determine whether the quality management system conforms to prior planned arrangements for realization	The audit shall determine whether the quality management system conforms to prior planned arrangements for realization
The audit shall determine whether the quality management system conforms to prior arrangements as set in the ISO 13485 Standard	The audit shall determine whether the quality management system conforms to prior arrangements as set in the ISO 9001 Standard
The audit shall determine whether the quality management system conforms to prior quality arrangements defined by the organization	The audit shall determine whether the quality management system conforms to prior quality arrangements defined by the organization
The audit shall determine whether the quality management system is implemented and maintained effectively	The audit shall determine whether the quality management system is implemented and maintained effectively
The organization shall establish an audit program that will cover processes of the quality management systems	The organization shall establish an audit program that will cover processes of the quality management systems
The program shall relate to the status and importance of processes, and will set the scope of the examinations	The program shall relate to the status and importance of processes, and will set the scope of the examinations
The audit shall relate to results of prior audits (internal and external) and evaluate their status	The audit shall relate to results of prior audits (internal and external) and evaluate their status
The organization shall define and document in a procedure: the required tests and methods for evaluations of the quality management system; the criteria and limits for the audit; the interval required to perform the audit; the authorities and roles to conduct the audit	The organization shall define and document in a procedure: the required tests and methods for evaluations of the quality management system; the criteria and limits for the audit; the interval required to perform the audit; the authorities and roles to conduct the audit
The auditor will be objective, qualified, and adequate to conduct an audit, and shall not audit his/her own work or processes on which he/she affects	The auditor will be objective, qualified, and adequate to conduct an audit, and shall not audit his/her own work or processes on which he/she affects
Records of the audit process and findings shall be kept and maintained. These records must be submitted to the records control process in the organization as required in subclause 4.2.4 (Control of Records)	Records of the audit process and findings shall be kept and maintained. These records must be submitted to the records control process in the organization as required in subclause 4.2.4 (Control of Records)
Nonconformities that were detected shall be referred. For each nonconformity, a decision and an action will be determined, ensuring that they will be handled and removed. The suitability and effectiveness of actions will be evaluated in a defined period of time, as required in subclause 8.5.2 (Corrective Action)	Nonconformities that were detected shall be referred. For each nonconformity, a decision and an action will be determined, ensuring that they will be handled and removed. The suitability and effectiveness of actions will be evaluated in a defined period of time as required in subclause 8.5.2 (Corrective Action)

(continued)

TABLE 8.4 (Continued)
Standard Requirements of Subclause 8.2.2

ISO 13485	ISO 9001
The top management is responsible for ensuring that all nonconformities that were detected during the audit, and their causes, shall be eliminated without delay	The top management is responsible for ensuring that all nonconformities that were detected during the audit, and their causes, shall be eliminated without delay
The organization may turn to the ISO 19011 Standard for guidance related to quality auditing	The organization may turn to the ISO 19011 Standard for guidance related to quality auditing

The Audit Program

The organization must maintain a documented program for conducting audits (internal as well as external). The goal of the program is to identify the required organizational elements that will be audited and determine an audit for them. The program must be documented. The program has five main objectives:

- The program shall introduce the auditor with the scope and objectives of the audit (fields, subjects, departments, locations, sites, products, areas, roles, processes, or the specific status of processes).
- The program shall specify the authorities and responsible parties that will participate in the audit (the auditor or audit team, employees, specific roles, management representatives, technical experts, etc.).
- The program shall detail the resources required for the audit (meeting rooms, records, products, production lines, etc.).
- The program shall give a description of the topics and issues that will be audited and discussed.
- The program shall indicate scheduled timeframes for the different audit' stages.

It is recommended that you publish and communicate the audit program. If you would like to perform "unexpected" audits, then define them on the program but do not publish them. Bear in mind that no matter how you schedule the program, all organizational units must be audited at least once a year.

The program can appear as a checklist or in a procedure. Below is a table for demonstrative purposes (Table 8.5).

Some organizations also include the details of the test and examinations that they conduct during the audit. I will refer to it as the "plan" of the audit. The audit program will ensure that the audits are conducted as planned. Employees and workers will understand that the internal audit is a part of the quality management system and not a capricious decision made by the top management. The program will be a controlled record under the records control process.

The Audit Plan

The audit plan's objective is to direct the auditor during the audit through specific areas, topics, and issues that must be audited, and to specify tests that need to be done in order to evaluate the situation. There are two types of audit plan—a general one and a specific one. The general one will refer to all the organizational units and will

TABLE 8.5
Example of an Audit Program

Time and Date: 8:00–12:00 12/12

Deportment: Assembly
Topics to be reviewed:
- Accomplishment of work instructions
- Accomplishment of cleanliness instructions
- Performance of training

Resources:
- All work instructions are to be available
- All required records are to be available

Time and Date: 13:00–17:00 12/12

Deportment: Warehouse
Topics to be reviewed:
- Accomplishment of work instructions
- Accomplishment of cleanliness instructions
- Performance of training

Resources:
- All warehouse employees are to attend the audit

ask to evaluate performance of procedures and work instructions, evaluating quality procedures, and sampling processes. Such a plan will be applicable to the entire organization.

The second type is a specific plan designed for one organizational unit. This plan was written in order to audit one unit alone, and is therefore not applicable to other units. The plan will refer specifically to processes related to this unit, will display the interrelations of this unit with other organizational units, shall present with the appropriate criteria for evaluation, examine specifically the quality requirements of this unit, and will ask to review records related to its processes. This plan is more effective; for example, if the auditor is auditing a warehouse, a specific plan will direct him to the appropriate processes and activities, support him/her with the right criteria, and describe to him/her the records must be seen. The ISO 13485 requires a few general topics to be audited:

- Quality plans for the medical device: Any requirement for product realization must be evaluated on whether it was performed as planned. The best way is to sample and evaluate against predefined criteria. Sample a product or an output of a process, review its quality plan, and check whether the product was realized according to the plan. Document the results.
- The ISO 13485 Standard requirements for quality processes include the documentation requirements (customer complaints, purchasing information, CAPA, training, etc). The examination must be conducted throughout the entire organizational units related to product realization, or are under the quality management scope. Any unit must be examined at least once a year. The examination shall indicate whether the organization implemented effectively the quality processes, continually meets the standard requirements, and whether the required documentation and records are maintained.

- The identification and implementation of international, national, or local regulations according to the ISO 13485 Standard requirements will be evaluated. The audit shall examine the identification of appropriate regulations, their introduction to the quality processes (such as management review, or integration in the training program), implementation throughout the realization processes, and maintenance of the appropriate records.
- Processes and procedures: The audit must evaluate whether the realization processes are performed as required. It could be a correlated with the quality plans. Generally speaking, an audit must sample processes and the outputs and evaluate their performances. The evaluation would refer to required results or predefined criteria.
- Quality objectives: The auditor must examine whether the organization has achieved its quality objectives. He/she evaluates the objectives (whether they are related to the product) and evaluates the results. If he/she reveals that the objectives have not been fulfilled, he/she must be presented with the causes and measures.
- Quality management system effectiveness: The audit must provide the ability to evaluate whether the quality management system is effective or not. The auditor may review the objectives and examine whether the expected improvement was achieved. If not, the auditor must be presented with the measures appointed.

The evaluation and review of data and information may be conducted in various ways:

- Interviews and questioning of employees or responsible parties
- Samplings of products or processes
- Observations
- Review of records
- Review of documents
- Review of corrective and preventive actions
- Review of audit follow ups

The three elements of the audit plan are: the purpose, the topics and issues, and the methods. You are required to create for yourselves an effective method to audit your organization. As a quality manager and consultant, I used to analyze all the organizational units and their quality objectives required to be audited. For each I listed the test and necessary examinations, and referred each test to a responsible party. I described the relevant records to support the test. This method proved itself to be quite effective in the long run; but it requires a fairly good acquaintance with the processes and units, along with continual updating until it stabilized and could be considered as effective.

The plan shall be documented. An audit will be considered as completed only when all the required tests and examinations from the plan are completed.

Criteria

In order to conduct effective tests, you need to assign and document criteria to each test. The objective of the criteria is to support decisions for judging, evaluating, and determining by facts, values, and data the compliance of the outputs to the requirements. The criteria will provide a successful validation by indicating whether the findings are accepted or rejected. The criteria will present a method for the evaluation and will refer not only to products, parts, or components, but also to realization processes and conditions for realization. Types of criteria include:

- Working instructions, test instructions, and procedures
- Drawing and specifications
- Quality plans
- Standards and technical specifications
- Regulations and directives
- Documented customer requirements

The audit plan shall refer each test to its appropriate criteria.

Audit Evidence and Findings

During the audit the auditor samples, observes, ask questions, and examines products and processes. The answers shall be translated and recorded as the audit findings. These shall then be compared to the predefined criteria and shall indicate the status of the processes or product; conformity or nonconformity, or opportunity for improvement. The findings include the evidence that the auditor reviewed (e.g., processes, products, records, etc.); for each, he may document what was presented or found, what is the requirement and its status against the criteria.

Each piece of evidence shall bear a classification—for example: good; opportunity for improvement; or corrective action is required (I will review this issue later). This is the most important part of the audit report. The findings generate the audit's conclusions, and specify what the auditor saw and revealed. The auditor must document the evidence as accurately as possible.

The Classification of Audit Findings

Any findings during the audit shall be indicated with one of three classifications:

- Conformity—the process or product sampled was in accordance with the relevant requirements and criteria.
- Opportunity for improvement (OFI)—in the auditor's opinion, an improvement can be applied to the matter, and the organization may or may not adopt take this opportunity.
- Nonconformity—the process sampled was not according to the requirements and audit criteria.
- If the manufacturer feels the need to add another classification suitable to its nature or processes he may do that but this will have to be documented on the procedure.

The Closing Report

Any audit report must have a summary. The auditor should gather all the information, data, findings, nonconformities, and opportunities for improvement, and process and present them together in one report. The goals are to provide the organization with a status report regarding the quality management system and for follow up during the next audit; to review the treatment and to verify that all nonconformities are closed. The report must specify:

- Who the participants were—it is required that you document who participated in the audit.
- The scope of the audit, the auditee, and the organization or functional units that were audited.
- The audit's objectives.

- General details and information that will support the evidence and shed light on the auditee or explain some findings (e.g., the amount of workers, special projects, special recent events, etc.).
- The audit findings that were sampled, observed, asked, and examined. This section will refer to the criteria that were used to evaluate the findings.
- Reference to prior audits and prior findings. The auditor must verify that all nonconformities that were revealed during the last audit are eliminated, the treatment is documented, and (most importantly) the treatment was effective and the nonconformities have not repeated.
- Recommendations—for every finding, the auditor may offer his/her recommendation.
- Nonconformities discovered during the audit—the objective is to concentrate all the nonconformities that were discovered in one list for the follow up in the next audit so that corrective actions can be initiated and the nonconformities are eliminated, and not repeated.

This summary will generate a corrective action report (which is a separate topic, and will not be discussed here).

Bear in mind, this report is designated for the top management and the function that is responsible for the auditee. The report is a tool for him/her to understand the status of the organization with reference to the requirements or the criteria. Therefore, it is recommended that the report be designed in a format that would be easy to understand.

Nonconformities Revealed in the Audit

Nonconformities are documented three times during the audit process:

- First—within the audit report along with the audit findings. We can also refer to it as the report itself.
- Second—where it is suitable, as nonconformities. Any audit report should contain a summary of the nonconformities at the end.
- Third—as an input for a corrective action.

When you reveal nonconformities, they should be applied to a controlled process. The ISO 13485 Standard specifically requires that for each nonconformity a decision and an action will be determined in order to ensure that they will be handled and removed. The goal is to verify that the nonconformities are removed or eliminated, and will not be repeated. The organization shall prove to the auditor that a corrective action was taken over any nonconformity (revealed during the audit) within the scheduled timeframe, the treatment was effective and the nonconformity did not occur again. In order to close the loop, you need to initiate the interface between the internal audit process and the corrective action process. Define and document the fact that audit findings may serve as inputs for the corrective action process. If you wish to be more creative and proactive, you may define that audit findings are also inputs to the continual improvement process (Subclause 8.5.1 (Improvement—General)).

A Documented Procedure

The standard requires a documented procedure describing the method of the audit; that is, a description of the process itself—who meets with whom; where; and what should everybody bring with them (e.g., procedures, documentation, samples, etc.). The procedure shall cover:

- The personnel that are to perform, manage, and participate in the audit
- The requirements for conducting an effective audit (an audit that will achieve its objectives, such as the objectives of the audits and tests)
- Reference the reporting methods and necessary records

There is a reason why I refer to the documented procedure at this stage—it is in order to present all the process stages first and then refer to a procedure.

Since the audit plan includes one part of the requirement of the procedure I suggest combining the plan requirements and the audit objectives with the other audit elements—the requirements for findings, the method for classifications, and the form of the closing report. This way you will describe the whole process and cover the requirement. If you have doubts, create an independent procedure. The procedure will be controlled under your documents control, as required in subclause 4.2.3 (Control of Documents) (Figure 8.1).

Top Management Responsibility

The top management is obligated to monitor the internal audit process. The top management will:

- Ensure and verify the conducting of the audits according to the program and plan.

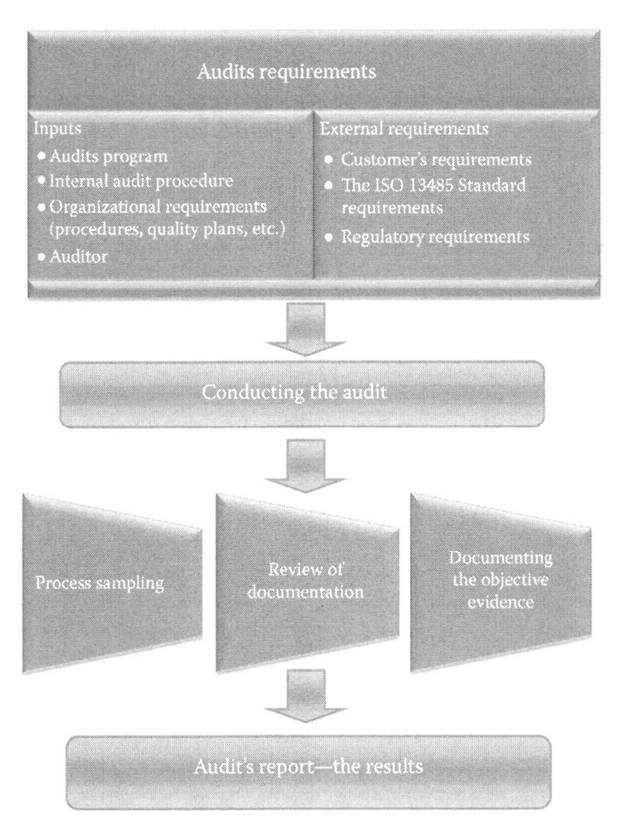

FIGURE 8.1 Internal audit process.

- Review and evaluate the results of the audit.
- Verify that all nonconformities detected during the audit are closed.

One way to implement this requirement (relating to the audit result on the management review) is specified in subclause 5.6.2 (Management Review Inputs).

Records

Records are the outputs of the audit process proving that activities were performed and the objectives of the audit were achieved. The records that are expected from the audit's process include:

- Audit program—the program is a record of the planning process.
- Audit plan—in case you are managing a dynamic plan that may change with time, it will be referred to as a record.
- The findings of the audit—the report that includes the documentation of the findings and evidence is considered a record.
- The closing report.
- The list of nonconformities for follow up.

The records are part of your quality management system and will be included under the process of records control as required in subclause 4.2.4; that is, they will be indicated, controlled, stored, and maintained.

8.2.3 Monitoring and Measuring of Processes

Measuring processes are mentioned many times throughout the standard: quality manual, quality objectives, management responsibility, and control of production and service provision. Until this subclause, the ISO 13485 Standard specified where it expects to find monitoring and measuring of processes and activities. In subclause 8.2.3 it specifies the objectives of the monitoring and measuring of processes, and how it expects us to perform these (Table 8.6).

TABLE 8.6
Standard Requirements of Subclause 8.2.3

ISO 13485	ISO 9001
The organization shall establish and implement appropriate methods for monitoring processes of the quality management system and, where applicable, use methods for the measuring of processes	The organization shall establish and implement appropriate methods for monitoring processes of the quality management system and, where applicable, use methods for the measuring of processes
The methods are to prove the ability of the processes to achieve desired results	The methods are to prove the ability of the processes to achieve desired results
When planned results are not reached, the organization shall introduce the processes to corrective actions, ensuring the achievement of the results	When planned results are not reached, the organization shall introduce the processes to corrective actions, ensuring the achievement of the results

Let us first look at the terms used:

- Monitoring—a continuous inspection throughout defined scope (for example, time intervals).
- Measuring—defining objectively a physical size and capturing a situation without any references to the significance.

The main ideas of the measuring and monitoring of processes are:

- Implementation of a systematic control of realization processes
- Identification of deviations in time and submitting them to a controlled process for treatment

This topic relates directly to the indications throughout this book; the ISO 13485 Standard requires that you maintain an effective quality management system. The assumption maintains that the effectiveness of a quality management system is accomplished through the control of its processes. We were required to define quality objectives, and now it is also necessary to control their achievement. Through the monitoring and measuring of processes, we can evaluate process outputs and compare them with our objectives. The objectives are: the quality objectives, quality plan specifications, customer requirements, device specifications, risk management outputs and regulatory requirements.

The monitoring and measurements shall prove conformity of processes to planned results, and the ability to deliver the desired medical device. Thus, the monitoring and measuring activities, methods, and reporting will be able to supply such proofs and provide the appropriate information about this ability of the processes. The processes are those that were described from chapter 4 to chapter 8 of the standard; quality and realization processes:

- Quality processes—management reviews, control of records and documents, control of training programs, control of nonconforming products, and CAPA processes.
- Realization processes—controls of substructures and work environments, fulfillment of quality plans, verifications and validations of realization processes, implementation of risk controls, preservation of customer property, and traceability activities.

You must derive from these the critical processes and define for them methods for monitoring and measuring necessary prove you that they have achieved their objectives. In order to make it easier to measure and analyze, set a quantitative criteria for the realization processes (in the appropriate cases). The data would be easier to collect and the report would be much clearer and more usable.

Note: When monitoring quality processes you are required not only to verify that they are defined and have been performed, but also to evaluate the results and whether processes have achieved their objectives. For example, when you are monitoring the management review process you are required to evaluate whether the decisions were carried out according to schedules. When you are monitoring a training program you need not only to verify the execution of training, but also its effectiveness.

Identification of Parameters

When planning control over the processes it is important to identify the core processes and the critical parameters that affect the quality of the medical device. It is useless to invest effort and resources in monitoring processes whose control will not contribute to the quality management system. Thus, define the important aspects in your processes in order to recognize the necessary parameters for monitoring and measuring. For example, if you are injecting a plastic part that will be assembled in the device, there are several production parameters that are responsible for the stability and reliability of the process, and thus the quality of the part: water pressure, moisture of the material, level of particles in the material, machine cycles, and so on. Such parameters are to be identified during the production process.

The next stage is identifying which data and information demonstrate these parameters. The identification requires analysis of the process flow and the data that it generates. At the same time, try to identify which process resources are related to the parameters (e.g., machines, human resources, materials, working tools, etc.). It will serve you later on if a nonconformity is detected. The resources will assist you in tracing the error back to its source.

Parameters are divided into various characters: length, costs, control over performance, achieving objectives, and level of quality. The last of these is the most significant. Common measurements include:

- Planned duration of processes compared to realized duration of processes
- Planned costs of processes compared to achieved costs
- Measurements of substructures and their performances—malfunctions, capacity, and utilization
- Measurement of resource utilization—material, rework, and human resources
- Deviations from production requirements—production cycles, technical parameters, resources, and scrap
- Control over measuring devices

A Defined Method

The monitoring and measuring shall be conducted according to defined methods. The methods are not required to be documented in procedures or work instructions. The defined method shall include the following issues:

- Identification of the monitored processes
- Definition of monitoring characters such as interval, sampling rates, batch loads, quantities, and stages during the process
- The activities for measuring each process
- The responsible party for conducting the measurements
- Results or criteria required for evaluation (the objectives)
- The documentation and reporting methods
- Action required in case of nonconformities

When planning your monitoring methods it is required that you enable an immediate comparison with the objectives. The simplest way to explain it is the performance test of a production machine where technical results are ranked in comparison with upper and lower limits. Such ranking immediately provides the status of the process—either within tolerances or not. The configuration of the data collection (forms, protocols, and databases) will be adjusted to type of the collected data and criteria of the process.

Defining a method for evaluation of quality processes can be confusing, such as monitoring the controls; but it is logical. These processes have a direct effect on the quality management system. Therefore, they must be monitored and measured. Each process has its objectives—training programs must be accomplished, corrective action must be closed in a defined timeframe and their effectiveness must be verified, and customer complaints must be handled according to a process and must be closed. Plan the monitoring activities according to these objectives. A statistical control is not required. Effectiveness is essential. Internal auditing is a terrific way to monitor quality processes, but you must try to be creative and design more frequent controls for these processes; for example, a digital chart or a periodic report that indicates the status of customer complaints.

The reporting of the monitoring and measuring is an integral part of the process. After collecting the data and comparing it to its criteria, it is time to report the situation to the appropriate party in order for them to evaluate it and make a decision. First, you must define how the data will be documented and reported—on a specific computer application, BI system, producing designated reports, manual test protocols, and so on. Then, define how the data will be distributed; e-mail, meetings, or notifications of alerts.

Advice: Organizations that manage their processes with a business process management (BPM) system may find it easier to meet the requirements of subclause 8.2.3 (Monitoring and Measurement of Processes). Such a system controls the production processes on specific points and collects and analyzes data regarding the performances of a process. The data is then distributed to appointed roles for control and maintenance; thus, the BPM system allows the effective monitoring and measuring of processes. If you are using such an application, then you must exert its utilities and possibilities in order to meet the standard requirements.

Evaluation and Submission to Corrective Action

It is required that you analyze the results and compare them with the planned objectives in order to identify deviations from the process specifications that might create quality problem in the medical device. The goal of the analysis is to analyze the deviations and to decide whether they are regarded as nonconformities and thus in need of corrective action. The ISO 13485 Standard requires a corrective action for every deviation from the planned results, as appropriate. You are not expected to initiate a corrective action for every minor deviation; this is not the purpose. There are rarely 100% stable realization processes; deviations are a daily matter. Not each deviation is critical and in need of corrective action. However, it is expected that you justify it: evaluate the severity of each deviation and decide if it is to be regarded as a nonconformity, and so in need of corrective action. This decision will be documented. As a quality manager, I used to report deviations to the production manager and document the notification in an e-mail with reference to the evidence (the test protocols). In return, he would answer whether the deviation affects the quality of the processes, and whether the process must be stopped and a corrective action must be initiated, or whether the matter is considered and no corrective action is needed. The answer was submitted with a justification. In any case, any deviation will be referred.

On the quality management side it is necessary to define the interface between the monitoring and measurement activities—the communication and report, and the decision to initiate a corrective action.

Documentation and Records

There is no requirement to document in a procedure the methods and processes of the measuring and monitoring. However, one issue is to be documented on the corrective action procedure—you must define when an input to the corrective action process is the result of monitoring and measurement activities. There is a requirement for available evidence proving that processes maintain conformity. The monitoring and measurement records relate to other standard requirements, such as subclause 7.5.1 (Control of Production and Service Provision) and 7.5.2 (Validation of Processes for Production and Service Provision), where there is a requirement to control records under the records control process.

8.2.4 Monitoring and Measurement of Product

8.2.4.1 Monitoring and Measurement of Product—General Requirements

In the last subclause, the ISO 13485 Standard related to the monitoring and measuring of processes. Now it is time to monitor and measure the competence of the medical device to its requirements as a product; that is, the customer, quality, risk and regulatory requirements. Monitoring and measuring activities of products are the necessary controls to ensure that the device performs as intended. The controls will be implanted throughout the realization processes and will apply product that the manufacturer produces as well as purchases. The standard demands that you control the product and to verify that (Table 8.7):

- Requirements specified by the customer are met.
- Requirements stated during the quality planning, and that are necessary for intended use, are achieved.
- Risk Management controls are effective.
- Statutory and regulatory requirements are met.

The organization is required to develop, conduct, control, measure, and monitor the product in order to ensure conformance with specifications. The standard guides us in the planning of the controls and demands that while we are planning the controls, we will consider two main elements of our quality management system—the quality planning, and the planning of the controls over the production and service provision.

Quality Plan and the Monitoring and Measurements of Products

Let us concentrate for the moment on the quality plan and its significance at this point. I want to consider the relation between the quality plan and subclause 8.2.4. Quality planning is the design and development of requirements, activities, and criteria that the organization must follow, fulfill, or achieve in order to deliver the medical device according to the requirements (quality objectives, product and customer specifications, regulations, activities for verifications and validations, documentation, and records).

TABLE 8.7
Standard Requirements of Subclause 8.2.4.1

ISO 13485	ISO 9001
The manufacturer will measure and monitor the characteristics of a product in order to ensure compliance with product specifications	The manufacturer will measure and monitor the characteristics of a product in order to ensure compliance with product specifications
Activities of monitoring and measuring of a product shall be conducted throughout the different realization processes at adequate levels	Activities of monitoring and measuring of a product shall be conducted throughout the different realization processes at adequate levels
The activities shall be planned considering, and corresponding to, the quality planning or quality plan as required in clause 7.1 (Planning of Product Realization) and the documented requirements as required in subclause 7.5.1.1 (Control of Production and Service Provisions—General Requirements)	The activities shall be planned considering, and corresponding to, the quality planning or quality plan as required in clause 7.1 (Planning of Product Realization)
Records and proof of a product's conforming to the requirements and criteria shall be kept and introduced to the records control process in the organization, as required in subclause 4.2.4 (Control of Records)	Records and proofs of a product's conforming to the requirements and criteria shall be kept and introduced to the records control process in the organization, as required in subclause 4.2.4 (Control of Records)
The records shall indicate the responsible party for releasing the product	The records shall indicate the responsible party for releasing the product
The release of the product and service activities will be authorized so long as all the requirements stated on the quality plan are fulfilled	

The monitoring and measuring activities of a product shall be planned in order to allow the manufacturer to examine whether the product is realized as planned. Therefore:

- A correlation between the quality plan and the controls of the product is required.
- The results and acceptance criteria of the product shall be planned according to the type of medical device and its intended use.

Just as quality planning covers all the realization process, so will the monitoring and measuring activities be implemented throughout all the realization processes and relevant elements: infrastructures, work environments, control of production and service provisions, and product validations. In practice, you will determine tests and set criteria to inspect the product during different realization processes, and evaluate how the parameters mentioned above affected the product and whether its requirements are being achieved.

Implementation of Monitoring and Measuring of Products during the Realization Processes

The activities of monitoring and measuring products are to be implemented throughout the realization processes. The ISO 13485 Standard refers us to subclause 7.5.1.1

(Production and Service Provision), where it is required that you maintain controls of the product realization processes. The controls will be documented, effectively implemented, and will include the methods and activities for monitoring and measuring the product. The activities and tests shall be defined and documented. There is no requirement in subclause 8.2.4 to do so; it is in subclause 7.5.1.1 that we find this requirement. This subclause demands that you specifically document all the controls. The monitoring and measuring activities are a substantial part of these.

For example, one of the controls designed for a component is the functionality test. Its documentation will include the set of operations and the criteria for an evaluation of results.

The scope of the activities is to include other realization actions that take place outside the organization's premises, such as service, maintenance, and installation activities. Sometimes certain product characteristics can be controlled effectively in certain conditions—for example, service, maintenance, or installation. The manufacturer needs to identify such activities and design appropriate monitoring activities.

Determining the Methods for Monitoring and Measuring the Product

The methods for monitoring and measuring the product are to be defined. The objective of the method is sampling and probing a product from a realization process and evaluating it against predefined criteria. When defining the method it is required that you take into account all the elements that are related to the product, such as:

- Identification of a specific product, part, component or medical device needed for the monitoring.
- The product characteristics that are to be measured.
- Tools, equipment, or software required to perform the test.
- The party responsible for performing the test must be defined (designated employees, a certain department, organizational unit, etc.).
- The exact realization stage where the product is to be sampled and controlled. The definition shall include the extent of the test; that is, the time interval and the sampling rate.
- The sequence of events in order to perform the monitoring and measurement activities. The conditions for the test are to be defined; such as room conditions, material conditions, and specific processes.
- The criteria needed for comparison of results and evaluations will be available.
- All the necessary data concerning the test will be available.
- The results of the monitoring and measuring activities.

Product Characteristics

The monitoring and measuring activities concentrate on product characteristics that reflect the status of the product and its compatibility. The characteristics are related to the requirements of the product; that is, the functionality, performance, intended use, safety, transportability, service, and maintenance. Inspecting and controlling these characteristics will ensure that the intended use will be achieved, and that medical device requirements and specification will be met.

The characteristics of a product will be monitored throughout the entire realization processes: storage of materials, productions, assembly, cleaning, sterilization, packaging, storage of finished goods, and (in certain cases) delivery.

Every characteristic will be checked with specific critical parameters that indicate the status of the product. Each parameter will be compared to its designated criterion.

When identifying the characters that need to be controlled, you must verify whether the customer requested control over a specific product's characteristics. A main objective is the early identification of nonconformities through the data gathered. The manufacturer will identify these characteristics and parameters and whether there are any deviations from them. Risks are an input when designing the control over the product. As a manufacturer, you shall use the outputs of risk analysis and requirements for controls in order to identify the required product characteristics to be monitored.

Setting Criteria

The criteria are needed for comparison and evaluation of results. In order to conduct effective tests you need to assign and document criteria to each product test. The objective of the criteria is to determine by facts, values, and data, the compliance of the product to the specifications. The criteria may be objective or subjective.

When you are required to set the criteria according to regulations, standards, or technical specification, these will be identified and implemented in your tests. When specific documentation related to the criteria is needed such as diagrams, calculation charts, tables, sample parts, or international standards, they will be defined and available during the test. When there is no standard or technical requirement for criteria, the manufacturer will determine and document criteria alone.

The criteria will be documented. In case you are implementing and using test protocols, the criteria will be documented or attached on these protocols or will at least be referred to. The criteria must be approved before submission for use. The following issues are to be considered when defining your criteria:

- The criteria shall refer to documented product requirements—material, functionality specifications, technical specifications, product characteristics, reference to drawings, and quality requirements.
- Where appropriate, the criteria will use statistical methods for validation.
- Criteria can be qualitative.
- Reference to the required information for evaluation against the criteria is to be defined—test data, findings, measurements.
- The criteria will be planned with relevance to the quality requirements.
- The criteria will be designed in order to provide alarms regarding the status of the product and to indicate when the results are regarded as nonconforming.

Monitoring and Measurement Activities

The activities of the monitoring and measuring shall be defined and documented. Documentation may appear as a procedure or a test instruction. The objective is to specify the sequence of events during the control, and verify that all the required details are being accounted for. The documentation of the activities will indicate all the elements necessary for the test:

- The identification of the product, parts, components, and materials that are required to be monitored
- Clear definition of the exact scope of the monitoring regarding the part—a certain area, a certain function and characteristic or activity (service or installation)
- Definition of interval for the control
- The responsible party or role that is required to perform the control
- The rate of the test for example, quantity that needs to be monitored
- Definition of required conditions for the test—temperature, humidity, light

- Requested tools, equipment, or devices
- The required activities necessary to perform the test including the different tests and references to the relevant criteria
- Reference to documents such as drawings, user manuals, documented criteria, standards, and technical specifications
- Methods for documenting the results
- Reporting the results to the responsible parties

The test must not be a quality assurance test. A production employee may inspect the product during the realization processes. However, such inspection is to be defined, documented, and recorded, as mentioned above. When regulations set specific activities per product or type of product, it is required that you verify that they were planned and implemented according to these requirements.

Traceability is the main tool that will allow you to track down a production disturbance and analyze it. In such a case, try to document as much data of the parameters that may affect the product as possible; for example, employees, material, work environment conditions, tools, and equipment.

Results and Records

All the necessary data concerning the test is to be defined and recorded. Records of the monitoring and measuring activities will include not only the results or the test, but identifying details of the test; that is, date, time, place, the employee who performed the test, batch number or any other production identifier, serial number of the part or purchased component, number and name of the equipment used for the test, and records of condition when the test was done such as room temperature or humidity (if required).

The results of the test are to reflect the status of the product compared with the specification; data against criteria. The records shall provide objective evidence of the medical device's conformance to the requirements. Therefore, it is necessary to define the results in accordance; that is, type of the data as well as the method for documenting the results (records). The evaluation of the data will supply the manufacturer with the acceptance approval on a certain realization point. If you are monitoring the functionality of a component with different functionality tests, the documentation of the test will be planned according to the results (whether the functionality is intact or not). If the test examines a product after a sterilization process, it is necessary to record the results that will prove the compatibility of the product according to the nature of the test; for example, levels of SAL on different surfaces of the medical device.

Bear in mind that the results of these activities are the inputs for the later analysis of data. In order to make it easier to measure and analyze your product, try to set quantitative types of data.

The ISO 13485 refers us to subclause 4.2.4 (Control of Records), which requires that these records are to be under the control of records in your quality management system.

Tools and Equipment

Tools, equipment, devices, or software that are required for monitoring and measuring will be defined. For each test the designated tool will identified. The tools will be controlled, qualified, and properly maintained according to the requirements in clause 6.3 (Infrastructure) and 7.6 (Control of Monitoring and Measuring Devices).

The definition shall include user instructions or activities on how one is to operate this equipment during the monitoring activities, and how one shall extract the necessary data. When a designated tool or a control gauge is needed, the method shall refer and identify it. When the customer has sent a control gauge for monitoring a product, a component, or part—for assembly or functionality—the use and operation of it will be documented on the method for monitoring and measurement. The documentation will be supported with criteria for evaluations. For example, it is possible to support it with photos or diagrams.

Training

The methods for monitoring and measuring are to be included in your training and certification program. The objective is verification that all responsible parties are aware of the importance of the issue and know exactly when and how the monitoring and measuring activities are to be conducted. For each role or job description involved in the realization processes, it is necessary to identify the monitoring and measuring activities and integrate them into the training program appropriately. The training shall also refer to the use and operation of monitoring and measuring devices.

The Release of the Medical Device

The activities of the release of the medical device shall be planned. The objective of the release activities is to inspect the product and ensure that:

- All the planned arrangements for the product realization have been conducted.
- All the results of the controls, verifications, and validations are accepted according to the specifications.
- All the required records and documents were reviewed and are available and appropriately maintained.
- The medical device fully conforms and all the requirements are in conformity with the acceptance criteria.

The release activities and tests shall be defined and documented. The definition shall indicate clearly what is to be checked and the evidence that is required in order to ensure that the medical device meets all the requirements and specifications, and the release is approved. The activities shall specify which issues are to be controlled before the release: labeling, packaging, results of process validations and tests, qualified personnel for certain processes, and execution of quality processes. The ISO 13485 Standard takes it one step further, and demands that the release of the medical device shall not be approved until all the predefined arrangements have been completed.

The scope of the release activities is to be defined, meaning what is to be released; one device, a batch, lot or production run. The release will set a new status to the process—products are finished and ready for the next stage. The exact release point will be identified. For example, if you are releasing a batch, the release activities will be done before delivery; that is, after realization and before transport to storage. If, however, you are releasing an installed device at the customer's premises, the release will take place after completion of the installment, and the execution of required training. After the release, the medical device shall be quarantined in a specific area. This segregation is necessary for the distinction between released and unreleased products. The acceptance sampling plan is an example; the manufacturer defines a plan for the sampling of products from a process in order to decide whether they are to be released or rejected. The plan defines the product, the process, the method for the technique and responsibility for the sampling as well as the rate and the methods for documenting and analyzing the data. The plan shall include the criteria for acceptance or rejection.

It is necessary that you identify—for each region or country where the product will be sold and distributed—what are the required release tests for the medical device, based on its type. For example, certain national regulations or standards require that devices that are in contact with circulating blood will be released with certain tests; such as, pyrogen or particle testing, depending of the region. Before the release of the medical device, the responsible party must verify that such tests were completed, and that the results comply with the specifications. Some local or national regulations may demand the presence of regulatory authorities during the release. When such authorities are requested, their visit and inspection must be documented. The same applies when the organization requires that certain specifications must be achieved before releasing the product; the function must verify that they were met and the results are satisfying.

The release of the medical device is composed of activities. The activities are to be designed with relevance to the device's nature. These will include references to the appropriate criteria. The criteria will be clear and indicate exactly when and how the devices will be released. The activities may be process verifications and validations:

- Process verifications are needed to verify that certain processes have been carried out, certain controls have been applied, and the required results were accepted.
- Process validations are tests that compare results to specifications and are to be conducted before the product is to be released.

For example, when cleanliness processes were determined at specific realization stages, the monitoring and measuring will verify:

1. That the processes were done as planned.
2. The results of the processes are required and the cleanliness level of the product is satisfying.

It has not been mentioned that the cleanliness process was before release because this does not make a difference. The process is to be verified whether it is before release or not—all predefined arrangements must be completed before release. The records of the release will supply the evidence that the release was conducted according to activities. The records are the approval and confirmation that the medical device fully conforms to the requirements. Plan your release method to examine and approve that all quality plans and arrangement were executed—only then will the device be released. Details to be documented on the release records include:

- Date of the release
- Identification of the medical device and identifiers
- Required documentation for the release (tests results or protocols, certifications, etc.)
- Clear identification of the authorized person that approved the release
- Identity of the person and a signature

The records may include records of earlier processes and required testing results, whose review and approval were necessary before the medical device could be released. The records may appear as a checklist of a file with certain documents, records, and approvals. It depends on the activities. I reviewed already release activities that were fully digital. Each production phase was documented on a computer system and at the end of the process a responsible function needed to verify the results on the system. Off

TABLE 8.8
Standard Requirements of Subclause 8.2.4.2

ISO 13485
The identity of persons or employees conducting the test, and inspections of any other kind of monitoring and measuring activity shall be recorded. The records will be submitted to the records control process as required in subclause 4.2.4 (Control of Records).

course he or she had to sample and view the devices but the documentations and records were with digital signatures.

The ISO 13485 Standard requires that only the organization may release the product—not the customer. The customer's approval is not sufficient in this case because it might not be objective, and therefore may omit some requirements. The ISO 13485 Standard cannot allow that.

8.2.4.2 Particular Requirement for Active Implantable Devices and Implantable Devices

When your organization realizes active implantable devices, or implantable devices, the identity of any individuals, roles, employees, or any other responsible parties that performed monitoring and measuring activities as mentioned in subclause 8.2.4.1 will be documented. Inspecting, examining, sampling, documenting, controlling, evaluating with criteria, and releasing will also be documented (Table 8.8).

In practice, the records that document your monitoring and measuring activities shall include the identity of the person involved, along with the test protocol, data charts, forms, and documented approvals. As well as name and identity, ensure that you document the date and obtain a signature. Table 8.9 is a basic table on implementation.

Add it to any of the records mentioned above. It can be printed in the form or appear as a stamp.

The main objective of this requirement is to ensure the qualification and certification of personnel that perform the monitoring and measurements activities.

The ISO 13485 refers us to subclause 4.2.4 (Control of Records). In other words, these records are required to be kept under the control of records in your quality management system. One option is that all the monitoring and measuring documentation will carry the identity of the persons. These records are already under control. A second (and less recommended) option is that the organization will plan designated forms to carry these identities. These forms will be then under the control of records control processes. This is less desirable because once you are managing

TABLE 8.9
Identification of Persons

Name	Date	Place	Signature

independent records for identities, they must refer to the performed test records, which can create unnecessary complications.

8.3 CONTROL OF NONCONFORMING PRODUCTS

As soon as nonconformity is detected within the organization, it must be identified, recorded, and controlled; and most importantly, it must be somehow treated. The objective is to prevent the release, delivery, or use of this product by customers. The process of identifying and controlling shall be documented in a procedure. The documentation of the treatment must include authorities and responsibilities (Table 8.10).

To clarify what we mean when we are referring to a nonconforming product—a nonconforming product is a product that has failed to meet its acceptance criteria or specifications, that is:

- Customer requirements
- Regulatory requirements

Nonconformity is nonfulfillment of a requirement; where a result was not achieved according to a specific requirement.

The main idea of controlling a nonconforming product is to separate it from the other conforming products, and to deal with independently, this includes:

- Identifying the nonconforming product
- Separating the nonconforming product from the other conforming products
- Eliminating the use or delivery of the nonconforming product

The control of nonconforming products extends from the purchasing processes and products to when products are delivered to the customer and service. Reasons for nonconformities include:

- The medical device failed to meet the design specifications.
- Procedures or processes were not accomplished.
- The medical device failed to meet regulatory requirements (e.g., directives or standard specifications).
- Realization processes did not meet validation criteria.
- Quality tests did not achieve their objectives.
- Service reports indicated nonconformity.
- Risks or residual risks are proved to exceed their levels of safety.

Responsibilities and Authorities

Before I start dealing with the standard requirements, there are some basic requirements that I need to discuss. The first is the need to appoint and certify authorities and responsible parties for controlling nonconforming products throughout the processes of handling them. It may be one individual or a number of people. The objective, however, is clear: at any given moment throughout the process, a responsible party will be appointed and qualified for detecting the nonconforming product or event and handling it. I recommend defining for each authority the process elements; that is, the

TABLE 8.10
Standard Requirements of Clause 8.3

ISO 13485	ISO 9001
The organization shall ensure that a product that does not meet its predefined requirements will be identified and controlled in order to eliminate its use or delivery	The organization shall ensure that a product that does not meet its predefined requirements will be identified and controlled in order to eliminate its use or delivery
The organization shall establish and maintain a documented procedure indicating the controls, authorities, and responsibilities when handling a nonconformed product	The organization shall establish and maintain a documented procedure indicating the controls, authorities, and responsibilities when handling a nonconformed product
Actions to eliminate the nonconformities will be established	Actions to eliminate the nonconformities will be established
Releasing a nonconforming product will be approved only with a concession	Releasing a nonconforming product will be approved only with a concession. An authorized person may give a concession. A customer may be defined as an authorized person for concessions
Concessions can be made only when all regulatory requirements are met	
Concessions can be made by an authorized person	
The identity of the person that approved the concession will be documented, and the records will be maintained under the records control process as required by subclause 4.2.4	
The organization must establish actions in order to prevent the use or application of nonconforming products	The organization must establish actions in order to prevent the use or application of nonconforming products
The organization is required to maintain records that describe the nonconformities detected and the following actions that were taken to eliminate them. The records are to be introduced to the records control process as required in subclause 4.2.4 (Control of Records)	The organization is required to maintain records that describe the nonconformities detected and the following actions that were taken to eliminate them. The records are to be introduced to the records control process as required in subclause 4.2.4 (Control of Records)
The organization shall maintain a documented procedure describing the activities required for controlling nonconformed products, authorities, and responsible parties	The organization shall maintain a documented procedure describing the activities required for controlling nonconformed products, authorities, and responsible parties
When a nonconforming product is reprocessed, it must be verified again to ensure that it meets the requirements (customer or regulatory)	When a nonconforming product was reprocessed, it must be verified again ensuring that it meets the requirements (customer or regulatory)
When nonconformity is detected after delivery of the product, it is required that you evaluate the influences and effects, and potential influences and effects, of the nonconformity	When nonconformity is detected after delivery of the product, it is required that you evaluate the influences and effects, and potential influences and effects, of the nonconformity

(continued)

TABLE 8.10 (Continued)
Standard Requirements of Clause 8.3

ISO 13485	ISO 9001
Rework of products must be documented in a work instruction. The rework instruction shall be reviewed and approved in the same process as the original work instruction	
It is required that you verify that all the required controls as specified in subclause 7.5.1 are identified and implemented	
The documentation of the rework must be controlled and introduced to the documents control process in the organization as required in subclause 4.2.3 (Control of Documents)	

communication channel, the inputs that it will receive, the reporting system, and the expected outputs. The definition will be documented—this may be done in the job description or in the documented procedure.

The authority for reporting and documenting nonconformity to a supervisor shall be granted to each role on the organizational structure. The issue will be implanted in each training program. This will ensure the timely detection and treatment of nonconformities.

Information concerning nonconforming items will be communicated to all defined parties, and when necessary actions are taken, it will be clear who is responsible for which action. The communication and responsibilities will be defined and documented in a procedure.

The Procedure of Handling a Nonconforming Product

The second basic requirement is the documentation of the process: the definition, documentation, and maintenance of a documented procedure describing precisely how a nonconforming medical device, or any other component of the medical device, shall be controlled once detected. The exact stages and actions for control and records must be identified. When a nonconforming product is detected it will be submitted to these actions. This procedure is one of the mandatory quality procedures. The process shall describe the stages of handling a nonconformed product; that is, the steps, activities, and records. Each requirement for activity or record will be defined and documented in this procedure. Of course, as in any other required procedure, the process of controlling nonconformed medical devices shall be submitted to the documents control process within the quality management system as required in subclause 4.2.3.

The topic of the procedure will be elaborated later on this chapter.

I will refer during this chapter to the issues of documented procedure the authorities.

Detecting the Nonconforming Products

In order to handle nonconforming products one must first detect them. Nonconformance can occur in raw material, components, finished goods or services. Nonconformance may occur in products that are in-process or in finished medical devices. In order to ensure thorough and effective detection, it is required that you implement systematic controls. These controls are already implemented throughout your quality management system:

- Monitoring and measuring of processes—during the monitoring it may be discovered that process parameters deviated, and thus products are nonconforming. Service and maintenance processes are also included here.
- Monitoring and measuring of products—during the monitoring it may be discovered that product characters deviated, and thus products are nonconforming.
- A customer complaint may indicate a malfunction in a product.
- Equipment failure during realization processes may account for nonconformity.
- A feedback activity may suggest that a product is nonconforming.
- An internal audit test may reveal nonconformance on processes or products.
- Verification of a purchased product may detect a nonconforming product.

The outputs of the processes mentioned above may also serve as inputs, and will ensure that detected nonconformities are submitted to the control of nonconforming products. These will be defined as the inputs of the process in the procedure. Their documentation in records will serve as the necessary quality evidence.

Deviations

Deviations may occur during the realization processes and are a departure from the specified requirements during product realization processes; namely, storing (environmental), manufacturing, packaging, releasing, or distributing. For example, say that a label was not correctly positioned on the medical device, or that cleanliness process parameters were above tolerances. The question is, when is a deviation considered to be a nonconformity? A deviation is considered a nonconformity when process specifications have not been met. There are, however, cases where the deviation is considered and accepted. Not every deviation will prevent the medical device from meeting its requirements. It is your responsibility to define a process for accepting and limiting such deviations. There are two kinds of deviations: planned and unplanned.

Unplanned deviations that occurred during the realization processes and that were detected will be regarded as nonconformities, and will be submitted to the controlling process.

Planned deviation is when a deviation is approved before it is implemented. In such a case you need to define and limit the deviation:

- Identification of the process and its specifications
- Identification of the related medical device, part, component, or material
- The reason for the deviation
- Review of the consequences and impact on the quality of the medical device
- Evidence (where appropriate) that the deviation will cause the medical device to not meet its specifications
- Allowed deviations from the specification—for example, value
- Limitations for the deviation (dates, batches, machines or equipment, a specific order, etc.)
- Approval of the deviation

The review will be conducted by several authorities in order to cover all the aspects and implications. The authorities that are permitted to approve deviations will be defined. The customer may also be involved. It is important to mention that deviations that relinquish regulatory requirements are not accepted. So the approval of the deviation must include a regulatory requirement review. The activities of planned deviation will be defined in the procedure. The review itself, and the approval, will be documented and serve as quality records.

Identifying a Nonconforming Product

The standards specifically demand the identification of nonconforming medical devices in an injective manner. That means that each nonconforming device will identified independently (physically as well as logically). One objective is to determine which products are involved in the nonconformity. The identification will be done according to realization process identifiers—production time intervals, batches, production machines, production areas, or products. If one defective medical device is detected, then the whole batch is becomes suspect. If you revealed a deviation in a process, you may then track down the time when the deviation occurred.

A second objective is differentiation and distinction of the nonconforming medical device from the conformed medical devices in an explicit manner. This ensures that the nonconforming devices would not contaminate the conformed ones. Defective medical devices may contaminate, pollute, infect, or trigger any other illness. Therefore, segregation from the conformed medical devices will be applied; that is, the nonconforming devices will be removed from the realization area to a specific controlled area. In case a component used in the assembly of the medical device, or a raw material used to realize it, has been detected as nonconforming, you will have to consider segregating the entire device. Processes of traceability and identification as planned according to clause 7.5.3 (Identification and traceability) will support the distinction of such products. The segregation may be physical or logical (in the case of software).

A third objective is ensuring, beyond any doubt or possibility, that the nonconforming product will not be used, applied, submitted to realization processes, or delivered to the customer. The status of the medical device must be changed in order to ensure this. The product's status shall indicate its conformance or nonconformance. In other words, the status shall indicate to the user or an employee whether the goods (medical devices or materials) are usable or not. The status shall be clearly identified using tags, stickers, signs, location of products, or serial numbers. Any employee could recognize the status at any given moment at any location—within the organization or at the customer's premises.

The issue is relevant to products that have already been delivered for distribution or are in use. Since you cannot physically identify products that are outside your factory, you need to identify them logically; that is, create a list with all the medical devices according to production identifiers that indicate these devices are nonconforming.

The activities of identifying and segregating will be defined in the procedure. The, tags, stickers, signs, or any other accessory will be considered as the quality records.

After detecting, identifying, segregating, and changing the status you must document the nonconformity and decide what to do next.

Documentation of the Nonconforming Product

The first level of documentation is the primary information gathered about the nonconformity and any information that would help you to investigate the nonconformity later on. The objective of the information is to assist you in mapping the problem and tracking down the root cause. Bear in mind that this documentation is the first step in a process that will later lead to a corrective action.

- Identification and detail of the medical device (e.g., product name, model, catalogue number, serial number, batch number, date of manufacture, etc.).
- Identification of the individual that detects it (employee, customer, supplier, regulatory authority, etc.).
- Identification of the individual that is responsible for handling the nonconforming product—it may be an individual or a committee.
- Type of nonconformity (production error, customer complaint, supplier error, etc.).
- Time and date of receiving or detecting the nonconformity.
- Quantities that were identified as nonconforming.
- Specific area where the nonconformity was detected or related to the product (department, production hall, machine, etc.).
- Description of the nonconformity (e.g., why it fails to meet the requirements—you can write here a literal description, or even attach other documents).
- Immediate treatment that was applied to the matter.
- Reference to documented evidence.
- Relevant procedures or work instructions.
- Categorization of the nonconformity—this is not required by the ISO 13485 Standard but is highly recommended and will assist you later with a statistical analysis.

The documenting of the nonconformity will be described in the procedure. When documenting the nonconformity, it is recommended that you record any characteristics of the medical device (or the service) at the time of the nonconformance. It will serve you later on when you evaluate the effects of the nonconforming product. The record can appear in any form: a paper document, excel chart, designated software, or an e-mail.

When designing the form I recommend designing it logically and chronologically—try to bear in mind that the form is a tool in the hand of the employee while gathering the information about the nonconformity and initiating an investigation concerning the nonconformity. You may combine records of customer complaints on the form.

Nonconformity in Delivered or Used Medical Devices

The manufacturer must define which actions are to be carried out once the detected nonconformity is in devices that have already been sent for distribution, or are already in use. The reporting method was discussed during chapter 7.2.3 (Customer Communication) and will be discussed later in chapter 8.5.1 (Improvement—General).

The first step is to identify customers that already purchased, or distributors that have already distributed the medical device. The second step is to identify the products that are nonconforming. There is the possibility that not all the used or delivered products will be nonconforming. Therefore, you must try to identify as accurately as possible the nonconforming products used by customers or delivered by distributors. This is an integral phase in the detection and identification of nonconforming medical devices.

After the detection and identification, it is necessary to define which action will be taken in order to deal with such products. There are several options:

- Withdrawing medical devices from sale and distribution for repair
- Delivering guidance and information regarding the nonconformance to customers and distributors
- Withdrawing medical devices from use (customers and distributors) for disposal

In some cases, regulatory bodies will demand specific actions for handling nonconforming products that were delivered or are in use. For example, maintaining a certain communication channel, providing evidence that notification was delivered, prescribing certain forms of data or specific information to be transferred to the customers concerning the possibility of adverse effects caused by the nonconformity. These requirements are to be identified and implemented in your process. The requirements may vary from one region to the other.

Immediate Action

Immediately after the nonconformity has been detected, it is necessary to initiate an urgent action in order to eliminate it in the short term:

- Separating the nonconforming and conforming devices
- Sterilization of the area
- Sorting out defective products, parts, or component
- Ordering new material
- Delivering a substitute shipment to the customer

The immediate action will be documented as a quality record.

Investigation of Root Cause

The nonconformity must be investigated. The investigation will lead to the root cause of the nonconformity. The objective is to analyze which elements of the process are responsible for the nonconformity, and to understand the chain of events that produced the nonconformity. It has already been suggested that you document all the parameters relevant to the nonconformity. This will now be of some use. The root causes are product or process parameters that did not meet their conditions; for example, functionality, performance, safety, or intended use. After identifying the parameters that led to the nonconformity, it is necessary that you analyze why they have not met their requirements. This investigation shall produce three main conclusions:

- The reason for the nonconformance that will need to be removed
- The severity of the nonconformance
- Which other product elements can be affected by this nonconformity

Risk management outputs may assist you in evaluating the severity and need for controls over the nonconformity.

The investigation, its findings, and conclusions will be documented. Once the reason was identified, all the relevant parties and authorities are to be notified in order to allow follow up treatment of the nonconformity.

Eliminating the Nonconformity

One of the main objectives of the control of nonconforming products is to develop activities for removing the nonconformities once they are detected, and to ensure that they will not reoccur. After investigating the nonconformity and detecting the root cause you can now treat the nonconformity and eliminate it. Elimination of nonconformity means the correction of a product or a process to fulfill its requirements, and the assurance that the nonconformity will not happen again. Elimination will be achieved with the definition of designated actions aimed at treating nonconforming factors.

The elimination of the nonconformity must be effective. This means that objectives for the actions of elimination are to be determined, and a control is to be implemented to ensure that they will be achieved. Initiating and implementing a corrective action is one example of eliminating the nonconformity; you are submitting the elimination of the nonconformity to a controlled process with objectives and verifications.

In principle, the standard requires for a detected nonconformity action to be taken in order to eliminate, correct, and prevent reoccurrence of the nonconformity. The standard's way of achieving this is through corrective action. There may be other ways of handling nonconformities, but I recommend submitting nonconformities to a controlled process—the CAPA. The decision for elimination and the actions decided upon will be documented.

Corrective and Preventive Actions

When action to eliminate the cause of nonconformity or other undesirable potential situations is required, it will be initiated as a corrective or preventive action. Once it is decided that a correction is needed in order to eliminate the nonconformity, the manufacturer will initiate a corrective action. Preventive action will be taken once a potential affect is detected and must be removed. The CAPA will be controlled via the appropriate processes and procedures as required in subclauses 8.5.2 (Corrective Action) and 8.5.3 (Preventive Action).

The relation between the two issues (handling nonconforming products and CAPA) is initiated due to the need for effectiveness. The organization needs to define the interface between the two processes. There is a debate on whether they are to be included under the same process. This will not be discussed here, but it is important to mention that there is a link between the two, and once the corrective or preventive process is updated the control of nonconforming products must be updated too. Therefore, if a corrective action was initiated as a result of nonconformity, the treatment of the nonconformity will be closed only when the corrective action is declared as closed and effective.

The ISO 13485 Standard allows combining records of two processes on one document. It means that you may document the nonconformity and the CAPA together on one form—this is possible and sometimes effective; but be careful—you must include requirements from both processes on the form and neglect nothing.

Disposal of the Medical Device

When required, the manufacturer will dispose of defective medical devices, parts, components, or materials as a corrective or preventive action. The activities of the disposal will be defined and controlled:

- The disposal activities will be defined and documented in a procedure or work instruction.
- The products, devices, parts, components, or materials are to be investigated and evaluated. Once it is decided that they are to be disposed, their status will be changed and they will be identified and quarantined.
- Segregation is important. The manufacturer will define a segregation area for devices that are to be disposed.
- When disposal is to be performed during service activities, the service technician will be certified for the disposal. When the supplier is to perform the disposal, the manufacturer must provide them with clear instructions.
- In case a medical device is disassembled, the process will be controlled and verified in order to ensure that defective parts are destroyed.
- The activities of the disposal will be recorded as quality records. The records will prove that the disposal was carried out according to the requirements (quantities, serial numbers, activities that were performed, and identities).

The objective is to ensure safety and that no confusion or mistakes occur, and that products designated for disposal will not entered into production or be delivered to customers.

Reworking Nonconforming Products

Corrections of nonconforming medical devices may be initiated as reworking or reprocessing. The rework includes the repair, rework, reprocessing, or adjustment of the medical device in order to eliminate the nonconformity and ensure that the product meets its specifications. Rework refers to parts, component, materials, or the entire device. Like everything else, parameters of the rework that may affect the quality of the medical device will be evaluated:

- Scope of the rework and identification of the medical device—each component or part of the medical device that requires rework will be identified.
- Objective of the rework—define which problem or nonconformity the rework will solve.
- Planning of rework activities—define which activities and actions are needed in order to achieve the objective.
- Risks—if there are controls that need to be implemented during the realization of the medical device due to risks, they will be applied on the rework too.
- Responsibilities—identify the roles and responsibilities that are to perform and approve the rework (certain roles, employees, and authorities). Implementation of the rework in the training plan is critical.
- Tool and equipment—determine which tools and equipment are needed to perform the rework.
- Materials, parts, and components—determine which materials are needed to perform the rework.
- Status—define the status of reworked devices (before rework, after rework, after revalidation).
- Necessary documentation—identify the necessary documentation needed for the rework (work instructions, diagrams, charts, drawings, etc.).
- Nonconformity—include a reference to the nonconformity that started the process.
- Tests, validations, and revalidations—the required controls are to be implemented in order to verify that the results are achieved.
- Revalidation—define revalidation tests to the medical device after the rework is done.
- Documentation—document the rework in a designated work instruction.
- Training—submit the rework to the training program in order for it to reach the appropriate roles.
- Statistical analysis—data related to the rework will be recorded and will serve later for product analysis.

Before submitting the devices to the rework, it is necessary to evaluate the feasibility and the effects (or potential effects) of the rework on the medical device specifications; that is, the functionality, performance, safety, and intended use, as well as other components in the medical device:

- Each person involved in the design and realization of the device will evaluate and give their professional opinion regarding the affect of the rework on the medical device; for example, engineering, design and development, quality department, manufacturing, and the customer.

- The review of the authorized roles will include the development of the rework activities. Each activity of the rework must be reviewed and approved by an authorized person. If you are replacing an electrical component in the device, the electrical department and its engineers must evaluate the replacement and its effects, and give their approval.
- This review will include the design of revalidation; each rework process and activity must be revalidated to ensure that the medical device will meet its specifications. The revalidation will include the regular product validations and tests that prove that the medical device meets its specifications, but also revalidation of the rework activities.
- The adverse effects that may arise as a result of the rework activities will be identified, reviewed, and their levels of the risk will be evaluated. You may be required for a risk analysis here.
- The rework may lead to the creation of a new version or configuration of the product. In such cases there is a need to implement controls as required in subclause 7.5.3 (Identification and Traceability).
- This review will be documented.

The organization will establish and maintain the rework on a document procedure identical to other work instructions included in your quality management system. The rework will be applied to the same controls:

- The rework instructions will be documented in the same form and manner of other work instructions.
- The rework instruction shall be reviewed and approved in the same process as the original work instruction before being submitted for execution.
- The document will be introduced to the documents control process in the organization as required in subclause 4.2.3 (Control of Documents).
- Each rework instruction will refer to a specific nonconformity.

Accepting of Nonconforming Medical Devices under Concession

Concession means allowing the use of the medical device for further realization or commercial use when it does not conform to its specifications or requirements. Concession may be regarded as release of nonconforming medical devices. The concession may minimize the costs of repairs, rework, or recall of the medical devices. The risk lies in cases where the manufacturer may not correctly assess the severity of the nonconformity, or may prefer to release a nonconforming product instead of investing resources in correcting the failure. Thus, before deciding and initiating a concession, two issues should be regarded:

- The first is that international, national, or local authorities may define criteria for concession. You must identify these criteria when considering a concession.
- The second is that concession may be initiated only when it is not relinquishing any relevant regulatory requirement. In other words, the conformity is to be examined and assured that it does not conflict with any regulatory requirements.

When determining the process or procedure for a concession, a few conditions must be kept in mind:

- The concession must be evaluated carefully for its effects and potential effects.
- The concession is to be limited, and limitations are to be defined (time, parts, products, models, components, etc.).

- The concession is to be approved by an authorized person.
- The concession and the decision are to be documented.
- The acceptance criteria that assisted in the decision making is to be documented or referred.
- The concession will be limited precisely to a batch, a medical device, production dates, a certain delivery, or a customer. The objective is to avoid "flowing" of the concession to other devices.

The review is to be documented as quality records. It is important to indicate that the documentation will include the identities of all the relevant individuals and authorities that participated in decision making and approval of the concession. You may involve the customer in the review and accept their opinion on the matter. However, the approval is to be conducted by the organization.

The main goal is to explain why the nonconformity is being approved. I suggest planning a form that guides the responsible parties through all the required stages, investigations, and questions. The main question will concern the reason for granting the concession. The review will first include the assurance that all relevant regulatory requirements have been fully met—all the regulations are to be specified and approved. Another objective of the review is to ensure beyond any doubt that releasing the medical device with the nonconformity does not risk users, patients, or their clinical environment. Thus, the review will include a reexamination of all records related to the nonconformity. The results and conclusions of reexaminations will be supported with scientific justifications (where appropriate) and will be documented. You are required to demonstrate, with evidence, that the nonconformity does not pose any risk, and that the medical device is safe for use.

After ensuring that the concession is not endangering or risking any users or patients, the manufacturer may submit the concession for evaluating whether a change in the design of the medical device is possible. Records of the reviews and concessions must be kept and included under the records control procedure (subclause 4.2.4).

Documentations and Records

As you have probably already noticed, documentation and records play a major role in the process of controlling nonconforming products.

The objectives of documentation include:

1. To provide clear definitions and guidelines to employees on what is to be done
2. To define the activities and responsibilities
3. To define the expected results
4. To submit and frame documented instructions and specifications regarding under control

Expected documentation:

- Responsibilities and authorities
- A documented and controlled procedure that defines the activities of handling and controlling the nonconforming medical device
- Activities for identifying and segregating nonconforming medical devices
- Activities for planned deviations
- Activities for dispositions
- Rework of nonconforming medical devices

The objectives of the records are:

1. To guide roles and responsibilities in performing the activities as required.
2. To prove that the process was conducted as planned.
3. To provide evidence that the treatment was effective and the nonconformity did not reoccur.

Expected records:

- Evidence that indicates nonconformity; such as customer complaints, results of monitoring and measuring of products or processes
- Records of nonconforming product identification and status
- Documentation of the nonconformity
- Evidence for immediate and urgent actions
- Notification to customers or distributors of nonconformance
- Decision for long-term actions
- Records required by regulatory requirements or directives
- Records of investigations
- Records of evaluation of the affect on other devices, components, or environments
- Decision of actions for elimination
- Decision of corrective and preventive actions with reference to the records of these actions
- Records of disposals
- Evidence of conformity after corrections were applied
- Authorization and approval of planned deviations
- Review and approval of the rework
- Review and approval of the concession

These records are considered quality records and must be included under the process of records controls as required in subclause 4.2.4.

8.4 ANALYSIS OF DATA

The ISO 13485 Standard requires collecting data from processes and activities and analyzing them in order to identify trends and pattern in your processes to verify a continuing suitability of the quality management system, and to control the effectiveness of the quality management system and maintain improvement (Table 8.11).

Some questions to ask when analyzing our quality management system include:

- Did we supply an appropriate medical device?
- Did we comply with the regulations?
- How long did the process last?
- How much raw material was used?
- How much scrap was there?
- How many times was the machine stopped?
- How many times did the customer complain?
- How many times did the customer call and said thank you?

Such issues can be analyzed over time with the information you have gathered. You must collect the information, examine it (by charts, by tables, or reports), and try to arrive at a conclusion.

TABLE 8.11
Standard Requirements of Clause 8.4

ISO 13485	ISO 9001
The organization is required to maintain a documented procedure describing the method of defining, collecting, and analyzing data proving the effectiveness and suitability of the quality management system	The organization is required to define, collect, and analyze data proving the effectiveness and suitability of the quality management system
The data analysis will allow examination of the effectiveness—and the improvements resulting from the effectiveness—of the quality management system	The data analysis will allow examination of the effectiveness—and the improvements resulting from the effectiveness—of the quality management system
The analysis shall refer to information and data gathered from various resources, and to monitoring and measuring activities included in the quality management system	The analysis shall refer to information and data gathered from various resources, and to monitoring and measuring activities included in the quality management system
Data and information generated from customer feedback shall, according to the requirements in subclause 8.2.1, be collected and analyzed	Data and information regarding Customer satisfaction shall be collected and analyzed
Data and information regarding the conformity of products to their predefined requirements shall, according to subclause 7.2.1, be collected and analyzed	Data and information regarding the conformity of products to their predefined requirements shall, according to subclause 7.2.1, be collected and analyzed
Data and information regarding products and processes characteristics shall be analyzed. The analysis will seize opportunities for preventive action	Data and information regarding products and processes characteristics shall be analyzed. The analysis will seize opportunities for preventive action
Data and information concerning suppliers' performances shall be analyzed	Data and information concerning suppliers' performances shall be analyzed
The results of the analysis will be documented, and the records will be maintained under the records control process as required by subclause 4.2.4	

The Effectiveness of Your Quality Management System

One of the main objectives of your quality management system is the systematic maintenance of its effectiveness; the setting of goals and their achievement. The data that will be gathered and analyzed shall demonstrate the effectiveness of the quality management system. In fact data analysis is one of the most efficient tools for measuring the quality management system's effectiveness. This is because you compare a clear numerical and quantitative status of your quality management system with your objectives: quality objectives, realization planning, customer and regulatory requirements. Effectiveness is the extent to which planned activities are realized and planned results achieved. Looking at the numbers you could say to yourself: "Our quality management system is effective because we achieved the next goals… ." You may also say: "We failed. Numbers are showing that we wasted our time and resources… ."

The difficult part of implementing the QMS is already behind you; you have defined and documented the objectives. Next you must link the methods and procedures of the analysis with these objectives.

Quality Objectives

Goals are quality objectives, as well as quality plans, for the realization of the product. The data analysis provides a status report regarding processes and their outputs (the products). The data analysis shall relate directly to quality objectives, such as:

- Harmonization with regulatory requirements
- Quality objectives as defined in your quality manual
- Customer requirements
- Quality planning for realization
- Objectives of design and development
- Human resource objectives
- Process objectives
- Product objectives
- Work environment specifications
- Supplier performances
- The success of improvements
- Risk management analytical needs

Throughout the standard there are requirements for implementing controls and goals. In subclause 8.4 the standard directs us on how to use these controls and presents guiding principles in defining and using the data.

Data analysis is one of the inputs for the management review. One of the goals of the management review is to continually examine the suitability, adequacy, and effectiveness of the QMS. Analyzed data is one of the most effective ways of persuading the top management about a particular matter. Trying to argue with charts and tables is more difficult than arguing with assumptions and claims.

Improvement

Another important aspect that the data analysis serves is the improvement of the quality management system. Improvement is a critical issue regarding your quality management system. Applying and implementing improvements demands an assurance that the goals were reached. Famous improvement activities include: CAPA, changes as a result of customer complaints, and advisory notices. Some of these activities require the use of data and its analysis in order to control them. Once an improvement has been initiated and implemented, the analysis of data is a tool that can be used to evaluate whether improvement activities have been successful and have achieved their objectives.

The systematic analysis of the data shall detect opportunities for improvement, or shall indicate situations that may need preventive actions. For example, trend analysis in customer complaints of service calls may suggest an unfulfilled need on the part of your customers or the product. Controlling and analyzing a supplier's performance may indicate their inability to comply with requirements. When a malfunction is detected in the product, analysis of production parameter may shed a light on the problem. When deciding upon data for analysis, data concerning improvements will be accounted.

Determining the Information Required

Let us discuss the strategy for identifying the data for analysis. The procedure will deal with the tactics. The data analysis shall relate to the subjects that are relevant to the performance of the quality management system. These will be the inputs for the data analysis. The requirements for data resources are the controls that were suggested throughout the standard; that is, human recourses, work environments, substructures, product quality planning, control of processes and products, design and development plans, risk controls performances of suppliers and purchased products, validations and verifications of realization processes, customer feedback, nonconformities, results of improvement, and CAPA. From these you need to identify which processes generate data that can be analyzed. The characterization of the data will lead to a status report that will answer the requirements above; for example, control of objectives, evaluation of effectiveness, and the detection and control of improvements and preventions. The analysis of the data will allow you to detect trends and patterns occurring on your processes that require attention. The trends and fluctuations will indicate your status regarding the objectives (e.g., progression or regression). First, you need to determine which kind of data will serve you best and then decide how it can be collected. The types of data will be defined on the procedure.

They include:

- Data generated from quality management processes
- Data concerning work environments and substructures
- Data regarding human resources
- Data generated from realization processes
- Data generated from purchasing processes
- Outputs of feedback activities

The data need not be statistical; it is expected, but qualitative data is expected also. There are processes that cannot be analyzed by numerical analysis. For example, the evaluation of customer satisfaction of the product is based on qualitative questions in the survey, or a review of the research and literature. Such analyses are purely qualitative.

Specific Requirements for Analysis

The ISO 13485 Standard specifies four issues that must be included under the analysis of data, though you are free to extend the scope of the analysis. However, data concerning these four issues must be collected, analyzed, and recorded:

- Feedback: The data generated from the activities of the feedback will be collected and analyzed—customer surveys, service calls, products reviews and audits, research, postmarket clinical evaluations, customers complaints, recalls of defective medical devices. The standard refers us to subclause 8.2.1 to indicate that the outputs of these activities will serve as an input for the data analysis.
- Conformity to product requirements: Data concerning requirements specified by the customer, requirements that were not specified by the customer, and additional requirements that are necessary for the realization of the process will be analyzed. In order to prove conformity to requirements related to the product, you need to supply objective evidence using analysis of data. Nonconformity reports, customers' returns or complaints, and service calls are status reports regarding the medical device's characteristics and specifications. Try to exert

this information and examine the level of the medical device's competence to meet its requirements, or which specifications were not achieved.

- The analysis shall enable the manufacturer to respond to trends, patterns, and fluctuations detected on the processes or products. This response is an integral aspect of maintaining your effectiveness. The data will support alerts, investigations, and inspections of nonconformities and potential nonconformities. These nonconformities (or potential nonconformities) were caused by process parameters or by a medical device's characteristics that did meet requirements. The analysis shall allow you to detect and react to situations with actions. The data collected will present the status of parameters or characteristics and enable the identification of root causes. The results of the analysis will be defined as one of the inputs for the CAPA processes.
- Suppliers' performances: Data regarding suppliers shall be collected and analyzed; such as the test results of incoming goods, evaluation of suppliers' performances, and returned goods. The analysis shall be conducted on a time scale. The objective is to detect trends regarding suppliers and their performances.

Documented Method on a Procedure

The ISO 13485 Standard requires a documented procedure that describes the data analysis method process:

- Definition of the appropriate data to be analyzed
- Identifying the sources and inputs
- Selecting the method for analysis
- Determining the method for collection
- Determining the method for records
- Evaluating the data for integrity
- Analysis of the data
- Submission of the data to responsible parties for actions or decision making

I met some quality managers in my life that included the procedure in quality management procedures. I persuaded them not to mess with the auditor and to document it on an independent procedure as requested. And then I responded: "Don't get too philosophical about it. Just do it and save us some rejections on our final report."

The procedure will relate to some basic elements that will ensure an effective process:

- Inputs: The sources, locations, and process elements of the information and data must be identified—including which documentation tools or means carry the data for analysis; such as specific forms, test protocols, specific processes, information systems, certain employees, machines, infrastructures, or control systems.
- Records: The documentation and records of the data will be determined.
- Documentation: Reference to necessary documentation is required (e.g., diagrams, work instructions, test instructions, documented criteria, etc.).
- Frequency: The interval of the collection will be defined. How frequently the data is gathered (i.e., daily, weekly, monthly, quarterly, or yearly).
- Integrity: The quality of the data must be reviewed. It is required that you evaluate the reliability and stability of the data sources. It is also required that you ensure that the data can be supplied for the long term, and that the data gathered is usable and contributive. It may occur that some processes or technologies will have to be changed in order for them to provide the appropriate data.

- Personnel: The responsibilities and authorities are to be defined; first for the gathering and then for the analysis. This is very important for the completeness and reliability of the data. Awareness of the matter is to be promoted in the organization. Each role in the organizational structure needs to know that the data that he/she is gathering is flowing in a certain direction and that some other role is waiting to use the data.
- Equipment: The tools assisting in the analysis of the data will be described; for example, computer systems, data analysis software, and paper forms.
- Analysis techniques for analyzing the data shall be determined.

Here are some examples for data sources that may be analyzed:

- Incoming acceptance records
- Customer complaints (internal and external)
- Quality records
- Service records
- Audit results (internal and external)
- Finished device acceptance records
- On process acceptance records
- Installation records
- Automation systems
- Manufacturing reports
- Supplier evaluations

The procedure may also appear as a process diagram that describes the sequence of events.

Advice: One difficulty that a lot of organizations face during audits is the claim, made by dissatisfied auditors, that the procedure is not practical, and thus a rejection follows. The main argument is that the procedure is too general and cannot be assigned to specific measurements. In such a case I recommend that you maintain a table and add it to the procedure (or refer to it) with the following fields: planned measurement, frequency, source of the data, location, responsible party, method for analysis, required tools, records, objective (or reference). The table will look something like this (Table 8.12).

The procedure will be controlled and submitted to the documents control process as required on subclause 4.2.3 (Control of Documents).

Analysis Technique

Method and techniques for analyzing the data shall be determined. The purpose of the technique is to objectively demonstrate through data that processes meet their specifications. The manufacturer will determine a method both suitable and relevant to the type of data. Using the method will provide an accurate status report regarding the processes:

- For each type of data, the appropriate method will be determined.
- The method will be determined in accordance with your analysis needs.
- The method will allow comparison to objectives and goals.
- The method will allow you to compare new data with old data.
- When international, national, or local standards for analysis techniques are demanded by your local authorities, they will be implemented.
- The use and instruction for implementing the method will be documented or referred.
- The need for records and documented results will be defined.

TABLE 8.12
Example of Documented Requirements for Data Analysis

Planned Measurement	Frequency	Source of the Data	Location	Responsible Party	Method of Analysis	Required Tools	Records	Objective (or Reference)
Supplier's evaluation	Every six months	Information systems, supplier evaluation forms	QA	Quality manager	Calculating a grade average	Excel	FO-003-44SP	Grade A or B
Health inspection	Once a year	Ministry of health	QA	Quality manager	Audit and review	N/A	External	Health certification

Common techniques include: SPC (statistical process control), Pareto charts, root cause analysis, statistical sampling, Taguchi methods, tolerance analysis, event tree analysis, fault tree analysis and screening experiments.

Records

The documentation and records of the data will be determined. The records will prove that the data was collected and analyzed according to your defined method. The records will include the results of the analysis. I am not relating the source from which the data has been extracted, but to the platform where the data will be transferred and saved for analysis. If you are analyzing service calls or repair reports, I am not referring the records of these processes, but to the records of the analysis and results; that is, the reports, test charts, data charts, test protocols, certain modules on the information system, and BI systems. In case you have determined in your process that a decision or action is to be taken and documented, the records will support this decision or action. This is important because roles that use the data for operative purposes need to know where to approach it in order to use the data. The means that the method of recording the data will be determined by the type that is to be recorded. The procedure will be controlled and submitted to the records control process as required in subclause 4.2.4 control of records.

8.5 IMPROVEMENT

8.5.1 Improvement—General

The ISO 13485 Standard requires the identification and implementation of the changes that are needed for improving the quality management system and maintaining its effectiveness through the use of implemented quality elements, such as quality policies and objectives. The standard adds descriptive definitions of cases that may suggest opportunities or which may serve as inputs for improvement (Table 8.13).

Improvement

The objective of improvement is the obtaining of a comparative advantage by improving the abilities and capabilities of the organization. The improvement will be obtained by developing a systematic identification of opportunities or needs for improvement, and submitting these cases to a controlled method of planning and controlling. This method shall be implemented on all levels of the organization:

- The importance and significance of the matter shall be demonstrated through training and certification of the relevant roles and functions on the different levels of the organization.
- Appropriate tools shall be planned in order to provide workers with the suitable platform to promote improvements (e.g., forms, meetings, reviews, motivation plans, competitions, incentives, etc.).
- The tools for the implementation of improvements shall relate to processes of the organization as well as their outputs (products), and the tools shall be planned with regard to the nature of these.

All levels of the organization refer not only to organizational levels, but to all products and services that the manufacturer offers as well as its suppliers agents and

TABLE 8.13
Standard Requirements of Subclause 8.5.1

ISO 13485	ISO 9001
The organization shall identify and implement the changes needed for the continued integrity and effectiveness of the quality management system	The organization shall maintain the integrity and effectiveness of the quality management system in a continuous manner
The changes shall be implemented using quality processes such as quality policy, quality objectives, internal audits, analysis of data, management review, and preventive and corrective actions	The changes shall be implemented using quality processes such as quality policy, quality objectives, internal audits, analysis of data, management review, and preventive and corrective actions
The organization shall maintain documented procedures describing the processes and activities of issuing, distributing, and publishing advisory notices. The procedure will be implementable in any given situation	
The organization shall maintain records regarding the investigation of customer complaints. The records are to be included under the records control process as required in subclause 4.2.4 (Control of Records)	
If it was determined that a customer's complaint was caused by activities performed outside the organization, or that such activities contributed to the complaint, the organization shall maintain a process of transferring the relevant information to the relevant external parties. See subclause 4.1	
When a customer complaint has not been followed by a corrective or preventive action, the reason shall be approved by an authorized person according to the specifications in subclause 5.5.1. Records of the approval shall be maintained and submitted to the records control process as required in subclause 4.2.4	
A documented procedure describing the reporting activities of adverse events—according to predefined reporting criteria—shall be defined and implemented, when such is demanded by regulatory requirements	

distributors. Another important aspect of the improvement is the assignment and definition of objectives; that is, for each improvement action that was introduced to the organization, a goal is to be set and defined. This objective will ensure that resources and efforts that were invested will realize the desired improvement. The next stage is evaluating the effectiveness of the improvement measure taken. The evaluation shall be carried out on two levels:

- Whether the objectives have been achieved
- Whether the desired improvements have been obtained

Identification of Improvement Opportunities

The ISO 13485 Standard expects the manufacturer to define which inputs and sources of information may indicate the need for improvement. The standard refers to well-known and used quality tools, and their outputs (which you will have already implemented as suggestions for improvements). The requirements are clear:

- Quality policy: Deviation of these general guidelines, intentions, and goals referring to quality may suggest that an improvement is required.
- Quality objectives: The purpose of quality objectives is to carry out the quality policy and implement it in the quality management system. These objectives are to be aimed, planned, and implanted for achieving improvement. Lack of obtainment of these objectives may suggest that an improvement is needed.
- Results of audits (internal or external): The audit is one of the most effective tools in identifying opportunities for improvements, since the outputs of the audit indicate whether a nonconformity (which is, by definition, a lack of achievement of objectives) or opportunity for improvement were detected.
- Data analysis: A quality activity that indicates the status of your quality management system in comparison to its objectives.
- Nonconformities: Nonconformity is an indication that the product has reached its specifications and thus may suggest a need for improvement.
- Risk management activities may suggest improvements relevant to the safety characteristics of the medical device.
- Corrective or preventive actions: There is a correlation between the improvement and the CAPA, since each of these may be considered an improvement. Therefore, these actions may be presented as improvements. However, there are cases where corrections or prevention are temporary, and thus a long-term action of improvement is required. The CAPA may then serve as an input.
- Management review: One of the outputs of the review is the suggestion for improvements and changes to the QMS and its processes.

The organization is required to initiate the interface between the quality activities mentioned above, and the systematical method for implanting improvements—that is, identify the relevant parties, processes, records and outputs of these activities, collect the essential data, evaluate the need for change, and decide whether an improvement is necessary or not. There is no requirement for a specific method for initiating and controlling improvements in the organization. I have decided to present one option since the ISO Standard supports it and suggests it as an effective method: the plan do check act (PDCA) cycle.

The Plan-Do-Check-Act Cycle

The PDCA cycle is not only related to the CAPA processes; it relates to the whole quality management system. The principle of the PDCA cycle exists in all of our daily business activities. We use it both formally and informally, and the PDCA cycle never ends. Its objective is to maintain continuous improvement.

Note: The PDCA cycle is not one of the ISO 13485 Standard requirements, though it is an efficient tool for achieving the improvement requirements.

The process approach promoted by the ISO 13485 Standard systematically identifies and manages processes that operate your quality system and maintain its interactions. This process model is actually based on the PDCA cycle, and thus could be implemented throughout all processes included in the QMS. The method combines planning, implementing, controlling, and improving the realization processes. Manufacturers will maintain continuous improvement once they implement the PDCA cycle in their processes—design, purchase, realization, storage, and distribution. The PDCA can be implemented at the core process, at a minor process, or even at several processes altogether. The PDCA is divided into four stages:

Plan: The planning stage is the starting point—planning is conducted according to information and inputs received after you raised questions regarding the improvement:

- Why is the improvement necessary? Indicate which objectives have not been fulfilled or what quality problem has raised its head.
- What needs to be done? Set the activities needed to achieve improvement.
- How much must be done? Set the objectives, goals, and targets that you would like to achieve.
- When must it be done? Set a timeframe in which you would like to achieve the improvement.
- Where must it be done? Set the scopes, areas, and processes.
- Who should do it? Set the resources required to achieve the results.

Planning should come after you have located exactly where you need the improvement. However, there is no defined way to plan. Each organization should plan according to its own environment. Ensure that you document the plan.

Do: This is the second stage—realization of your plan. During this stage you set the plan for the relevant participants for execution on the adequate areas or scope in the organization. This is the hard part—putting words into action. Therefore, try to make the plan as clear, concise, and detailed as possible. Consider writing the plan with the participants themselves; they may provide appropriate inputs and set effective activities. Try to make the "do" part easier for them to perform.

Check: The third stage—monitor and measure the activities that you have planned and evaluate their progress according to the objectives of the plan. Then, you must report the results. This part is crucial. For every question presented above you must deliver results. Depending on the results and conclusions of the "check," you would then advance to the next stage—"act."

Act: The fourth stage—take measures and activities for improving the performance. At any points where you are not satisfied with the results of the plan's progress, review your plan and improve it. Examine in which parameters you failed to reach the objectives and try again, or in another way. This is how you maintain constant improvement.

The PDCA is not a complicated process to implement, but to achieve maximum effect you must conduct it correctly and permanently. The Figure 8.2 presents graphically the PDCA process and its continual cycle.

Advisory Notice

Advisory notice regards cases where any malfunction or deterioration in the characteristics of the medical device occurred, or may potentially occur. The cases relate to any deviations from the medical device's requirements—intended use, safety, functionality, and performance. The issue refers to all elements that include or construct the medical device: the functions, parts, materials, and even inadequacy in the labeling or user instructions. For example, suppose that the manufacturer discovers (through a complaint) that certain components on the medical device may present a risk of burning due to a connector failure. The problem occurs due to the nature of the connector and its physical link to other components of the medical device. The result is an error

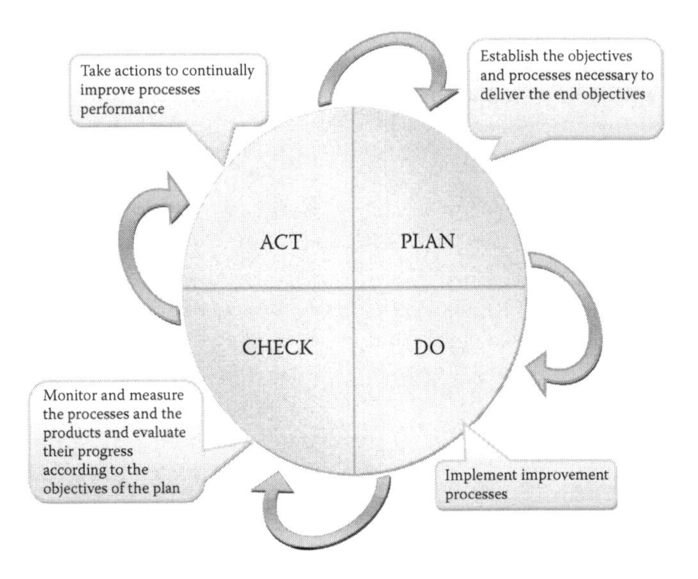

FIGURE 8.2 The Plan Do Check Act process.

message on the screen. In such a case, the manufacturer is required to issue an advisory notice. The objective is:

- To draw attention to the issue in a systematic way
- To provide structured information and data regarding the problem and its nature
- To suggest safety measures in order to eliminate or reduce the problem by as much as possible
- To improve the safety and health of other users or patients that use the medical device

There are four cases that may initiate the need for an advisory notice:

- Provision of information regarding the use of the medical device
- Provision of information regarding the need for a change or correction in the medical device
- The requirement for disposal of medical devices
- Initiation of a medical device recall

For each region that you are active in, it is required that you investigate what are the definitions and regulatory requirements of an advisory notice and what are the necessary activities. The organization is required to maintain a documented procedure describing the manners and methods of how these advisory notices shall be communicated to the relevant parties:

- The manufacturer shall define what inputs and sources of such incidents or events require an advisory notice; for example, customer complaint, feedback activities, or application of the local authorities.
- The procedure shall define the responsible parties of the different stages of the process. This may involve different parties from different aspects of the organization. The definition shall relate to the authority in the organization that will decide whether to issue an advisory notice.

- Importance shall be given to the handling and investigation of the matter—receiving the inputs, examining and analyzing them, suggesting measures for the elimination of the problem, documenting the issue, and issuing the notice. The method shall relate to the interrelations with other quality processes or procedures, such as control of nonconforming products, corrective and preventive actions, follow ups, modifications to the medical device, and disposals or recalls.
- The required documentation and data sources must support the investigation, and their availability shall be defined: technical data and information (DHF), regulatory requirements, production records (DHR), risk management inputs (Risk Management File)—the documentation needed to support the investigation of the matter, and the identification of an effective solution or measure. The type and extent of the information is depended on the life cycle phase of the medical device.
- The procedure shall define the target groups that are to receive the advisory notice: users, patients, distributors, local authorities, and suppliers. The matter is to be defined according to the requirements in subclause 7.2.3 (Customer Communication), where you are required to develop and implement communication channels with your customers.
- The procedure shall indicate what reporting activities need to be initiated: the required records, responsibilities, and communication channels. In case regulations, where the medical device is being marketed, require specified reporting criteria and methods, and these shall be identified and implemented. For example, some regulations may require publishing the presence of some materials or components in the medical device itself as an advisory notice. Usually such regulatory requirements indicate exactly how the reporting shall be done: a structure, target group, content, and period of time.
- The procedure shall relate to the outputs and records of the investigation: records of meetings, reviews, and evaluations; and the documentation of the advisory notice itself.
- The procedure will be submitted to the documents control process as required in subclause 4.2.3 (Control of Documents).

The advisory notice itself shall be planned, and will include:

- Identification of the manufacturer and the organization
- Date and place where the noticed was issued
- Target audience or group (customers, users, operators, distributors, local authorities, etc.)
- A full identification of the medical device which the advisory notice refers to (name, model, catalog number, manufacturer, batch number, serial numbers, date of manufacture, etc.)
- Purpose of the notice referring to scopes and areas in the medical device that are on the spot (certain components, a process, a function on the medical device, etc.)
- Description of the functions and uses of the medical device to be referred to
- A description of the problem (or possible hazard) and its cause
- Background information
- Reference to users or patients that the problem may relate to
- Measures or actions to be applied or taken, and, if applicable, the verifications
- Reference to other documentation supporting the issue

When describing the actions and measure to be applied you must be as specific as possible. The advisory notice shall be a controlled record, and will be submitted to the control of records as required in subclause 4.2.4.

A final issue on the topic concerns the creation of a process that can be executed at any situation even when no personnel are available. I will use the worst case scenario to explain: if death or the unanticipated and serious deterioration in a state of health is seen to result from the use of the medical device, the advisory notice shall be issued immediately and without consideration of working hours or holidays. This is why the communication channels, the documents to be issued (the form and structure of the notice), and the means of communication (e-mail, fax, telephone, and through a website) should all be available and clear. The topic must be clear to the parties that receive and investigate the issue. They should have access to all means of issuing such notices without delay.

Recall

Recall refers to a specific case of an advisory notice. The term is not related in the ISO 13485 Standard due to the fact that it has several meanings and implications in several areas with different authorities. The main objective is public protection—for example, suppose that the manufacturer has detected a problem that may pose a hazard to the user. After evaluation, the manufacturer decides that the problem is a safety threat to users or operators. As a result they conclude that removing the medical device from the market is necessary to correct, inspect, or dispose of the medical device. The tactic is to dictate to the customer what has to be done with the medical device. In principle, the term "recall" relates to the methodical removal of medical devices that do not meet their requirements (functional, safety, performance, and intended use) and thus must be removed from the market for:

- Correction—for example, the replacement of components
- Further inspection—the application of further tests
- Change—for example, relabeling of the product
- Disposal of the medical device

The inspection, correction, or application of a change will usually be carried out by the manufacturer or their agents, and thus must be collected by them. The disposal, however, can also be done by the customer under instructions and restrictions (provided in the advisory notice). However, as indicated, the definition may vary from one region to another. This is why it is important for the manufacturer to identify the exact regulations applicable to their medical device. Executing a recall would require posing a few questions, such as:

- Where is the device sold?
- Who uses the device?
- How many were released?
- How may I contact the end users or patients?

Thus, you need to ensure that the information that will provide answers to the questions above is maintained. Recalling a product involves:

- Implementing the policy for initiating a recall
- The processes of gathering the data and evaluating the need for a recall
- Identifying the responsible parties, authorities, and clients (internal and external) involved in the process (organizations, customers, distributors, agents, or local authorities)

- Planning and verifying effective communication activities with the customers; maintaining details for communication, defining the type of communication and the communication channels
- Issuing advisory notices with a definition of the content
- Planning removal activities
- Defining verification activities of the recall
- Defining termination activities of the recall
- Identifying and incorporating regulatory requirements

Defining a plan for recall is an effective way of implementing the issue in the quality management system. An important aspect is the verification of the respective recall activities, verification that all the addressees received the notifications, and that these notifications were acted upon as instructed. Another verification is that the devices that are returned to the organization are properly introduced to the designated action; correction, inspection, change, or disposal. After verification of the recall, it is necessary to define its termination; that is, the activities and the authority. In many external audits, the organization is required to present a test proving the effectiveness of the plan. The effectiveness of the plan may be evaluated by a simulated recall and examination of the plan activities, and the parameters involved—communicating with customers, examining the response, and performing a dummy removal of devices from the market. Such simulation will help identify any potential errors in the plan.

Identifying the applicable regulations is crucial to the plan and its definitions. For example, it is possible that the notification of the advisory notice differs from one region to the other. In some regions, it is obligatory to feed a local system in addition to the notices sent to the customers. When regulations demand the establishment and maintenance of a documented procedure for the notification of the authorities, the procedure will be implemented and submitted to the documents control process as required in subclause 4.2.3. Records of recall activities shall be submitted to the control of records.

Investigation of Customer Complaints

A customer's complaint is seized and recorded in the organization according to the requirements in subclause 7.2.3. In subclause 8.5.1, the standards expect you to conduct an effective investigation of the complaint, evaluate its severity, and decide whether it is necessary to submit the complaint to an improvement activity, such as a corrective or a preventive action. A customer's complaint suggests that a released medical device might have not met its requirements. It would be well investigated once you submit the complaint to a controlled process. The investigation of complaints may serve as a statistical database for the analysis of trends and fluctuations regarding the quality of the medical device. The investigation might lead to a conclusion that the complaint is justified and requires a corrective or preventive action. The ISO 13485 Standard demands the maintenance of investigation records. You must decide which details you need to record:

- Details: The required data and details regarding the complaint shall be gathered (e.g., product, model, batch number, delivery date, service, and any other production details that would identify the product and assist later on). Naturally, the data is supposed to be recorded during the recording of the complaint. The objective of the information is to assist you in mapping the problem and tracking down the root cause. The details shall be sufficient to ensure that you reach the right conclusions and administer effective treatment.

- Findings: Evidence related to the complaint will be recorded and analyzed (e.g., returned devices, or samples taken from the customer).
- Responsibilities: It is necessary to define the relevant parties and authorities that are to conduct the investigation of the complaints. These could be department or development managers. However, it is important to assign parties that have the necessary qualifications to evaluate the information, and to reach the right decisions. It is not sufficient to assign treatment to the quality manager as he or she may not have the required tools to evaluate the matter.
- Root cause: The complaint will be evaluated and analyzed, and the root cause will be recognized and documented (e.g., a certain realization process, design of the medical device, the package, the delivery, etc.). The evaluation of a nonconformity and its root cause shall assess whether the product design failed or that it is a user fault.
- Decision: The decision that was made and accepted—based on the investigation and the identification of the root cause—will be recorded. When a decision not to pursue the matter further to a corrective or preventive action has been accepted, it will be documented, explained, and justified. The identification of the approver is also to be recorded.
- Follow up: Where applicable, subsequent activities and responsibilities shall be defined and documented.

The standard demands a documented definition of the persons and authorities responsible for conducting the investigation, reviewing the complaint, and reaching a conclusion. It refers us to subclause 5.5.1 (Responsibility and Authority). There it is required that you appoint and hire persons for the performance of certain roles and functions, as set out by the regulatory requirements. In relation to the requirements of subclause 8.5.1, you must verify that regulations refer to the issue of review and the approval of customer complaints. When such regulations demand the nominations of such functions, as mentioned above, the organization shall hire them or their services for the activities of approving customer complaints. The matter may be documented in the appropriate procedure or documentation (e.g., a job description, procedure of handling a nonconforming product, corrective and preventive actions, or feedback).

Improving the Control of Outsourced Products and Services

When the investigation of a complaint reveals that the root cause of the problem lies in activities that were performed outside the organization, the manufacturer will communicate with the relevant parties and notify them about the nonconformities. The parties outside of the organization that could contribute to the occurrence of a complaint include:

- A supplier of materials, parts, components, or services
- A distributor of the medical device
- An agent of the manufacturer

The standard refers us to subclause 4.1 (Quality Management System—General Requirements). I refer to the specific subclause indicating that the organization shall maintain the appropriate controls of outsourced elements (products or services) that are used to realize the medical device, and that may affect its quality. Such controls are to be incorporated and implemented in the QMS. Subclause 8.5.1 verifies that the controls of outsourced products and services are effective. A complaint is one way to locate problems in outsourced products and services. When it is detected that a source for complaint is an outsourced product, it means that the controls must be improved. For example, one specific purchased component in the medical device controls various other functions in the device. A complaint was received in the organization, claiming that some functions in the medical device did not operate correctly. The investigation revealed that the malfunction originated in this controlling component. The conclusion: the control and verification of the purchased product (the controlling component in the example) are insufficient and require submission to an improvement process.

Adverse Events

When using the medical device, adverse events may arise. In most regions and countries such events, caused from the use of the medical device, must be reported to the local authorities in a specific manner and in a specific timeframe. These are usually defined in the regulations. When such are required, the organization is to establish and implement a documented procedure.

An adverse event is any side effect or adverse change in health that occurs in a person who uses or operates the medical device. The event may occur during the operation and use of the medical device, or within a specified period of time after the use or operation. An adverse event is considered as such when any harm (or potential harm) that may be related to the use of the medical device, its influence on the patient or operator, or on the environment in which it is active, exists. For example, adverse events may occur as: death, life-threatening events, illness, damage to the patient, injury, infection, or the need for hospitalization. There are several sources that may serve as inputs and supply details regarding adverse events:

- Customer complaints
- Clinical evaluations
- Feedback activities
- Postproduction activities
- Local authorities reports

In most cases, events that were caused by the use of the medical device must be reported to the local regulatory authorities in a specific manner and in a specific timeframe. In order to implement an effective reporting system, you must initiate the interface between the two processes—the inputs mentioned above, and the organizational unit that is responsible for the reporting. The manufacturer must identify the regions in which the device is marketed and used, and what the adverse event reporting regulations are. Normally the function in the organization that responsible for the matter is referred to as regulatory associate. The regulations for reporting may be variously characterized:

- The manner and method for reporting—it is required that you identify the reporting methods required by the authorities in order to plan the appropriate tools and implement them in the quality management system. For example, the FDA demands certain obligatory reporting methods, but it manages a computerized information database for gathering and monitoring information regarding new adverse events. Such system initiates the distribution of reported in adverse event databases based on experience of other manufacturers. This system is not obligatory and is maintained in addition to the reporting requirements. Designated forms may be downloaded from the web, sent to you by the authorities, or you may need to register as a manufacturer.

- Timeframe—it is required that you identify the timeframe in which an adverse event must be reported.
- Details and information—the necessary details and information for the reporting are to be defined; for example, product, product type, date of the event, details, clinical evaluations, required attachments, descriptions of the event, the effects, the (actual and potential) harms and damages.
- Responsibilities—the parties in the organization responsible for the reporting are to be defined.
- The address for the report—the details of the reporting address are to be identified and documented in the organization; for example, a website, a call center, a specific office, or a specific authority.
- The need for approval of the notification—when an approval is given after the notification, it shall be mentioned in order to control that it has been received.

The ISO 13485 Standard demands the establishment and maintenance of a documented procedure in order to implement the issue effectively. The procedure shall cover all of the issues mentioned above, and will be submitted to the documents control process as required in subclause 4.2.3 (Control of Documents).

8.5.2 Corrective Action

Corrective action is one of the foundation elements of quality management, and is essential for sustaining improvement of the quality management system. The main concept of corrective action promotes a systematic analysis of quality problems that have already occurred, and the elimination of any root causes of nonconformities through the implementation of controlled measures (Table 8.14).

The main principle of corrective action is to eliminate any cause of nonconformity in order to prevent such from occurring again. The initiation of a corrective action in an organization is not to be submitted or assigned to one person, role, function, or department, but it is an issue that relates, covers, and involves all levels of the organization—management, design and development, purchase, production, assembly, quality, service, and logistics.

A Documented Procedure

The process of evaluating and investigating nonconformity and applying a corrective action will be implemented in the organization in a methodical way through a documented procedure. The objectives of the procedure are:

- Identification of nonconformities
- Determination of responsibilities and authorities
- Definition of a method for the analysis of root causes
- Promoting a systematic evaluation of root causes and identification of appropriate solutions
- Evaluation and review of risks—and the consequences of actions—that may affect the realization processes or the medical device
- Planning of the necessary actions
- Implementation of the actions
- Review of the effectiveness
- Definition of the expected records

TABLE 8.14
Standard Requirements of Subclause 8.5.2

ISO 13485	ISO 9001
For any nonconformity that was detected, the organization shall take measures to eliminate it and prevent its reoccurrence	For any nonconformity that was detected, the organization shall take measures to eliminate it and prevent its reoccurrence
The actions and measures taken shall be suitable for the type and character of the nonconformity	The actions and measures taken shall be suitable for the type and character of the nonconformity
The organization shall maintain a documented procedure describing the activities of handling nonconformities and submitting them to a controlled process	The organization shall maintain a documented procedure describing the activities of handling nonconformities and submitting them to a controlled process
The organization shall review nonconformities and refer to customer complaints as well	The organization shall review nonconformities and refer to customer's complaints as well
The organization shall perform activities for the identification of factors and root causes of nonconformities	The organization shall perform activities for the identification of factors and root causes of nonconformities
For any cause that was detected, the organization shall evaluate and determine whether a corrective action is required	For any cause that was detected, the organization shall evaluate and determine whether a corrective action is required
After determining the need for a corrective action, the organization shall determine an action plan and its implementation. When needed, the relevant documentation shall be updated according to subclause 4.2	After determining the need for a corrective action, the organization shall determine an action plan and its implementation
The corrective action and its effectiveness will be reviewed periodically	The corrective action will be reviewed periodically
Records and evidence of the corrective action, the investigation that followed, and the results of the action taken must be documented. The records shall be submitted to the records control process as mentioned in subclause 4.2.4 (Control of Records)	Records and evidence of the corrective action and the results of the action taken must be documented. The records shall be submitted to the records control process as mentioned in subclause 4.2.4 (Control of Records)

Figure 8.3 to describe the process in general.

The procedure shall include all of the stages and activities mentioned in this chapter (when applicable). The procedure shall be submitted to the process of documents control as required in subclause 4.2.3.

Inputs for the Process

The identification of a quality problem is the starting point of the corrective action process. However, as with any other quality process designed according to the ISO 13485 Standard requirements, the matter is expected to be structured and defined; and the inputs that will drive the organization to initiate a corrective action are to be identified. Here are some examples of quality activities that may produce inputs for a corrective action:

- Monitoring and measuring of product or processes—results of validation studies, quality tests, and so on

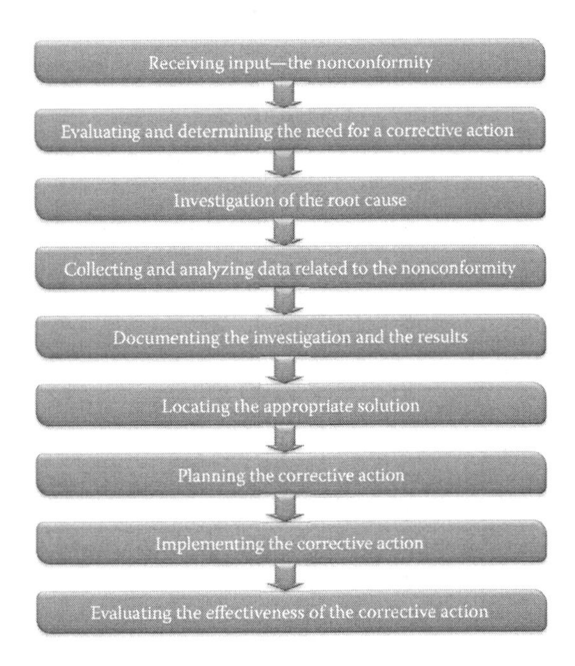

FIGURE 8.3 Corrective action process.

- Feedback activities—customer survey, research and clinical evaluations, and recalls
- Need for revalidation
- Data analysis
- Nonconformities and faults
- Customer complaints
- Purchase problems
- Results of management review
- The lack of achievement of organizational goals and objectives
- Results and findings of audits (internal and external)
- Service feedback

The need for revalidation may indicate, in certain situations, where process parameters have not met their requirements and a corrective action is therefore required. The matter is discussed in details in subclause 7.5.2 (Validation of Processes for Production and Service Provision).

All of the above are topics and issues that are already planned. What they have in common is this: they are structurally controlled, evaluated, and they provide an output. In some cases this output might be the input for the corrective action. In practice the documented procedure will define what the inputs of the process are, and will define the interface between the processes and activities and the submission to a corrective action. This is where the responsibility to the corrective action comes in.

Evaluation and Determination of Need for a Corrective Action

Each nonconformity shall be evaluated in order to determine whether a corrective action is needed or whether it is sufficient to provide only a local correction for the problem. The stages of the evaluation include:

- The review of the nonconformity
- Identification of affected devices and recipients of the devices
- The identification and location of the root cause
- Identification of all the quality documentation related to the nonconformity
- Identification of all regulations, standards, or directives that may set requirements for the review
- Evaluation and analysis of risks affecting other elements, scopes, areas, or functions of the product

The objective of the review is to measure the severity of the nonconformity, and to decide whether a corrective action is required. You may set the criteria, a checklist, or perform an independent review of the matter in order to reach a decision. An effective review is one that gathers all the relevant information and evaluates it, using the right tools and functions (or roles) to help determine the meaning of the data. This is why the activities and inputs related to the nonconformity must be defined.

Evaluation of the Root Cause

The source of the nonconformity may occur in various elements throughout the quality management system—product, process, machine, worker, supplier, or service. The objective is to identify all the elements in the realization process that have deviated from their requirements and might have caused the nonconformity, or might have affected the quality of a process or product. Here is where the traceability assists. The next step is to evaluate their influence and relation to the nonconformity. The goal is to find something wrong and correct with the objective of eliminating it forever. The investigation is based on few basic principles:

- All the required data and information regarding the nonconformity is available, reliable, and, where necessary, verified.
- The methods for analyzing the data are defined.
- The decision is finalized using these two elements: the adequate data and the use of analysis tools.

You may implement and use different methods for identifying the root cause: histograms, fishbone diagrams, statistical analysis, correlation diagrams and so on. The analysis of the root cause shall be accompanied with different documents, such as:

- Description of the investigation, including activities, tools, equipment, and participants
- Statistical analyses results
- Data and information from process observations or product tests

These are all to be documented and controlled in order to be able to trace and join all the relevant evidence in one dossier. For example, if you performed a statistical analysis of a process as part of the investigation, the ISO Standard expects to see a report including all the details mentioned above, with a reference to the relevant nonconformity.

Once the cause for the nonconformity is identified, you are required to plan a solution with the objective of eliminating the root cause permanently. The solution will relate to all product or process elements that may have been affected. Let us assume, for example, that nonconformity was reported, and the investigation determined that the package is the root cause. A conclusion of the investigation claims that a new package is to be implemented. Before submitting the solution for planning and implementation, it is necessary to evaluate the feasibility of the solution:

- Influence of the solution on packaging processes
- Influence of the solution on other realization processes, such as transportation and delivery
- Influence of the solution on the product requirements; that is, the functionality, intended use, performance, and safety
- Compatibility with local or international regulations regarding packages
- Compatibility with risk management requirements
- Cost benefit analysis, in order to justify the investment of resources

One last thing before we move on to the next issue: there is room for experience and intuition when making a decision regarding the need for a corrective action. A situation may arise that, on paper—and according to the data analysis—requires a corrective action; but an experienced or intuitive review may report that such action is unnecessary. When the decision is based on these, try to justify it with records of previous similar cases.

Planning and Implementing Corrective Action

For each element that is to be corrected the organization is required to determine a plan according to the following questions:

- Which corrective actions or activities are to be taken?
- Who is responsible for the execution and implementation?
- What are the necessary tools and equipment?
- What are the training needs?
- What are the timeframes?
- What are the operative objectives and actions to be implemented, tested, and approved?
- Which controls need to be implemented in order to test the effectiveness of the corrective action?
- What are the required results that will prove that the corrective action is effective and the root cause is eliminated?
- Which documents must be updated?

Reaction time may be a factor for consideration. It may be necessary to implement an action or a short-term correction immediately.

In practice, the planning of the corrective action is to be documented, and will serve as a quality record. Although the standard does not specify what the exact details to be documented are, here are some of the necessary details:

- Statement of the starting date
- The team that participates and is responsible for the planning and implementation of the corrective action
- Description of the of the relevant nonconformity or reference to documentation and evidence of the relevant nonconformity (you may include internal classification for future statistics)—customer complaints, quality tests, audit findings
- The nonconformity details: customer's name, affected product, catalogue number, name of the employee that detected the nonconformity (any information that would help you to identify and review the corrective action later on)

- Description of immediate or short-term corrective action (if undertaken), its results, and reference to the relevant records
- Identification of all relevant organizational documentation
- Reference to the results of the root cause analysis investigation and the conclusions
- Description of the solution and corrective action to be taken with reference to the relevant factors; for example, departments, products, processes, packages, tools and equipment, monitoring and measuring devices, and controls. In general each defined action is to be approved before release or implementation
- Reference to human resources
- The objectives of the actions taken, including timeframes

The record may appear as a work plan, a project plan, or refer to such dossiers. However, the principle demands a specification of activities or milestones assigned to responsibilities and framed with objectives of time and results. Useful documentation of the plan will also include the results of the implementation.

Review of the Corrective Action Results and Effectiveness

The manufacturer is required to review and verify the effectiveness of the corrective action. This is a target performance analysis with the goal of indicating or defining the status of the corrective action—opened, in-process, or closed:

- The corrective action was suitable to the nature of the nonconformity.
- The corrective action could be introduced to the necessary elements and be properly implemented.
- The objectives of the corrective action have been achieved.
- The corrective action is effective and the nonconformity did not, and will not, reoccur.

The review shall consider also the results: success or failure; or perhaps more time or other actions are required to examine its effectiveness. The results of the review are to be recorded.

Closing the Corrective Action

Closing the corrective action is to be recorded as well. The corrective action may be closed for various reasons:

- The corrective action achieved its objectives effectively.
- The product is no longer produced.
- New data and information were received; a reevaluation of the situation is needed.

The identification of the approver who concluded the corrective action is to be recorded. When a corrective action was closed but was found to be ineffective, it is recommended that you open a new one. This is not required by the ISO 13485 Standard, but an unsuccessful or ineffective corrective action indicates the fact that the root cause of nonconformity has not been eliminated (which is forbidden by the ISO 13485 Standard).

Updating the Relevant Documentation

In case the corrective action taken has triggered any changes or updates to any of your quality management documents, these documents must be updated. The objective here is to verify that changes initiated by, or resulting from, the corrective action in quality elements (such as quality policy, objectives, or documentation) are controlled and implemented. The standard refers us to clause 4.2 in order to specify where changes may occur: quality policy, quality objectives, quality manual, quality procedures, work procedures, work instructions, specifications, and documented requirements. The standard demands that these documents also be evaluated, since these have a part in the realization processes. The changes will be initiated and controlled according to the control of documents requirements. Changes and updates may be expressed in various aspects of the document:

- The information and content on the document
- The structure of the document
- The coverage of all the medical device requirements (customer, regulatory, safety, etc.)
- The distribution of the document
- The media of the document
- The approval of the document

Advice: In order to maintain this requirement, I would suggest including on the corrective action plan the review of the relevant documentation, and to determine whether a change has been made as part of the implementation. This would ensure the required control.

The Corrective Action Records

Records and evidence of the corrective action process will be submitted to the records control process as required in subclause 4.2.4 (Control of Records). The main goals of these records are supervision and control. The records that are expected include:

- The nonconformity—this is supposed to have been already documented as part of clause 8.3 (Control of Nonconforming Products). You do not have to record it again. You may refer to the appropriate documentation.
- The root cause investigation—the records of the investigation depend on the type of method you are using for identifying the root cause of nonconformity.
- Evaluation—the review and evaluation of the need for corrective action will include details such as the performer of the evaluation, the date, the considerations, and conclusions or reference to the relevant documentation.
- The corrective action—if case a corrective action is taken it shall be specified and documented.
- Review and effectiveness—the review and evaluation of the corrective action will include data and evidence that the nonconformity did not reoccur.
- The closing and approval of the corrective action.

There are a lot of different solutions for documenting the corrective actions—from the simple traditional forms to sophisticated designated software. The questions, however, remain as follows:

- What suits you as a manufacturer?
- Who is supposed to detect and document a nonconformity?
- What are the types of data to be recorded?
- Who are the addressed parties of the process?
- Who is required to update and review the process?
- Who is required to approve the results?

8.5.3 Preventive Action

What is the difference between corrective and preventive action? Corrective action deals with existential nonconformities—that is, a nonconformity occurred, and was detected and submitted to a treatment and a process. Preventive action is a quality tool for protecting the devices from nonconformities—that is, evaluating risks and potential events that may affect the quality of the medical device. By defining inputs for analysis, the organization develops an ability to detect processes or process elements that may deviate from their requirements at some point, if a change will not be applied. The nonconformity has not yet occurred, but you know that it may—this is the time to capture and submit it to a controlled process (Table 8.15).

The main principle of the preventive action is as follows: the organization shall promote the liability and credibility of its processes and products by establishing a methodical system for the detection of potential nonconformities—and for the elimination of their root cause—in order to prevent them from occurring. Applying such

TABLE 8.15
Standard Requirements of Subclause 8.5.3

ISO 13485	ISO 9001
For any potential nonconformity that might come about, the organization shall take measures to eliminate it and prevent its occurrence	For any potential nonconformity that might come about, the organization shall take measures to eliminate it and prevent its occurrence
The actions and measures taken shall be suitable to the type and character of the potential nonconformity	The actions and measures taken shall be suitable to the type and character of the potential nonconformity
The organization shall maintain a documented procedure describing the activities of handling potential nonconformities and submitting them to a controlled process	The organization shall maintain a documented procedure describing the activities of handling potential nonconformities and submitting them to a controlled process
The procedure shall describe the activities for the identification of factors and root causes of potential nonconformities	The procedure shall describe the activities for the identification of factors and root causes of potential nonconformities
For any cause that was detected, the organization shall evaluate and determine whether a preventive action is required	For any cause that was detected, the organization shall evaluate and determine whether a preventive action is required
After determining the need for a preventive action, the organization shall determine an action plan and its implementation	After determining the need for a preventive action, the organization shall determine an action plan and its implementation
The preventive action and its effectiveness will be reviewed periodically	The preventive action will be reviewed periodically
The preventive action, the investigation that followed, and the results of the action taken must be documented. The records shall be submitted to the records control process as mentioned in subclause 4.2.4 (Control of Records)	The preventive action and the results of the action taken must be documented. The records shall be submitted to the records control process as mentioned in subclause 4.2.4 (Control of Records)

an approach may shorten the reaction time and extent of quality problems. The initiation of the preventive action will not be coincidental, but systematic and structured. By using traditional methods of identifying problems early, you will implement systematic quality tools that may ensure the liability and dependability of processes and maintain the quality of the medical device. The initiation of a preventive action in the organization is not to be submitted or assigned to one person, role, function, or department—it is an issue that relates, covers, and involves all levels of the organization: management, design and development, purchase, production, assembly, quality, service, and logistics.

A Documented Procedure

The process of detecting a potential nonconformity and applying a preventive action will be systematically implemented in the organization with the help of a documented procedure. The objectives of the procedure are:

- Definition of inputs that may indicate nonconformities
- Determination of responsibilities and authorities
- Identification of potential nonconformities
- Definition of a method for the analysis and evaluation of root causes
- Planning of appropriate solutions
- Evaluation and review of risks and the consequences of actions that may affect the realization processes or the medical device
- Planning of the necessary actions
- Implementation of the actions
- Review of the effectiveness

Figure 8.4 describing the process in general.

The procedure shall include all the stages and activities mentioned in this chapter. The procedure shall be submitted to the process of documents control as required in subclause 4.2.3.

Inputs for the Process

The identification of a potential quality problem is the starting point of the preventive action process. However, as with any other quality process designed according to the ISO 13485 Standard requirements, the matter is expected to be structured and defined, and the inputs that will drive the organization to initiate a preventive action are to be identified. Here are some examples of quality activities that may produce inputs for a preventive action:

- Monitoring and measuring of products or processes (e.g., results of validation studies, quality tests, evaluation of process capacity, or performances)
- Data analysis
- Feedback activities (e.g., customer surveys, research and clinical evaluations, recalls, etc.)
- Purchase problems
- Need for revalidation
- Results of management review
- The lack of achievement of organizational goals and objectives
- Results and findings of audits (internal and external)
- Service feedback

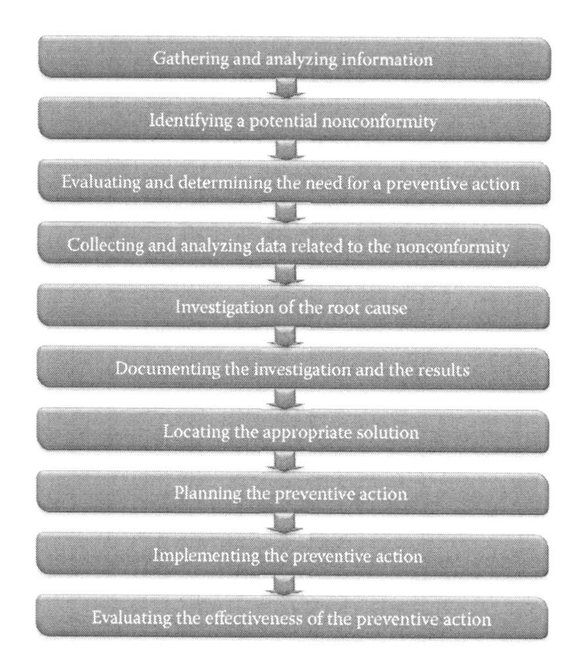

FIGURE 8.4 Preventive action process.

The need for revalidation may indicate certain situations where process parameters have not met their requirements and thus a preventive action may be required. The matter is discussed in chapter 7.5.2 (Validation of Processes for Production and Service Provision).

The above are activities that generate data to be analyzed. Throughout the realization processes there are implemented controls and alarms that gather and evaluate process outputs. In practice, the documented procedure is to define what the expected inputs of a process are, and to define the interface between the control activities and the submission to a preventive action.

Evaluation and Determination of Need for a Preventive Action

Each potential nonconformity shall be evaluated in order to determine whether a preventive action is needed. The stages of the evaluation are:

- The review of the potential nonconformity
- Identification of devices, processes, or areas that might be affected by the potential nonconformity
- The identification and location of root causes
- Identification of all the quality documentation related to the nonconformity
- Identification of all regulations, standards, or directives that may set requirements for the review
- Evaluation and analysis of risks affecting other elements, scopes, areas, or functions in the product

The objective of the review is to measure the severity of the potential nonconformity and decide whether a preventive action is required. You may set criteria, a checklist, perform an independent review relating to the matter, or consider the matter as a cost-effective issue. An effective review is one that gathers all the relevant information and evaluates it, using the right tools, functions, or roles to interpret the meaning of the data. This is why activities and inputs related to the potential nonconformity are to be defined. Initiating preventive action bears costs: human resources, time, new equipment, new processes and so on. The right way to examine a potential nonconformity and to determine whether it is a cost-effective way to carry out the action is reserved for you as a manufacturer. Sometimes it would be too expensive (and thus not worthwhile) to implement a preventive action. The organization would rather live with the potential nonconformity—as long as critical requirements are being maintained: regulatory, risk, and customer. However, you must provide a documented justification of the fact that you detected a potential problem, examined it, and subsequently decided to withdraw.

Evaluation of the Root Cause

The process of evaluation of a root cause of a potential nonconformity is identical to the evaluation of a root cause of an occurred nonconformity (see chapter 8.5.2 for further details.)

Planning and Implementing the Preventive Action

For each element that is to be prevented, it is required that you determine a plan according to the following questions:

- Which preventive actions or activities are to be taken?
- Who is responsible for the execution and implementation of them?
- What are the necessary tools and equipment?
- What are the training needs?
- What are the timeframes?
- What are the operative objectives and actions to be implemented, tested, and approved?
- Which controls need to be implemented in order to test the effectiveness of the preventive action?
- What are the required results that will prove that the preventive action is effective and the root cause has been eliminated?
- Which documents must be updated?

Reaction time may be a factor for consideration; it may be necessary that you implement an action or short-term prevention immediately. The difference from the corrective action is that the nonconformity has not yet occurred. But in order to prevent it, it is in your responsibility to perform simulation of the preventive action and to verify that the nonconformity would not occur.

In practice, the planning of the preventive action is to be documented and serve as a quality record. Although the standard does not specify what the exact details to be documented are, here are some of the necessary details:

- Statement of the starting date
- The team that participates and is responsible for the planning and implementation of the preventive action
- Description of the of the potential nonconformity or reference to the relevant documentation, findings, and data: analysis of data, quality test, audit findings, reports of purchase

- The potential nonconformity details: affected product, catalogue number, name of the employee that detected the nonconformity (any information that would help identify and review the preventive action later on)
- Description of immediate or short-term preventive action (if undertaken), its results, and reference to the relevant records
- Identification of all relevant organizational documentation
- Reference to the results of the root cause analysis investigation, and the conclusions
- Description of the solution and preventive action to be taken with reference to the relevant factors: departments, products, processes, packages, tools and equipment, monitoring and measuring devices, and controls
- Reference to human resources
- The objectives of the actions, including timeframes

The records may appear in a work plan, a project plan, or refer to such dossiers. However, the principle demands a specification of activities or milestones assigned to responsibilities and framed with objectives of time and results. Useful documents of the plan will also include the results of the implementations.

Review of the Preventive Action Results and Effectiveness

The organization is required to review and verify the effectiveness of the preventive action. This is a target performance analysis with the goal of indicating or defining the status of the preventive action; that is, opened, in process, or closed:

- The preventive action was suitable to the nature of the nonconformity.
- The preventive action could be introduced to the necessary elements and be properly implemented.
- The objectives of the preventive action have been achieved.
- The preventive action is effective and the nonconformity will not occur.

The review shall also consider the results: success or failure—or perhaps more time or other actions are required to examine its effectiveness. The results of the review are to be recorded.

Advice: One way of reviewing effectiveness is the presentation of presumable situations—that is, using data, indicating what will happen if the preventive action was not implemented. After a defined period of time, examine the status and check whether the nonconformity occurred or whether the situation remained static and the nonconformity was prevented.

Closing the Preventive Action

Closing the preventive action is to be recorded as well. The preventive action may be closed for various reasons:

- The preventive action achieved its objectives effectively.
- The product is no longer produced.
- New data and information were received; reevaluation of the situation is required.

The identification of the approver of the preventive action is to be recorded. When a preventive action was closed but found to be ineffective, it is recommended that you open a new one. It is not required by the ISO 13485 Standard, but an unsuccessful or ineffective preventive action indicates the fact that the root cause of the potential nonconformity was not eliminated (which is forbidden by the ISO 13485 Standard).

The Preventive Action Records

Records and evidence of the preventive action process will be submitted to the records control process as required in subclause 4.2.4. The main goals of the records are supervision and control. The expected records are:

- The potential nonconformity or reference to appropriate records.
- The root cause investigation—the records of the investigation depend on the type of method you are using for identifying the root cause of the nonconformity.
- Evaluation—the review and evaluation for the need of preventive action will include details such as the performer of the evaluation, the date, the considerations, and conclusions or reference to relevant documentation.
- The preventive action—if a preventive action is taken it shall be specified and documented.
- Review and effectiveness—the review and evaluation of the preventive action will include data and evidence that the nonconformity did not occur.
- The closing of the preventive action.

As mentioned already in chapter 8.5.2, there are a lot of different solutions for documenting and controlling preventive actions—from the simple traditional forms to sophisticated designated software. As a manufacturer you need to find the appropriate solution for your organization and the nature of your processes. When doing so, consider the following issues:

- Who is supposed to detect and document a potential nonconformity?
- What are the types of data to be recorded?
- Who are the addressed parties of the process?
- Who is required to update and review the process?
- Who is required to approve the results?

Index

E

F

H

I

M

R

S

T

W